Home Health Care

Second Edition

Allen D. Spiegel, Ph.D.

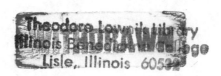
Home
Health Care

Second Edition

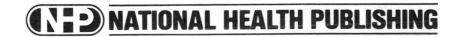
(NHP) NATIONAL HEALTH PUBLISHING

Copyright © 1987 by
Rynd Communications
99 Painters Mill Road
Owings Mills, MD 21117
(301) 363-6400

Printed in the United States of America
First Printing
ISBN: 0-932500-63-3
LC: 87-62021

Contents

List of Exhibits .... *viii*
Foreword .... *xvii*
Preface .... *xix*
About the Author .... *xxiii*

Chapter 1

Beginnings Of Home Health Care: A Brief History 1
    The Beginning 1
    Developing a Homecare Industry 1
    Expanding the Need for Home Nursing 2
    The Birth of Modern Homecare 3
        Establishing Guidelines *4*   Home Health Care Under
        Medicare *5*   Today's Home Health Care System *5*
    The History of the Homemaker-Home Health Aide 6
        The Establishment of Visiting Housewives *6*   Organizing
        Visiting Housekeepers *7*
    Summary 8

Chapter 2

Ins And Outs Of Home Health Care 11
    Caring and Home Health Care 12
    Public Awareness of Homecare 13
    Consumerism 14
    Patient Education for Postinstitutional Homecare 14
    A Suitable Home 15
    Homecare Defined 16
    Levels of Care 21
    Elements of the Homecare System 23
    What are Homecare Services? 24
        An Alphabet of Services *25*
    Coordination--A Must in Homecare 26
    Persons Benefiting from Homecare 30
    Alternative Choices 33
        Day Care, AFDA, and Group Living *24*

Advantages and Disadvantages of Homecare 35
    Advantages for Patient and Family *35* Advantages for the
    Hospital *36* Disadvantages for the Hospital *37*
Inappropriate Institutionalization 38
Typical Homecare Programs 41
    National Survey Data *41* Hospital Homecare Programs *43*
    Disease/Condition Homecare Programs *44* Specific
    Population Groups Homecare Programs *47* Foreign
    Homecare Programs *48*
Homecare as a Business 49
    Hospital/Home Health Agency Relations *50* HMO and
    Homecare Relationship *50* Management Aspects of
    Homecare *51* Corporate Restructuring *51* Operational
    Management *53* Management Survival Strategies *55*
Malpractice and Homecare 56
Ethics and Homecare 57

Chapter 3

DRGs Stimulate High Technology and DME Services 65
    PPS/DRGs 65
        Quicker and Sicker *66* Differing Views on Quicker and
        Sicker *68* Enter Home Health Care *68* DRGS as a
        Reason for Discharge *69* Studies Supporting Increased
        Homecare *69* Discharge Planning, DRGs, and Homecare
        70 PPS/DRGs for Home Health Care *71* DRG Impact
        Summary *73*
    DRGs Spur High Technology Use in Home Health Care 73
        What is High Tech? *74* Issues Common to High Tech at
        Home *75* Reimbursement Commonalities *76* High Tech
        Growth Factors *76* Marketing Analysis *77* Safety and
        Training *79* Standards for High-Tech *79* High-Tech
        Impact Summary *80*
    Durable Medical Equipment (DME): Keeping Pace in
    Home Health Care 80
        DME Defined *80* DME Historical Overview *81* DME
        Growth and Potential *82* Marketing DME *84* DME
        Wheeling and Dealing *86* Reimbursement--The Root of It
        All *88* DME Impact Summary *95*
    DRGs, High Tech, and DME--An Overview 96

Chapter 4

Need Assessment In Homecare 103
 Measuring the Need 103
  Public Hearings on Need *106* Factors in Need
  Determination *107*
 Homecare Need Assessment Methods and Techniques 107
 Application of the Nine Formulas 109
 Consensus Patterns in Need Determination 111
 Hospital-based Need Determinations 113
 Need Determination by Attending Physicians 114
 Patient Assessment/Classification for Need Determination 115
 Inappropriate Placements in Need Calculations 116
 Resource Allocation for Homecare 119
 Reasoned Needs Determination 121

Chapter 5

Long-term Care, Homecare, And The Elderly 125
 Toward a Better Understanding of the Issues 125
  Facts and Figures *126* Impairment Status *130* Semantics
  132 Health Care or Social Care? *132* Quality of Life for
  the Elderly *134* Public Policies on the Elderly and Long-
  term Care *136*
 Continuing or Long-term Care 143
  Nursing Home Care *147* Homecare *148* Family Caregiv-
  ing and Long-term Care *150* Homemaker-Home Aide:
  Essential Services for the Elderly *151*
 Professional Education and the Elderly 151
  Physician Education *152*
 Planning and Research 155
 Long-term Care Overview 157

Chapter 6

Funding Homecare; Governmental And Other Sources 163
 Reimbursement Basics 166
 Funding Sources for Homecare 167
 Public Health Values and Reimbursement 167

Medicare 169
  Medicare Overview *169* Definitions *171* Budget Stimula-
  tion *176* Reimbursement Expenditures *180* Waiver of
  Liability for Home Health Agencies *180* Denials *185*
  Medicare's Future *186*
Medicaid 187
  Medicaid Homecare Expenditures *188* Section 2176
  Waivers *189*
Social Services Block Grant--Title XX 192
  Services *193* Funding and Expenditures *193* Impact *195*
Older Americans Act 196
  Services *196* Funding and Expenditures *197* Impact *198*
Government-funded Projects 199
Private Funding of Homecare 199
  Insurance Companies *201* Blue Cross Plans *201* Prepaid
  Group Health Plans *202*
Reimbursement Variations 202
Fraud and Abuse 203
Funding and Homecare: Impact 206

Chapter 7

Does Homecare Curtail The Costs? 211
  General Approval 211
  Basic Premises 212
    Cost-Effectiveness *213* Cost-Benefit Analysis *215*
    Substitution or Add-on *217* Cost and Impairment Level
    217 Cost Evaluation Problems *219*
  Homecare Cost Comparisons 220
    Inpatient Hospital Care vs. Homecare *220* Nursing
    Homecare vs. Homecare *224*
  Cost Comparisons 225
    Hospice Care vs. Homecare *230*
  Cost-saving Strategies 232
  Cost-Saving and Social Policy 233

Chapter 8

The Quality Of Homecare 237
  Quality of Care Generics 238
  Homecare Industry and Quality of Care 238
  Impediments to Quality Homecare 239

Recurring Themes in Quality Homecare 241
Rights of Patients 242
Standards, Norms, and Criteria for Quality Care 243
Homecare Accreditation 244
    Accreditation Defined *245* Existing Homecare Accredita-
    tion Organizations *246* Accreditation in the Future *253*
Licensure 253
Certification 257
    Certified via Medicare Conditions of Participation *257*
Regulation via Certificate of Need 260
Quality Assurance Programs 261
    Joint Commission and Quality Assurance *261* Internal and
    External Review *262* Drawbacks to Quality Assurance *262*
    Homecare System Characteristics *262* Pennsylvania
    Assembly Quality Assurance Project *264* Problem
    Oriented Medical Record *265* Patient Appraisal *265*
    Structure, Process, and Outcome Measures of Quality Care
    268 Utilization Review *270* Medical Records--Key to
    Quality Care *272*
Personnel Standards and Quality Care 273
Physicians and Quality Homecare 275
Win or Lose with Quality Care 276

Chapter 9

A Variety Of Homecare Workers: Professionals And Others

A Variety Of Homecare Workers: Professionals And
Others 283
Physicians 284
    Role of the Physician *285* Medical Education *286*
    What's Ahead *288*
Nursing 288
    Nursing Responsibilities *288* Nursing Education *289*
    Trend to Independent Practice *291* LPN and LVN
    291 Aides and Orderlies *292*
Home Health Aide 292
    Different Titles *293* Tasks *293* Worker Traits of
    H-HHAs *293* Profile of a Typical H-HHA *294* A
    Model Curriculum *294* Personnel Issues *295* Future
    of H-HHAs *296*
Physical Therapist 296
    Patient Referrals *297* Image of Physical Therapist *298*
    Quality Assurance *298* Adequate Personnel *299*
Occupational Therapist 299

OT Functions *299*   OT Training *300*   Uniqueness of
OT Homecare *300*   Standards of Practice *301*
Medicare and OT *302*   Future Concerns *303*
Medical Social Work 303
Tangible or Intangible Services? *304*   Special Areas
304   Planning and Policy *305*
Communication Services 305
Utilization of Personnel *306*   Ethics and Business *307*
Pharmacist 307
Role of the Pharmacist *308*   Reimbursement Impact
308   Independent Prescribing Authority *308*
Dietitian and Nutritionist 309
Typical Tasks *309*   Dietitian *310*   Nutritionist *310*
What's Ahead *311*
Dental Care 312
Volunteers 312
Program Examples *313*   Typical Volunteer Tasks *313*
Family Members 314
Public Policy and Family Homecare *314*   Homecare
Problems for Family Members *316*   Homecare While
Working Full-time *316*   Support Groups for Family
Caregivers *317*   Hospice and Family Caregiving *318*
Respite for Family Caregivers *318*   Females, Families
and Homecare *319*
Personnel in the Homecare Team 320
Future Homecare Personnel 321

Chapter 10

The Growth Of Homecare 329
Growth Rationales 329
Awareness of Homecare *329*   Self-Testing at Home *330*
Market Research Forecasts *330*   Inhibiting Growth Factors
331
Marketing Homecare 332
Basic Marketing Issues *332*   A Marketing Plan *334*   Ten
Marketing Rules *335*   Marketing in the Future *335*
Homecare Trade Associations 336
Joint Ventures for Growth 337
Advantages and Disadvantages *337*   Not Lucrative? *338*
Key Role of Physicians *338*   Caveat Emptor *339*   Typical
Joint Ventures *339*   Legal Aspects of Joint Ventures *340*
Hospital-based Homecare 341

Proprietary Homecare Growth 342
Voluntary Nonprofit Agency Growth 344
Utilization as a Measure of Growth 344
    Early Growth *344* Home Health Agencies from 1966 to
    1985 *345* Variability in Growth by State *345* Growth of
    Home Visits *347* Utilization Impact *357*
Barriers to Homecare Growth 359
Physicians and Homecare Growth 361
Referrals--The Touchstone of Homecare Growth 362
Homecare--Growing! Growing! Growing! 363

Chapter 11

Homecare Evaluation 367
Homecare Evaluation Questions 367
Specific Areas for Homecare Evaluations 368
Cost Containment and Evaluation 369
What is the Best Evaluation Method? 370
Evaluation Defined 371
Homecare Evaluation Study Characteristics 371
Political and Other Evaluation Pitfalls 373
Data Collection 375
    Uniform Basic Data Set *375* Deterrents to Data Collection
    and Use *376*
Evaluation Using Five Ds 377
Typical Homecare Evaluations 378
    Reviews of Evaluations in the Literature *379* Descriptive
    Evaluations *382* Survey/Polling Evaluations *383* Evalua-
    tions Using Personal Interviews *385* Evaluations Using
    Data Analysis *386* Comparison Evaluations *388*
Participant Observation 393
Evaluation Constants 393

Chapter 12

The Future Of Homecare: Trends, Issues And Dilemmas .. 399
Trends 399
    Early and Developing Homecare Patterns *399* Current Pat-
    terns *399* Future Patterns *401* Impact of Trends *402*
Issues 403
    Quicker and Sicker *403* Saving Money or Lives *403*
    Vantage Viewpoints *404* Government Actions Initiating Is-

sues *404*   Constancy of Homecare Issues *406*   Is a National
Homecare Policy Missing? *406*   Suggested Resolutions *407*
Dilemmas 408
Dilemmas Linked to PPS/DRG *408*   Medicare Dilemmas
and Reforms *412*   Long-term Care Dilemmas *413*
Homecare/Long-term Care Reforms *416*   Legislation to
Resolve Dilemmas *418*   Quality: The Bottom Line
Dilemma *421*   Impact of Trends, Issues and Dilemmas *422*
Laws of Physics and Homecare 422

Index 427

List of Exhibits

2-1   Homecare Levels by Patient Characteristics and Services

2-2   Perceived Need for Homecare Services within the Past Five Years as Seen by a Rural Elderly Population

2-3   Federal Funding Sources and Services for the Elderly

2-4   Where Do You Stand in the Homecare Debate?

2-5   Indicators for the Assessment of Institutionalization

2-6   Average Home Health Agency Employees by FTEs, Contract FTEs, Home Visits, Visits per Employee and Percent of Agency Visits

4-1   Limitation of Activity Due to Chronic Conditions by Degree of Limitation and Selected Age Groups, 1981

4-2   Comparison of Formulas Used for Need Determination

4-3   Service Checklist in Assessment Form

4-4   Medicaid Subsidizes Nursing Homecare for Individuals Ineligible for Community-based Coverage

4-5   Trends in Home Health Care Visits under Medicare, Selected Years, 1969-1984.

4-6   Medicare Persons Served by Number of Home Visits and Visits per Beneficiary, 1984

5-1   U.S. Population (in millions) All Ages and 65 Years and Over Selected Years, 1900-2000

5-2   Living Arrangements of Persons 65 and Over, by Sex, 1984

5-3   Number of Persons Who Need Homecare per 1,000 Adults 45 Years and Over, by Type of Measure and Age, U.S., 1979-1980

5-4   People Needing Assistance with ADL or IADL Activities, by Percentage of Age Group

5-5   Americans 65 and Older in Need of Long-term Care by Nursing Home or Community Care, 1980-2040

5-6   Homecare Services Required at Various Impairment Levels

5-7   Summary of Home Equity Conversion Plans

5-8   Long-term Care Services, Providers, and Settings

6-1   Major Federal Programs Funding Homecare Services: Services Covered, Eligibility, and Administering Agency

6-2   Percent of Individuals with Paid Care, by Payment Source and Limitation Level, U.S., 1982

6-3   Medicare 1987 per Visit Limits for Home Health Care Agencies and Add-on Amounts for Hospital-based Agencies

6-4   Medicare Utilization of Home Health Agency Services, Total Medicare Reimbursement, Reimbursement for Home Health Services, and Number of Home Health Visits, Selected Years 1969-1984

6-5   Medicare Home Health Agency Services: Reimbursement by State, 1984

6-6   Medicare Home Health Agency Services: Visits and Charges by Type of Visit and Type of Agency, 1984

6-7   Medicaid Medical Vendor Payments for Home Health Services by Locality, Fiscal Year 1984

6-8   Social Service Block Grant Estimates of Funding by State, by Percent of Total, by Homecare Allocations, and by Percentage, 1985

6-9   Visit and Hourly Charges by Provider to Private Pay Patients

7-1   Cost Inclusions Necessary for Comparison of Home Health, Skilled Nursing Facility/Health Related Facility, and Acute Hospital Care

7-2   Homecare Costs vs. Nursing Home Costs as a Function of Service Requirements

7-3   Assigned Average Monthly Percentage of Cost per Person by Impairment Level

7-4   Cost Comparisons for Nursing Home Without Walls Patients in New York City for May 1984

8-1   Status of State Licensure and Certificate-of-Need Laws

8-2   Characteristics of the Health Care System, Definitions

8-3   Criteria to Assess Quality of Home Health Care Rendered to Patients with Diabetes Mellitus, on Insulin

8-4   Examples of Components of a Structure, Process, Outcome Evaluation Measurement

10-1   Medicare Certified Participating Home Health Agencies, Selected Years 1966-1985

10-2   Medicare: Participating Home Health Agencies by Locality, by Type of Agency, December 1985

10-3   Medicare Home Health Agency Services: Persons Served and Visits by Region, Selected Years, 1975-1984

10-4   Medicare Home Health Agency Services: Visits by State, Selected Years, 1975-1984

10-5   Medicare Home Health Agency Services: Visits (in thousands) by Type of Agency and Type of Visit, Selected Years 1975-1984

10-6   Medicare: Home Health Aide Utilization by Type of Agency, 1984

10-7   Medicare: Persons Served, Number of Home Visits, and Average Visits per Beneficiary by Type of Agency, 1984

11-1   Possible Subjects for Homecare Evaluation Studies

11-2   Evaluation Dos and Don'ts

12-1   Examples of NAHC's Position on Various Homecare Issues

Foreword

Allen Spiegel has brought together in one book the history of home care and the range of home care issues that face this country as we move into the twenty-first century. We clearly need to develop a more expansive home care system to meet the postacute care needs of patients. This is especially true since the adoption of the prospective payment system, which has meant that hospitals release patients earlier and sicker than in the past.

Expanded homecare is also an essential element of our long-term care strategy. A New Jersey constituent wrote me recently about her personal struggle to provide home care for her 91-year-old mother. She said her mother was "mentally alert but extremely feeble," and she was no longer able to pay for the constant assistance that she required. "To have some-one come once a week and give me a whole day to myself would give me a new lease on life. We thought about a nursing home, but just couldn't do it after examining a few. Even mother says she has lived too long, but there has to be another answer besides nursing homes!"

Even more alarming is the plight of elderly people who have no family to take care of them, or whose families are simply unable to help because of financial, social, or psychological constraints. What happens to these older people? Many find themselves trapped--some at home with no support sys-tems and others inside hospitals and nursing homes--isolated, in a lonely en-vironment and deprived of their independence and dignity.

The lack of a home care alternative to institutionalization is a serious problem for many elderly today, but unless we take action, it will become a more serious problem in the years ahead. The increased life expectancy of individuals, the dominance of chronic disability in older individuals, and the "shrinking" of the American family all point to a growing need for ex-panded home care.

Between 1968 and 1979, two years were added to the life expectancy of a 65-year-old American, more than in the 50 years from 1900 to 1950. By the year 2000, the over-85 population in this country will be 60 percent larger than it is today. The increasing lifespan and aging of the population, as well as continuing medical advances, will leave even more older in-dividuals suffering from chronic illness such as cancer. It is estimated that by the year 2000, over 15 million older Americans will suffer from chronic disease that will limit their daily activities, a 50 percent increase over 1980.

Finally, our older Americans also are facing increasing difficulties get-ting needed care from other family members because the extended American family is "shrinking." People are marrying later. Families are much more mobile now. There are more divorces. More women are working, and couples are having fewer children. All of this means that direct family care for those in need is much less available than it was in the past.

There are no easy solutions, but in many cases life would be a lot better for many elderly people and concerned families if this country developed a comprehensive approach to providing more health care services at home. Families could be kept intact, and many elderly persons would no longer be forced into institutions, as they are now because federal programs don't pay for needed treatment outside of an institution.

The current health care delivery system views institutional care as the norm and home-based care as a promising alternative care system. We need to turn this around. Home care should not be viewed as an alternative. Home care should be the norm and institutional care should be the alternative only when home care is not feasible.

But even if acceptable financing mechanisms become available for home care, the problems will not end. Patients who receive services in the home are particularly vulnerable to poor quality of care. And the federal government's oversight of home care agencies does little to prevent this. Federal requirements focus only on the home care agency's capacity to provide care, rather than the quality of services actually provided. The fact is that quality concerns have taken a back seat to more visible cost concerns. Despite the growing need for home care, government and consumers simply do not know what level of quality they are getting for their money.

Clearly, we need to develop a health care system that first and foremost provides quality health care in the least restrictive setting. This will not be easy, but I believe that America is up to the task. Dr. Spiegel shows us where we have come and what the issues will be in the future. It is up to us to have the foresight and courage to adopt solutions.

Bill Bradley
United States Senator
New Jersey

Preface

Having finished the manuscript for *Home Health Care: Home Birthing to Hospice* in June 1983, I quickly responded in the affirmative when my publisher asked me to revise it in 1986. I thought, foolishly, in retrospect, that I would update the statistical exhibits and add bits and pieces while redoing the last chapter on trends and issues; most of the book would still be intact. After all, the material was only three years old!

As we became immersed in our research, the realization rapidly sunk in that the volume of literature on homecare had not abated--if anything, it had increased. Based on our analysis of the accumulated material, this revision turned into an almost entirely rewritten book--very little remains from the prior edition.

Combining ordinary hard work with advanced computer capabilities to produce this book, we believe that this volume can increase public and professional knowledge of the width and breadth of homecare activities. Since homecare may also be a neglected area in professional schools, this book should prove useful in curriculum development for future providers. We also anticipated that busy practitioners would be able to pick and choose those sections that concern them to keep up-to-date and to save time by having references handy. Finally, the public audience, including volunteers and family members, may wish to learn more and to educate others to create an awareness of homecare concerns.

A major impetus to the burgeoning of home health agencies was the federal Medicare program's implementation of the prospective payment system (PPS) using diagnosis related groups (DRGs), on October 1, 1983. In addition to the growth of home health agencies, there was a concomitant increase in the use of high technology care and durable medical equipment (DME) in the home.

An entirely new chapter deals with the impact of DRGs on the homecare industry. Chapter 3 examines the ability to create a minihospital at home with the combined sophistication of high technology care and scientifically advanced durable medical equipment. Antibiotic infusions, parenteral and enteral nutrition, oxygen therapy, and respiratory/ventilator support are examples of procedures now routinely administered in the home. Patients may be discharged from the hospital "quicker and sicker" and require a higher degree of intensive homecare.

Consumerism and public awareness are part of the rationales explaining the ins and outs and the advantages and disadvantages of homecare. National survey data on home health agencies fills an informational gap while detailing aspects of typical homecare providers. Additionally, Chapter 2 cites numerous examples of hospital homecare programs, such as a senior care network, a hospital coalition, and a hospital-based agency; disease/condition activities for victims of AIDS and Alzheimer's Disease; and specific population oriented programs, such as pediatrics, services in rural areas, and long-term care. Furthermore, this chapter discusses homecare as a business, covering corporate restructuring, marketing, relations with hospitals, and interactions with health maintenance organizations (HMOs). Finally, the sticky issues of malpractice and ethics are addressed.

In a chapter on need assessment, more than nine formulas for calculating homecare need are detailed, with a consensus analysis of the common elements. Techniques used by hospitals and physicians are also explained, along with consideration of inappropriate placement. Resource allocation links to need assessment may create a "chicken or egg first" dilemma when pondering homecare services for the community.

Chapter 5 on long-term care, homecare, and the elderly devotes considerable attention to innovative approaches to public policy recommendations on topics such as heath care vs. social care, impairment status, semantics, and quality of life. A dominant factor bringing a sense of urgency to the long-term care problem is the "graying of America." People are living longer than ever, with the "old-old"--those over 85--having the greatest population growth. It is apparent that there is a direct relation between advanced age and the utilization of health care resources. Policymakers advocate homecare as a viable alternative to institutionalization for the resolution of long-term care needs. Other options elucidated include long-term care insurance, life/continuing care communities, and home equity conversion. Care by family members continues to constitute an overwhelming portion of long-term care services while nursing home care continues to be the facility used most often.

Reimbursement for homecare services is being subjected to severe buffeting by governmental, especially Health Care Financing Administration (HCFA) policies and procedures. Chapter 6 discusses the bitter interactions relating to interpretations of eligibility for homecare services and definitions of "homebound, part-time intermittent care and skilled nursing care" by HCFA and fiscal intermediaries as denials of claims mount. The waiver of liability presumption that offers providers some protection for services rendered in good faith is also under attack. In addition, home health care cost caps have been imposed by discipline, and not in the aggregate as previously. These actions create a "Catch 22" situation, wherein the cost containment DRGs stimulate the need for homecare services while the HCFA restricts and reduces the funding for homecare reimbursements.

Chapter 7 responds to the question of homecare curtailing the costs of health care. Specific comparisons look at homecare vs. inpatient hospital care, vs. nursing home care, vs. hospice care, as well as other alternatives.

Particularly telling, from a cost saving viewpoint, are those involving the use of high technology at home compared to such therapy in the hospital. Of course, there are disagreements about whether or not homecare merely substitutes a more frequent but less expensive service for an expensive infrequent service. Nevertheless, it is illuminating to consider the recommended cost saving strategies and the social policy aspects of the cost containment mentality of the U.S. health care delivery system.

Quality of care, according to some analysts, is now a marketable commodity in the competition for the health care dollar. Chapter 8 discusses the bottom line issue: Can there still be high quality homecare services in an environment of cost containment and restriction? Attention is given to accreditation, licensure, certification, and professional standards, norms, and criteria. In addition, the impact of state certificate-of-need requirements raises issues related to restraint of trade and costs added to services. A number of quality assurance mechanisms are described, including patient appraisal (PA), utilization review (UR), patient oriented medical record (POMR), internal and external review, and the structure/process/outcome technique. Impediments to quality homecare are enumerated, including the major difficulty with evaluating care delivered in a home setting.

Chapter 9 discusses the role of a variety of homecare providers, including physicians, nurses, home health aides, physical therapists, occupational therapists, medical social workers, speech and hearing therapists, pharmacists, dietitians and nutritionists, dentists, and volunteers. Services rendered by family members receive special attention because of the volume of care delivered and its importance. Even working family members contribute significant hours to the care of impaired parents and/or relatives. Feminism is also an issue in family care, since females appear to be actually rendering the majority of the services in the home.

Joint ventures and marketing get considerable attention in Chapter 10 on the growth of homecare. Simply put, joint ventures involve agreements between organizations, such as hospitals and home health agencies, to form a new agency to offer homecare services. PPS/DRG seems to have stimulated joint ventures, as organizations seek additional sources of revenue to offset losses. At the same time, and for the same reason, agencies are increasing their efforts in marketing services to the public. Although there are legal pitfalls, such as antitrust violations, the growth of organizations providing homecare services continues at a rapid pace, almost doubling in two years.

Chapter 11 cites specific examples of homecare evaluations utilizing a variety of methods. Of concern in evaluation is the relation of cost containment policies and the outcomes of investigations. What is the best evaluation technique in that situation? What are the barriers to evaluation? How can worthwhile data be collected? These and other generic evaluation questions are considered at length in this chapter. Finally, evaluation constants are identified, pointing out guideposts for those concerned.

Starting with a philosophical overview, Chapter 12 reviews the actions and reactions, the policies and reforms related to the homecare industry. Areas under discussion include HCFA policies and procedures, recommendations for changes in Medicare, long-term care dilemmas, homecare policy patterns over the years and into the future, and legislative initiatives. While there is much stirring of the pot, the soup is yet to be finished and served. Ingredients are constantly being added by a variety of cooks; and it remains to be seen whether or not too many will spoil it.

It would be remiss not to mention the many people who were most helpful in speaking with me and sending me material. Not wishing to offend anyone, I thank them *in toto* for their generous assistance. Research associates included Gerard Domanowski, M.D., Rhonda Osborne, M.D., Albert Riddle, M.D., Marc B. Spiegel, and Cheryl Thomas, M.D. This intrepid group followed the library trails and found the articles, the books, and the reports that contributed to the comprehensiveness of this study. Medical librarians at the SUNY Health Science Center at Brooklyn translated our requests into interlibrary loans and computer literature searches that struck pay dirt. Jack Lubowsky, Ph.D. of our Scientific Computing Center and the staff of our Computer Information Center arranged for us to converse with the electronic brains that turned green tracks on cathode screens into printed words.

Additionally, Kay Dobson, Lois Hahn, Constance Jones, Molly Kessert, Cheryl Moore, and Maureen Roaldsen assisted with the typing and assorted tasks. Sincere thanks to all, for the realization is obvious that a book as comprehensive as this was not the work of a single individual.

About the Author

Allen D. Spiegel is a Professor of Preventive Medicine and Community Health, College of Medicine, Health Science Center at Brooklyn, State University of New York. Previously, he was a special research fellow at Brandeis University, a health education associate with The Medical Foundation, Inc. in Boston, and chief of the radio and TV unit of the New York City Health Department.

His education includes degrees from Brooklyn College (A.B.; B.S. Equivalent), New York University (Special Diploma in Radio/TV), Columbia University (M.P.H.), and the Heller School at Brandeis University (Ph.D.).

Dr. Spiegel is active as a consultant and speaker to a wide variety of medical, health, and social welfare organizations on topics such as community mental health, health planning, public/patient/physician/health communications, medical sociology, and health care administration.

A prolific author, Dr. Spiegel has more than 100 articles to his credit, in addition to over 20 books; including: *Perspectives on Community Mental Health; Medicaid: Lessons for National Health Insurance; the Medicaid Experience; Curing and Caring; Basic Health Planning Methods; Rehabilitating People with Disabilities into the Mainstream of Society; Medical Technology, Health Care and the Consumer; Home Healthcare: Home Birthing to Hospice; and Cost Containment* and *DRGs: A Guide to Prospective Payment.*

Chapter One

Beginnings of Home Health Care

A Brief History

The Beginning

Care of the ill and infirm in the home is not new. In some prehistoric cave, someone probably sipped spoonfuls of hot dinosaur soup as a remedy for a fever of unknown origin. Even as late as the mid-1900s, people were still receiving a fair portion of their medical care in their own homes. Physicians still made visits to apply hot or cold compresses and to render personal tender loving care. This was an expansion of the attitude toward drug usage expressed by Dr. Oliver Wendell Holmes (1962, 176) at a Massachusetts Medical Society meeting in 1860: "I firmly believe that if the whole *materia medica* as now used could be sunk to the bottom of the sea, it would be better for all mankind--and all the worse for the fishes." A hospital was a pest house into which you walked on two feet and came out of flat on your back in a casket.

To some extent, this remains so. Norman Cousins (1976, 29) noted the feeling when he recovered from a serious illness--a recovery in which he played the major role in his own therapy regimen. During his confinement he "had a fast-growing conviction that a hospital is no place for a person who is seriously ill."

As history is often cyclical, we are seeing a resurgence of care provided to the sick in their own homes. This time the motive appears to be economic and is subsumed under the rubric of "cost containment." This alternative, however, does include attention to maintaining the quality of care rendered at home as well as the anticipated money savings.

Developing the Homecare Industry

A founding principle established by the Boston Dispensary in 1796 spoke to the home health care issue: "The sick, without being pained by separation from their families, may be attended and relieved at home" (Irwin 1978, 4). At this time well-to-do patients rarely went into the hospital for care. Physicians came to their homes and families often accepted the responsibility for day-to-day care. When the Boston Dispensary created the first homecare program, an enlightened idea at the time, the Overseers of the

1

Poor stated, "Those who have seen better days may be comforted without being humiliated, and all the poor receive the benefit of a charity. The more refined as it is the more secret" (Moynihan 1981). As a result, the Boston Dispensary home health care program avoided the welfare stigma attached to hospital care while sick people were able to be helped at home.

In the late 1800s, home nursing services were organized and administered by lay persons. These agencies provided skilled nursing care and taught cleanliness and home care techniques to the ill and their families. In 1877, the Women's Branch of the New York City Mission was the first group to employ a graduate nurse to care for the sick at home. A voluntary agency was established in 1885 in Buffalo, New York, to provide home nursing care. In 1886, other voluntary agencies providing patients with similar home health care services emerged in Boston and Philadelphia. These would later become Visiting Nurse Associations (Hanlon 1974). Stewart (1979), in her book on home health care, notes the fact that graduate nurses were hired by the Los Angeles County Health Department in 1898 to make visits to the sick poor. This was the first governmental health department to set up such services.

Home nursing care also became part of the benefits offered by life insurance companies. In 1909, the Metropolitan Life Insurance Company was the first to offer such a service to its policyholders. Home nursing became so popular that by 1928, Metropolitan was affiliated with 953 organizations that provided visiting nurse services; Metropolitan itself employed 592 nurses to carry out the program. Other insurance companies adopted the idea and the programs lasted until the 1940s, with emphasis on promoting health rather than curing the sick (Stewart 1979).

With the advent of antibiotics, immunization programs and improvements in nutrition, sanitation, and housing, health care problems shifted from communicable diseases to long-term illnesses. Hospitals became overcrowded, so ways were sought to alleviate bed shortages. In 1941, Syracuse University (New York) initiated a program to provide medical care for the discharged hospital patient, indicating that there was important medical value attached to caring for patients in the home after hospitalization (Jensen, Weiskotten, and Thomas 1944).

Expanding the Need for Home Nursing

By this time, the home health care providers included governmental agencies, voluntary health associations, private insurance companies, and hospital-based programs. At times agencies combined to offer services. The National Organization of Public Health Nursing (1946) established a nationwide committee to investigate the most desirable method of rendering public health nursing services for family care. Three patterns of home nursing care were recommended:

- An all-public health nursing service, including care of the sick at home, to be administered and supported by the health department--the most satisfactory pattern for rural communities.

- Preventive services sponsored by the health department, with one voluntary agency working in close coordination with the department and having responsibility for bedside nursing and some special fields--at present the most common type of organization in large cities.

- A combination service jointly administered and financed by official and voluntary agencies, with all field service rendered by a single group of public health nurses--most desirable in smaller cities because it provides more and better service for each family.

The committee's recommendations had little effect, however, and home health care programs continued to develop haphazardly.

The Birth of Modern Homecare

Dr. E.M. Bluestone founded a prototype hospital-based homecare program at Montefiore Hospital, New York City in 1947. Finding that many indigent people with chronic illnesses were hospitalized for longer periods than necessary, Dr. Bluestone pioneered the "hospital without walls" or "extramural program." Montefiore's home healthcare program was revolutionary in that services were not limited to the poor or the elderly. Dr. Bluestone envisioned the same hospital staff tending the patient in home care, the same record system and the same services rendered: "If you have a 500-bed hospital and 50 patients on homecare, you have a 550-bed hospital" (Ryder 1967).

Dr. Martin Cherkasky (1949), homecare executive of the Montefiore program, delineated the following homecare services:

- medical service
- social service
- nursing
- housekeeping service
- transportation

- medication

- occupational therapy

- physical therapy

In enunciating the philosophy of the Montefiore home health care program, Dr. Cherkasky said, "When we think about a patient, we should think about him not only as an organic and spiritual whole, but also as a whole in society. It is no more fair or useful to separate a man from his environment than it is to divide him into separate and independent parts."

Establishing Guidelines

Professional interest was reflected in material appearing in medical and public health journals. A symposium in the *American Journal of Public Health* included reports on homecare projects in Gallinger Municipal Hospital (Shindell 1953), Washington, D.C.; in New York City municipal hospitals (Kogel 1953); in the Richmond, Virginia, Health Department (Holmes 1953); and in the Massachusetts Memorial Hospital--Boston University Medical School Service (Bakst 1953). In the same year, the *Journal of Medical Education* published a "Symposium on Extramural Facilities in Medical Education" under the editorial leadership of Dr. James M. Faulkner. These articles included material from medical schools at Cornell University, University of Tennessee, University of Pennsylvania, Boston University, and Montefiore and New York Hospitals (Bakst 1953; Barr 1953; Cherkasky 1953; Hubbard 1953; Packer 1953; Reader 1953). The professionals were urging the teaching and use of homecare services.

After about ten years of organized homecare activity, the Surgeon General's National Advisory Committee on Chronic Disease and Health of the Aged suggested that a conference be convened on the subject. Following up on this recommendation, the Chronic Disease Program of the U.S. Public Health Service (1958) held a "Conference on Organized Homecare" in Roanoke, Virginia. Four elements were considered necessary for an organized homecare program: administration, personnel, community resources, and evaluation. Standards were presented for hospital-based and community-based homecare programs. Of necessity, the conference addressed funding issues and there was considerable discussion of prepayment insurance plans. Criteria for the selection of patients for homecare programs were expansive rather than restrictive. Moving on to the required service, conference participants expressed concern about the lack of dental and nutritional services, while they listed a comprehensive roster of health professionals as necessary consultants. Also discussed were respite services so that family members could have freedom for recreation and coordination of care, with particular emphasis on records and referrals. Finally, suggestions were made for areas of research and study, including the collection of information for insurance companies to gain experience rating data for premium calculations, staffing patterns and case loads, and the preparation of a guide for organized homecare programs.

As early as 1961, the Community Health Services and Facilities Act authorized the Surgeon General to make project grants to public or non-profit agencies for the development of outside-of-the-hospital health services. These were defined as those which prevent, detect, or treat disease and disability, and improve care for persons who are not patients in a hospital. Services included nursing care, homemaker services, physical therapy, occupational therapy, nutritional services and social services. During the six years of the Act's authority (from 1962 to 1967) $42 million was used to support nearly 300 projects. About 15 percent of the funds was used for home health care activities. Most of the homecare projects continued beyond this period and became eligible for Medicare reimbursement.

Home Health Care under Medicare

The passage of Medicare in 1965 greatly influenced the expansion of home health care over the next two decades. Federal definitions required home health care agencies to have nursing service and one additional service such as physical therapy, occupational therapy, speech therapy, medical social services, or home health aide service. Yet even that minimal "nursing plus one" requirement was more than many of the existing nursing agencies were providing. The guideline fell far short of the comprehensive pattern known as Coordinated Homecare. Of the 1,100 agencies offering nursing care for the sick at home in 1963, only 250 could have qualified for Medicare participation (Warhola 1980). Therefore, the federal government appropriated funds to assist home care agencies in raising their levels of care. After the expenditure of approximately $16 million, 1,275 home health agencies were certified for Medicare participation by October 1966. This number continued to rise dramatically for the next few years.

Today's Home Health Care System

Medicaid programs did not require the provision of home health services at first; such services were optional at the state level. However, in 1971, home health care benefits were made mandatory. While the number of Medicaid dollars spent on homecare increased more than 25-fold, the percentage of total Medicaid expenditures for in-home services still remains at about 1 percent (Warhola 1980).

Homecare services are also available under Title XX of the Social Security Act, the Older Americans Act and as part of the Public Health Service and Health Care Financing Administration activities.

Recently there has been a rather large-scale entrance into the homecare field by several proprietary organizations that operate free-standing homecare agencies. In fact, the for-profit companies have become the major suppliers of homecare personnel in the nation.

The History of the Homemaker-Home Health Aide

In Europe, the first program organized to provide health care services in the home was established in Frankfurt, Germany, in 1892. This was quickly followed by a similar group in London in 1897, which sent "home helps" to assist the ill (Lowe 1976). In the early 1900s, American charitable agencies concerned with the care of young children developed the first specialized homecare services. "Substitute mothers" took over when the child's mother was hospitalized, the father had to go to work, and no relative or neighbor was available to help.

The Establishment of Visiting Housewives

In 1903, an annual report of the Family Services Bureau of the Association for the Improvement of the Condition of the Poor in New York City noted as an addition to nursing services "employing four women for the purpose of lifting temporarily the simple everyday burdens from sick mothers" (Werner 1965, 31). At first, the women were called "visiting cleaners," and later, in the 1904 report, "visiting housewives." Their duties included taking care of the children as well as the house. In its 1908 annual report, the agency said that these workers "helped in the renovation and restoration of homes." The annual report of 1912 noted that the women were "demonstrating the art of good housekeeping." Reports from 1918 to 1925 said that the women were "caring for children where the mother by reason of illness is temporarily unable to do her own housework."

With the shift in emphasis toward child care, the Jewish Welfare Society of Philadelphia began the first organized homemaker program in 1923 (Hunt 1971). This program hired women primarily to care for young children when the mother was incapacitated. While Jewish social agencies in Chicago and Baltimore followed suit, growth of this type of service remained slow until the beginning of the Great Depression in the 1930s. A program was developed by the Works Progress Administration (WPA) to employ women as "housekeeping aides," usually on a contract basis with organized services. Housekeeping aides were to attend families with overwhelming problems and hopefully prevent family breakups. By the early

1940s, when the WPA was discontinued, there were 38,000 homemakers in the nation (Department of Health and Human Services 1980).

Organizing Visiting Housekeepers

In 1937, actions of the U.S. Children's Bureau led to a "National Conference on Visiting Housekeeper Services." In its announcements, the Children's Bureau "recognized this service as one of the essential tools to prevent unnecessary foster care placement" (Hunt 1971). Two years later, the National Committee on Homemaker Service was formed; it held annual meetings from 1939 through 1957. At an early meeting, the group came up with "supervised homemaker service" to replace the old term.

A national survey on home health care was conducted in 1958. Responses showed that 143 agencies in the United States employed 1,715 part- and full-time homemakers. About 50 percent of the agencies restricted their services to children (Stewart and Smith 1958). Furthermore, one or more persons were ill in more than 80 percent of the households receiving homemaker services. A national conference was convened in 1959 to find ways to stimulate the development of additional services, while another conference was sponsored by the National Health Council in 1960 to discuss personal care. The latter came forth with guidelines for the kind and amount of personal care that homemakers could give to the ill and disabled. Additional guidelines ensued for the training and supervision necessary to ensure efficient and safe care (Department of Health and Human Services 1980).

Representatives from 26 national organizations and eight federal bureaus met in 1961. A formal request was made to the National Health Council and the National Social Welfare Assembly for the creation of an independent national homemaker agency. In 1962, the national Council for Homemaker Services was incorporated. Functions of this newly created agency included stipulation of homemaker services generally, setting standards for the field, provision of consultation to agencies, conduct of research when needed, and dissemination of information about the need for and impact of homemaker services.

In 1971, the name of the agency was changed to the National Council for Homemaker-Home Health Aide Services, to reflect the usefulness of one service to both the health and social service fields. Standards as well as a monitoring system were formalized in 1972. The agency subsequently became the National Home-Caring Council.

Summary

Currently, the home health care movement appears to be in an era of growth and increased utilization as it becomes an integral part of the health care delivery system. Lists of professional articles in the standard reference books such as *Index Medicus* reveal the variety and volume of the scope of homecare. In addition to professional attention, we have seen the advent of consumer groups emphasizing self-help and other forms of individual effort to strive for an improved health care system expressing the age-old humanistic qualities of homecare.

In conclusion, it is worthwhile to consider Hippocrates' comments on this approach in the Aphorisms: "Life is short, and the Art long; the occasion fleeting; experience fallacious, and judgment difficult. The physician must not only be prepared to do what is right himself, but also to make the patient, the attendants, and externals cooperate."

References

Bakst, H.J. 1953. Domiciliary medical care and the voluntary teaching hospital. *American Journal of Public Health* 43:589-595.

Bakst, H.J. 1953. Medical care. *Journal of Medical Education* 28(7): 40-43.

Barr, D.P. 1953. Extramural facilities in medical education. *Journal of Medical Education* 28(7):9-12.

Cherkasky, M. 1949. The Montefiore hospital home care program. *American Journal of Public Health* 39:163-166.

Cherkasky, M. 1953. Prolonged illness. *Journal of Medical Education* 28(7):15-20.

Cousins, N. 1976. *The anatomy of an illness as perceived by the patient.* New York: W.W. Norton.

Department of Health and Human Services. 1980. Bureau of Community Health Services. *A model curriculum and teaching guide for the instruction of homemaker-home health aides.* Washington, DC: Government Printing Office Pub. No. HSA 80-5508.

Hanlon, J.J. 1974. *Public health administration and practice.* 6th ed. St. Louis: C.V. Mosby.

Holmes, O.W. 1962. The young physicians in *The good physician* edited by W.H. Davenport. New York: MacMillan.

Holmes, E.M., K. Nelson, and C.L. Harper, Jr. 1953. The Richmond home medical care program. *American Journal of Public Health* 43:596-602.

Hubbard, J.P. 1953. Observation of the family in the home. *Journal of Medical Education* 28(7):26-30.

Hunt. R. 1971. *Homemaker-home health aide in Encyclopedia of Social Work.* Washington, DC: National Association of Social Workers.

Irwin, T. 1978. *Home health care: when a patient leaves the hospital.* New York: Public Affairs Committee.

Jensen, F., H.G. Weiskotten, and M.A. Thomas. 1944. *Medical care of the discharged hospital patient.* New York: The Commonwealth Fund.

Kogel, M.D. 1953. Some aspect of the home care program conducted by the New York City Department of Hospitals. *American Journal of Public Health* 43:584-588.

Lowe, J. 1976. The alternative to hospitals. *Modern Maturity* 19(2):29-31.

Moynihan, D.P. 1981. Remarks on S.861. *Congressional Record* 127(54):53356.

National Organization for Public Health Nursing. 1946. Desirable organization of public health nursing for family service. *Public Health Nursing* 38(8):389.

Packer, H. 1953. General practitioner supervision. *Journal of Medical Education* 28(7):12-15.

Public Health Service. Chronic Disease Program. 1958. Report of the Roanoke conference on organized home care. Washington, DC: Government Printing Office.

Reader, G.G. 1953. Comprehensive medical care. *Journal of Medical Education* 28(7):34-40.

Ryder, C.F. 1967. *Changing patterns in home care.* Washington, DC: Public Health Service. Pub. No. 1657.

Shindell, S. 1953. Preliminary report on Gallinger home care study. *American Journal of Public Health* 43:577-583.

Stewart, J.E. 1979. *Home health care.* St. Louis: C.V. Mosby.

Steward, W.H., and L.M. Smith. 1958. *Homemaker services in the United States.* Washington, DC: Public Health Service. Pub. No. 644.

Warhola, C.F.R. 1980. *Planning for home health services: A resource handbook.* Washington, DC: Department of Health and Human Services. Pub. No. HRA 80-14017.

Werner, A.A. 1965. *Homemaker-home health aide services in Encyclopedia of Social Work.* Washington, DC: National Association of Social Workers.

Chapter 2

Ins and Outs of
Home Health Care

In joining the celebration of National Home Care Week, President Ronald Reagan (*Caring* 1985a) expressed views that aptly describe basic tenets of the ins and outs of home health care:

> Health care in the home is as old as medical treatment itself. Today, it presents Americans with important opportunities. As an integrated part of our health care system, the home setting can offer the comfort of familiar surroundings and the flexibility of personalized treatment. It can preserve the dignity and independence of individuals and prevent or postpone institutionalization for millions of patients each year. In a significant number of cases, homecare can even reduce the cost of medical treatment.

These comments speak to points often made about the rationale for home health care: history, integrated care, benefits of care at home, avoiding institutionalization, and containing costs.

Speaking at his Congressional confirmation hearings, HHS Secretary Otis Bowen, the first physician to hold that office, also supported home health care (*Long Term Care Management* 1985). He told the Senate committees that people should be treated in the least restrictive setting possible and that home health care should be encouraged by government programs. However, Bowen also warned that the rapidly growing home health care services under Medicare have to be reviewed to prevent abuse and overutilization.

In an in-depth review, the Heritage Foundation (1984, 103) had rather pertinent things to say about the basis for promoting home health care services:

> The keystone of long-term health care policy should be a comprehensive program fostering home services. . . . To temper the cost of building and maintaining new nursing homes, the elderly and disabled should have the option of being cared for in their own homes. . . . Allowing patients to remain in their own homes is an antidote to an ominous wave of depersonalized institutional medical care.

Recommendation: Widening use of home health programs included under Medicare/Medicaid, the Public Health Service Act and other laws would reduce cost considerably.

Home health care is an efficient and yet humane health service program for handicapped citizens and the elderly and infirm who do not wish to be institutionalized. It remains an increasingly popular concept and an alternative to institutionalization.

Even the *New York Times* endorsed home health care. Jane Brody's Personal Health column (1986) noted that "Home health care fosters a greater sense of wellness and provides the opportunity to remain as independent as possible and involved with life. In general, patients heal faster and feel better when they are cared for in a home setting."

These few references by the President of the United States, a family physician who is also HHS Secretary, a respected policy research and analysis organization and a prominent science writer all emphasize the principles that have been expounded for years to stimulate the development of home health care services.

Caring and Home Health Care

Dr. E.M. Bluestone (1954), an originator of the prototype extramural function of homecare at Montefiore Hospital in 1947, spoke to the caring aspects of homecare in his early articles on the subject. He cites two motivating factors that spurred the implementation of homecare services: the rebellion against the cold, impersonal, mechanical services of ward care doled out over a strictly limited period of time, and the consequent need for discovering a way to give a sense of personal importance to each patient. Implicit in Dr. Bluestone's statement is a caring attitude and belief in the need for personal attention by health care professionals.

Shortly after the organization of Montefiore's homecare program, Dr. Martin Cherkasky (1949) pointed out elements he believed vital to an understanding of the homecare idea:

When we think about a patient, we should think about him not only as an organic and spiritual whole, but also as a whole in society. To understand what caused this patient to become sick, it is necessary to know what sort of family he has, where he lives, what kind of employment he has, and how he reacts to these factors. To the doctors on the program it has brought a new realization of the importance of social factors in disease.

Today, these expressions from pioneers in the home health care movement easily fit into the prevailing, caring, humanistic philosophy.

Public Awareness of Homecare

If there is so much verbal support for home health care and if the services are so beneficial, why are so many people still unaware of what homecare is all about? Part of the answer may come from a survey of 1,200 telephone interviews conducted from June 17 to July 8, 1985. Cetron (1985) reported that only 38 percent of the people were able to name any home health care services. Of the group that identified a service, nursing scored highest in awareness with 26 percent, while the other five services scored only from 2 to 7 percent. Few Americans saw advertisements, read articles about home health care services or agencies or watched special programs on the subject -- only 34 percent during the past year. Of the 465 people who knew about home health services, the information came from a family member's usage (35 percent), mass media stories (23 percent) or health care professionals (18 percent). Among those who had any awareness, 85 percent had a very positive image of homecare. "Homecare is preferred by 72 percent of the American public over nursing homes for the care of those persons who need frequent medical and housekeeping assistance." In conclusion, Cetron stated that homecare is "supported most by upper income, highly educated, slightly younger Americans rather than by many of its beneficiaries -- older Americans." Although very supportive, Hispanics and Blacks were often less aware of the services than the general population.

Val J. Halamandaris (1985a), President of the National Association for Home Care (NAHC), expressed the opinion that Congress has a positive image of homecare in a special issue of *Caring* devoted to a celebration of National Home Care Week held during the first week of December, 1985. Resolutions were passed in both the Senate and the House; introduced by Senator Orrin Hatch and Representative Leon Panetta (*Congressional Record* 1985). Numerous Congresspersons voiced support of home health care. Flashenberg (1985) presented a how-to-do-it publicity kit for home health agencies with suggested special events, sample mass media materials, and assorted creative ideas for community activities to promote awareness. In addition, case studies from 10 communities across the nation described efforts in prior years as further motivation (*Caring* 1985b). Yet, despite all the effort, Halamandaris (1985a) felt that ". . . home care still remains the best kept secret in health care."

Consumerism

In an attempt to spread the word, Coleman (1985) prepared *A Consumer Guide to Home Health Care* for the National Consumers League. that booklet defined home health care, described services, listed resources, discussed standards and funding along with problem areas, and presented a checklist for potential consumers to use to evaluate agency problems. Similarly, the Council of Better Business Bureaus, in cooperation with the National HomeCaring Council (1983) produced *All About Home Care: A Consumer's Guide*. That booklet covered the same material and included a homecare Bill of Rights for consumers. Early on, before Diagnosis Related Groups (DRGs), the Public Affairs Committee (Irwin 1978) published *Home Health Care. When a Patient Leaves the Hospital* to educate the public about noninstitutional care. This booklet addressed the issues of pressure for early discharge to cut costs and the changing role of hospitals. Additional material dealt with matters similar to the other consumer-oriented material, citing patient education within the hospital to prepare the individual and family for homecare programs.

Nassif's (1985) book is labeled "a complete consumer guide to the home health care solution." Advice is given on funding sources, special services, quality of care, homecare alternatives, and case management. A useful resource guide and a number of checklists also help the consumer through the insurance maze, tax deductions, and self-help organizations. Friedman (1986) and Murphy (1982) also wrote books intended to help patients and their families deal with the home health care situation.

Patient Education for Postinstitutional Homecare

Noting that homecare "remains an area of patient education that has not yet been maximized," Logue (1984) describes a 10-point patient education protocol for a patient with cancer. Beginning with the number of reimburseable days, a timeframe is set, with homecare educational goals calling for the patient and family members to demonstrate whatever skills will be required for homecare. Arrangements for referrals to community agencies and for special equipment are made by the social worker shortly before discharge. All professionals in the facility participate in the discharge plan, review it with the attending physician, and go over any appropriate teaching materials to be used by patient and family. On the home visit, the nurse again reviews all procedures and resolves problems. Should readmission be required, the homecare agency coordinates it with the facility to maintain continuity of care. In another patient education effort with cancer patients, Coyle (1984) commented that "relieving patient anxiety has been one of the major successes of the program."

A featured article in *Patient Care* (Borders 1985a) addressed the practice of preparing for posthospital homecare, reporting on a roundtable discussion on programs at Saint Joseph Hospital in Denver and at New York University Medical Center. Saint Joseph Hospital has a patient education coordinator who utilizes preoperative teaching packets and focus sessions with the private practice office nurses to improve continuity of care; gives diabetes teaching records to patients prior to appointments; and uses discharge teaching sheets for cardiac patients. This patient education program succeeds because top hospital administrators support the effort and the physicians cooperate. Physicians have to believe in the importance of patient education, be willing to share the educational tasks and allow their office staff the time to teach.

New York University Medical Center allows a close relative or friend to move into the hospital to receive education along with the patient. In a Cooperative Care Center, the patient and family are prepared for living at home after discharge by specific hospital educational and clinical groups. Obviously, the patient and the family must be ambulatory and be able to handle the emotional and physical demands. Borders (1985a) states that "most patients and their partners find the experience overwhelmingly positive."

While consumerism and patient education attempt to resolve many difficult areas, there is a possibility of patient abuse in homecare situations. Tamme (1985) identifies a number of hypotheses, including dependency of the impaired person, stresses upon the caretaker, family dynamics, the impaired caretaker, and an older person being viewed with contempt or as a burden. Despite all states having laws that may apply in these homecare situations, the patients may rarely seek aid because of their dependency. However, the consumer material does provide advice on handling problems and complaints.

A Suitable Home

Consumerism and patient education can prepare the individual for homecare, but there must be an appropriate environment -- not every home is suitable. A Pennsylvania Home Care Information Consortium (Russell 1977) arrived at the following attributes for a suitable atmosphere for homecare:

- Is it a quiet home? A sick person can be extremely sensitive to excessive noise.

- Are there stairs leading to the home or inside? For some people stairs can pose a serious problem, but they can be replaced by a ramp, banister lift, or other device.

- Will the person have a private room? One near a bathroom and dining facility is ideal.

- Will the doors and walkways accommodate a wheelchair or walker? Plenty of room is needed for maneuvering.

- Are there small children in the home? Youngsters cannot be expected to remain quiet all the time.

- Is there an adult nearby during the day? At night? Not all persons receiving homecare need constant attendance, but a relatively hapless person will be safer and happier with someone else there.

- Does the individual have easy access to a telephone or emergency response system? This is essential for morale and a sense of self-sufficiency.

- Is a television or radio available for the person's room? These help to pass the time and keep the person in touch with the outside world.

- A major ingredient for a suitable homecare environment is that intangible TLC factor: Tender Loving Care. TLC should be lavished upon the patient by family and friends.

- With an awareness of homecare services, an understanding of the caring concept, proper education and preparation and a suitable home environment, homecare has a much greater probability of succeeding.

Homecare Defined

Definitions of homecare usually include the words "home health care" in the initial phrase. Yet, as the definition continues, the meaning expands to include care other than that strictly related to health. Blum and Minkler (1980) consider the range of services and the involvement of the total family unit in devising their preferred terminology:

For this reason, we suggest the broader, more encompassing term, "homecare" instead of the sometimes misleading designation "home *health* care" (authors' emphasis). Our policies and programs should provide an array of services that foster not only health, but also activity and independence in one's normal environment. The term "home health care," with its links to existing medical reimbursement patterns and regulations, needs to be broadened.

Even within the existing use of home health care terminology, it is worth noting that the definitions cite undefined services, expanding the interpretation. Typically, the AMA (Weller 1978) states, "Home health care is any arrangement for providing, under medical supervision, needed health care and supportive services to a sick or disabled person in his home surroundings."

Trager (1972) reported to a Senate Special Committee on Aging and established a foundation for the expansive view. Under medical supervision, home health care was described as follows:

An array of services which may be brought into the home singly or in combination in order to achieve and sustain the optimum state of health, activity, and independence for individuals of all ages who require such services because of acute illness, exacerbations of chronic illness, long-term, or permanent limitations due to chronic illness and disability.

Definitions are as varied as the perspectives of the agencies producing them. Some stress services, others emphasize reimbursement, and still others concentrate upon quality of care. A federal intradepartmental work group developed an operational definition of home health care, seeking to bridge the gaps between providers and payers. Using materials prepared by the then existing agencies: the Assembly of Ambulatory and Home Care Services of the American Hospital Association (AHA), the National Association for Homemaker-Home Health Aide Services, Inc., the Council of Home Health Agencies and Community Health Services of the National League for Nursing (NLN), the American Nurses Association (ANA), the National Health Council, the American Medical Association (AMA), and the Work Group (Department of Health, Education and Welfare 1976) arrived at the following definition:

Home health care is that component of a continuum of comprehensive health care whereby health services are provided to individuals and families in their places of residence for the purpose of promoting, maintaining or restoring health, or of maximizing the level of independence, while minimizing the effects of disability and illness, including terminal illness. Services appropriate to the needs of the individual patient and family are planned, coordinated, and made available by providers organized for the delivery of home health care through the use of employed staff, contractual arrangements, or a combination of the two patterns.

Home health services are made available based upon patient care needs as determined by an objective patient assessment administered by a multidisciplinary team or a single health professional. Centralized professional coordination and case management are included. These services are provided under a plan of care that includes, but is not limited to appropriate service components such as medical, dental, nursing, social work, pharmacy, laboratory, physical therapy, speech therapy, occupational therapy, nutrition, homemaker-home health aide service, transportation, chore services, and provision of medical equipment and supplies.

That expansive definition also included points relative to the key phrases. Although the definition was produced in 1976, long before PPS and DRGs, it should prove illuminating to read while considering holistic care concepts, cost containment initiatives, and today's health care delivery system.

Home Health care is that component of a continuum of comprehensive health care . . . .

Homecare if often viewed as a substitute for, or a "second best" to needed care in an institution. On the other hand, some advocates go to the opposite extreme, viewing homecare as a panacea for overutilization and high cost of medical care. In actuality, homecare is neither a "cheap" substitute nor a panacea, but a legitimate form of care for some persons at strategic times during the course of their illnesses. It is that component in the continuum of health care in the community that should be provided only when an individual does not need intensive, full-time care or supervision in an institutional setting yet cannot, without undue effort, get to such services on an ambulatory basis. Then homecare can and should be delivered on an intermittent basis. As part of a continuum, homecare can, as need dictates, precede or follow institutional care in a hospital or long-term care facility, or be given in combination with ambulatory care or care in a long-term facility.

. . . whereby health services are provided to individuals and families in their places of residence . . .

In the delivery of homecare, two phrases from the definition are often forgotten or too narrowly defined -- family and place of residence. When coordinated homecare programs were first established in this country, great emphasis was placed on the physical surroundings of the patient. Home environment was felt to be extremely important to proper care, and the availability of a private room on the ground floor with adjoining bathroom was considered essential. This re-creation of a hospital-like setting in the home eventually took on a lesser role. It was found that even when these requirements were filled, good care was not possible without a "caretaker" who could provide the necessary support and maintenance between visits of professional persons. Today the emphasis is on the caretaker and the word "home" has taken on many meanings -- from the person's own residence, whether it be a single family dwelling, apartment, trailer, room in a boarding home or home for the aged, to a foster home or congregate-living facility. "Caretaker" has similarly been more broadly defined as any individual, family member or not, who can take responsibility for supervision and personal care of the individual receiving home health service.

. . . for the purpose of promoting, maintaining, or restoring health. . .

In keeping with its definition as an active component of community care, homecare has multiple functions. Homecare is useful for an individual recuperating from an acute illness, helping him to be restored to full function. In terms of long-term illness, homecare services provide the support necessary to maintain that individual in the community and prevent premature admission to an institution. For all individuals on homecare, regardless of age or physical condition, health promotion is also a possibility. Recognizing this, home health agencies have included such diverse activities as immunization, prenatal care, nutritional guidance, accident prevention in the home, health education, and screening tests for chronic diseases.

. . . or maximizing the level of independence . . .

One level of prevention alleviates dependency through rehabilitation services. These services are usually viewed by care providers as most effective for the younger individual where independence means return to a job, school or homemaking role. More emphasis must be placed on the older individual's need for "habilitation" services to restore her to the highest level of independence possible. Even if that level is only a chair and bed situation, as long as the individual can carry out his personal care needs himself and can communicate to others those needs he cannot meet, he is independent. Homecare is not long-term care but long-term living.

. . . while minimizing the effects of disability and illness . . .

Homecare cannot be limited only to passive support of older persons who need long-term care. For any age group, the prevention of disability or of complications of illness is possible when homecare is active and aggressive. Much of the disability seen in long-term illness is preventable when the homecare program views it role in such a positive manner.

. . . including terminal illness.

Early homecare programs failed to meet the needs of the terminally ill. A few programs began to care for them at home and found positive acceptance of the services, particularly from the family. Today, more homecare programs are making an effort to reach the terminally ill.

Services appropriate to the needs of the individual patient and family . . .

Homecare offers a unique opportunity to tailor care to exactly what the patient and his family require. In homecare, scheduling of visits is very flexible, and can be increased or decreased in number or modified by type, e.g., physical therapy visits changed to nursing, or nursing to home health aide service, as the needs of the patient change. Thus, the danger of overcare can be minimized. In addition, the strengths of family members can be utilized to supplement and reduce professional care, just as their weaknesses can be supported by professional assistance when they are in need of respite from care.

... are planned, coordinated and made available ...

The concept of patient care management establishes a system of patient appraisal, care planning and care evaluation. Although this concept is basic to all good medical care, it is not a process that has been applied formally and consistently. Frequently in homecare, appraisal of patient needs may be limited to the disease process. An added benefit of patient care management is the enhancement of continuity of care. All care providers describe the patient in identical terms and appropriate services can be readily provided and tailored to changing needs as the patient moves between institution and home.

... by providers organized for the delivery of home health care ...

Since the first organized program of homecare was started, many types of organizations have established programs, including hospitals, health departments and VNAs. Of the providers presently administering home care programs there are four general types:

1. Public agencies -- all agencies operated by state or local units such as health and welfare departments.

2. Nonprofit agencies -- nongovernmental organizations such as VNAs or agencies located in hospitals, skilled nursing facilities or rehabilitation facilities, as well as private nonprofit agencies organized and operated by an individual.

3. Proprietary agencies -- all privately owned profit-making agencies.

4. Combined agencies -- those agencies operated by an organization with dual sponsorship by a governmental unit and a voluntary agency, e.g., a health department and a VNA.

... through the use of employed staff, contractual arrangements, or a combination of the two patterns.

Not all the services identified in the full definition are reimbursable under governmental and/or insurance plans. As a result, the number and kinds of services provided by home health agencies today varies greatly. As community needs were identified, some services were supplied more frequently than others. For example, physical therapy and home health aide service is provided in at least 75 percent of the agencies. Occupational therapy, speech therapy, and medical social services are offered by fewer agencies, and these mainly in urban areas. Some agencies employ service personnel such as nutritionists and psychologists, but charge them to administrative costs. Whether full- or part-time, nursing personnel are generally permanent members of a home health agency staff. In contrast, therapists and medical social workers are more often employed in another agency (e.g., hospital, clinic, rehabilitation center) and provide services to patients in the home under contractual arrangements or on a fee-for-service basis.

Except for variations in the types of providers, much of the explanatory material seems to have stood the test of time rather well.

Levels of Care

Homecare service levels can range from high technology (similar to hospital inpatient care), to help with the activities of daily living (ADL) such as housecleaning and meal preparation. Concentrated medical care activities could occupy most of the in-home program or the effort could be a maintenance one of mostly social and supportative services with little health and medical attention. A diverse number of organizations and a variety of homecare workers could be involved in each individual's plan for homecare services. In essence, each person's homecare program is tailored to fit and to match needs with appropriate services. Levels of homecare can be intensive, concentrated, intermediate, maintenance or basic, as follows:

- *Intensive homecare*--provided to persons with serious illness whose medical condition is unstable and who require concentrated physician and nursing management. Such patients would normally require in-patient care if the professional, technical, ancillary medical services, personal care and environmental supportive services needed were not readily available and professionally coordinated by the appropriate primary providers.

- *Intermediate homecare*--provided to persons whose medical condition is not expected to fluctuate significantly as rehabilitation is achieved or the disease progresses. Such patients require professional health services and may also need personal care and other environmental supportive social services.

- *Maintenance homecare*--provided to persons whose primary needs are usually for personal care and/or other supportive environmental and social services. The medical condition of such persons is generally stable and requires only periodic monitoring to ensure maintenance of an optimum state of health.

While not differing greatly in general description, (HHS) also describes three levels of homecare. "Intensive" is now "concentrated" and "maintenance" is now basic:

- *Concentrated or intensive services*--for those individuals who otherwise would need to be hospitalized but who can benefit from multiple professional, diagnostic, therapeutic and supportive services under professional supervision and coordination on an intermittent basis.

- *Intermediate services*--a less concentrated array of home health services for individuals who need convalescent care from acute illness or have a temporary disability related to chronic illness.

- *Basic services*--a simple combination of health supervision and maintenance designed to maintain individuals who have long-term care needs in their own home, thus preventing or postponing the need for institutionalization.

The Blue Cross Association (1978) also defines structures of services for an effective home health care system in its model benefit program. These characteristics are displayed in Exhibit 2-1. In the description, the point is made that maintenance care is "sometimes inaccurately referred to as 'custodial care'."

Exhibit 2-1 Homecare Levels by Patient Characteristics and Services

Level of Homecare	Patients and Their Needs	Service Types
Intensive	Seriously ill/unstable disease or injury Physician and nursing concentrated services Professional coordination and administration Otherwise inpatient care needed	Hospital inpatient type services Ambulance or similar transportation
Intermediate	Disease or injury controlled Lesser physician care Mainly nursing care and rehabilitation and health aide services	Range of health and social services provided by home health agencies singly or in combinations
Maintenance	Condition stable At rehabilitation plateau Monitoring and assessment periodically Mainly help with activities of daily living	Range of social and supportive services in addition to some health services

Source: *Home Health Care. Model Benefit and Related Guidelines.* Chicago: Blue Cross Association, IL, June 1978, pp. 3-5.

Hennessey and Gorenberg (1980) also indentified three levels of care: preventive, supportive, and therapeutic services. Level one (preventive) aims to prevent further physical or mental deterioration; level two (supportive) helps people with chronic illnesses able to be discharged to community services; level three (therapeutic) provides assistance to people in need of more professional help along with community services.

Generally, all the descriptions of levels of homecare are similar. This uniformity means that professionals and administrators can be reasonably sure they are in agreement when discussing different care levels. This consensus has ramifications for reimbursement calculations and for the preparation of treatment plans that can be carried out without misunderstandings.

Elements of the Homecare System

Because homecare consumers can be subject to exploitation, appropriate professional personnel must prepare a written plan of action, ensure that the tasks are carried out and see that all concerned comply with established standards. Continuous evaluation should find gaps and devise actions to satisfy unmet needs. Consumers should be able to interact with the professionals and be assured that their input will be considered.

A joint committee of representatives from the Assembly of Ambulatory and Home Care Services of the AHA, the NAHHA, the National Council for Homemaker-Home Health Aide Services, Inc., and the Council of Home Health Agencies and Community Health Services of the NLN (1978) prepared a prospectus for a national homecare policy. Their document mandated that homecare systems must incorporate at least the following six elements:

1. Homecare services, which include:
   a) professional assessment of health and social needs;
   b) establishment of a plan of care;
   c) professional preventive, treatment, and maintenance services;
   d) professionally supervised personal care, environmental, and other supportive services; and
   e) centralized professional coordination of all services included in an individual's plan of care when multiple services and/or providers are involved;

2. Formally arranged administrative and operational links among provider organizations participating in the homecare system;

3. Uniform guidelines for both the designation and role of the primary provider according to the individual's condition and plan of care,

and for the primary provider organizations' professional and administrative responsibilities;

4. Participation of health care institutions, community health and social agencies, and individual professional practitioners to provide the full scope of preventive, treatment and maintenance services;

5. Administrative policies that adhere to nationally recognized accreditation/certification standards; and

6. Arrangements for external monitoring and evaluation of the appropriate utilization, quality, and the cost of the services provided, according to established professional standards and prudent fiscal policies.

These mandated elements of a homecare system are broadbased in their interpretation, but do rely on a professional understanding of what the terms mean. To most professionals, the six elements indicate a comprehensive homecare organization.

The Blue Cross Association (1978) listed 12 characteristics of an effective home health care system. Their model plan called for coordination by a professional nurse, complete medical records, central administration, contractual arrangements, standards for quality care, patient care planning, utilization review, data collection and analysis, no restriction by age, sex or source of payment, and flexible but standardized administrative and professional policies. Even with the third-party bias in mind, the document is very similar to that produced by the joint committee, emphasizing that all elements in a homecare system aim to establish a comprehensive program providing continuity of care in a professional and humane manner.

What are Homecare Services?

Based on these definitions of homecare, it is obvious that a wide variety of specific services will exist. In fact, Connecticut Community Care, Inc. (1985) contracted with more than 165 agency-based service providers to meet the needs of 5,000 + people in their various programs during 1985. Hayslip, et al. (1980) studied the homecare needs of the rural elderly over a five-year period and identified a diversity of perceived needs (see Exhibit 2-2).

Reporting on a six-year Wisconsin investigation, Seidl et al. (1981) cautioned that the provision of homecare services may be subject to political agenda and advocacy pressure groups. In fact, the researchers felt that homecare agencies may be forced to displace their official goals related to the delivery of services. It is sometimes difficult to comprehend how political squabbles could interfere with supplying needed services. Yet, since that

Exhibit 2-2 Perceived Need for Homecare Services within the Past Five Years as Seen by a Rural Elderly Population

Heavy Household Tasks
Scrubbing floors
Moving furniture
Lifting
Lawn care
Window washing
Cleaning

Light Household Tasks
Dusting
Vacuuming
Making beds
Washing clothes
Fold/iron clothes
Dishwashing
Preparing meals
Putting away groceries

Human Services
Personal counseling
Telephone reassurance
Telephone hotline
Protective services

Personal Maintenance, Medical Supervision and Rehabilitation
Personal hygiene
Bathing
Eating
Getting in/out of bed
Exercising
Taking medicine
Taking temperature
Reinforce/change dressings
Give/remove bed pan
Change position in bed
Climbing stairs
Live-in home aide

Social and Community Services
Medical transportation
Personal transportation
Grocery shopping
Meals on wheels

Source: Adapted from Hayslip, B., Jr., Ritter, M.L., Oltman, R.M., and McDonnel, C. Homecare services and the rural elderly. *The Gerontologist* 20(2):192-199, 1980.

appears to be the reality, homecare organizations should be alert to the possibility of such interference.

An Alphabet of Services

In his report on the pioneering Montefiore Hospital homecare program, Cherkasky (1949) listed the eight services provided: medical services, social services, nursing, housekeeping services, transportation, medication, occupational therapy, physical therapy. An alphabetical list of recommended services to be provided in home health care programs has been developed by the ANA and the NLN (Stewart 1979):

Audiologic services
Barber-cosmetology
Dental care

Education or vocational training
Handyman
Home-delivered meals

Housekeeping and heavy cleaning	Physical therapy
Information and referral	Physician services
Laboratory	Podiatry
Legal	Prescription drugs
Medical supplies and equipment	Prosthetics/orthotics
Nursing	Protective services
Nutrition and diet therapy	Recreational service
Occupational therapy	Respiratory therapy
Opthalmologic services	Social work
Pastoral services	Speech pathology
Personal contact services	Translation service
(friendly visitor, telephone	Transportation & escort service
reassurance)	X-rays

Other organizations have prepared their own listings of homecare services, the only variation being in the number of items.

Lancaster (1985) identified at least four major components reflecting the changes in homecare: personal services, equipment, high technology services, and self-or family care. Also in speaking about innovations, Stitt (1985) got right to the point of what homecare service is all about. "A house is not a home and homecare is more than house calls."

What emerges from a comparison of the various listings is the broad spectrum of services that can fit into a homecare program. There seems to be no aspect of human life that cannot be covered under the aegis of homecare. This could be a blessing as well as a curse -- blessing because help would be available for almost any problem; a curse because third party payers would have to be wary of reimbursing any program with such an amorphous appetite, able to absorb countless dollars in benefits.

Coordination -- A Must in Homecare

With the variety of home health care services and the numerous health and social care workers coming in and out of the individual's home, arranging for continuity of care is an absolute necessity. Professional case managers must ensure that equipment shows up in the right place in working order, as well as keeping track of the network of homecare providers destined for specific clients. These homecare coordinators can explain the total plan to all concerned, monitor daily activities, evaluate services, solve problems, and act as liaison between clients and agencies (*Forum* 1978).

Stewart (1979) comments on continuity of care, in particular about the difficulty of achieving a flow of harmonious, coordinated, continuous care. She also notes that the staff of homecare agencies are functioning independently in the client's home and not a central location with colleagues.

To maintain continuity of care of each individual served by homecare agencies, Stewart (1979) suggests the following five actions:

1. Informal discussions among individual staff members.

2. Formal discussions among individual staff and/or their supervisors.

3. Informal group or team discussions (for example, over lunch).

4. Formal team conferences; and/or

5. A written care plan.

Reporting on a number of surveys of coordinated homecare programs, Ryder (1967) noted a more than doubling of agencies between 1961 and 1964: from 33 to 70. Coordination was defined as including central administration by a single organization, physician directed patient services and coordinated planning, education and follow-up. Calling the changes a "new look," the authors commented on the shifts in administration from hospitals to health departments, VNAs and independent homecare agencies.

Working within the existing health and social care delivery systems, Trager (1980) commented on the obstacles to coordination in home health care, including the following:

- Variations in agency philosophy re service provisions.

- Differences in the assessment of patient's needs.

- Separate, and often conflicting, plans for care.

- Differing perspectives on the kind and amount of services required, and the type of personnel best suited to render those services.

Obviously, individuals could spend countless hours and much energy trying to be their own contractors, building coordinated homecare programs -- time ill-spent spinning wheels.

Weller (1978) proposed six solutions to fragmentation and coordinated obstacles:

- There should be a coordinated single locus of service.

- The management mechanism should be coordinated. Thus, the community would receive a single assessment, eligibility, prescription referral, coordination, follow-up and advocacy mechanisms.

- There should be formal interagency contracts to permit patients to enter and move through the system on the basis of need.

- Homecare must be given greater attention as an integral part of the overall planning for community health and social care delivery systems. There should be coordination between nursing homes and homecare agencies, for example.

- Uniform funding sources are necessary and could provide a single source of uniform eligibility under various governmental funding programs.

- Improved data collection at local levels is important to document cases and cost, making for a more efficient system.

Exhibit 2-3 demonstrates the criss-crossing between federal funding sources and service needs of the chronically impaired elderly. Fragmentation, duplication and a lack of coordination have to result from the diagrammed interagency program conflicts. Lee and Stein (1980), in their Guale project study report, concluded that fragmented funding leads to duplication and artificial separation of social and health care services.

In Boston, the Massachusetts General Hospital (Tolkoff-Rubin, Fisher, O'Brien, et al. 1978) Home Care Program is under the central administration of the Boston VNA. A Home Care Coordinator, a visiting nurse assigned to the hospital, is the pivotal person in that homecare service. A two-fold emphasis exists in this program that is similar to most coordinated homecare efforts:

- To bring to bear the coordinated services of a wide variety of community agencies to maintain the patient within the family environment.

- To ensure the ongoing evaluation of the effectiveness of the individual patient's health care plan.

Frasca (1981) reported on a homecare program that offered comprehensive, coordinated services to an average of 3,000 patients daily. South Hills Health System (SHHS) Home Health Agency is one of the largest multihospital-based health care programs in the nation, involving eight hospitals and one skilled nursing facility in a four-county area of western Pennsylvania. South Hills Health System includes a 400-bed acute care hospital, a 78-bed nursing facility and an active ambulatory care program integrated within its non-profit corporation status.

While Friedman and Kaye (1979) reassert that the case manager is a vital cog in a coordinated homecare system, they do note problems. Stress factors in the interactional aspects of the coordinated homecare system do exist and can cause friction. Stress can come from within the organization providing the services, from clashes between the personalities of the workers and the clients, and from differences in role perceptions of members in the homecare relationship.

Exhibit 2-3 Federal Funding Sources and Services for the Elderly

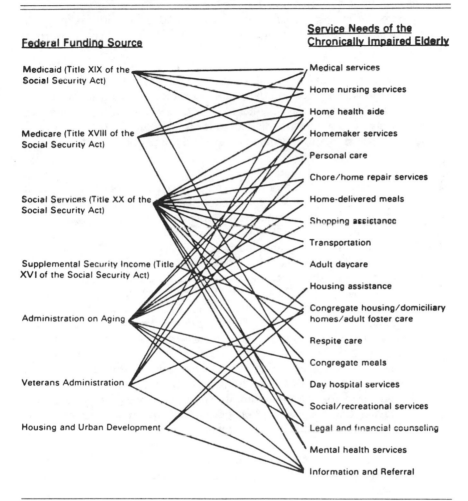

Source: General Accounting Office. Nov. 26, 1979. *Entering a nursing home. Costly implications for Medicaid and the elderly.* Washington, DC: Government Printing Office. Pub. no. PAD 80-12, p. 74.

Reif's (1980) analysis of nine comprehensive homecare agencies elicited characteristics of those agencies most successful in establishing well-coordinated services. Successful agencies had staff that collaborated and worked as a team with good communication, were able to use existing funding sources effectively while reducing overhead costs, and were able to obtain additional funding from grants and through waivers. Leadership, training, and staff support were also mentioned.

Despite the strong plea for coordination and continuity made by experts and illustrated by examples, Roberts (1978) does speak a word of warning:

> Always there has to be an adjustment between professional ideals of care in individual cases and the proper demands of "the system." Thus there is conflict between the idea of a "patient-centered" approach and the reality of community-wide demands on services; and between the idea of professionally coordinated care and the people's right to reject it.

Incorporated in September 1982, the American Association for Continuity of Care (AACC) aims to make coordination an essential component of the health care delivery system, with emphasis on discharge planning and access to an educational and supportive network. Agnes C. McBroom (1985), President of AACC, summed it up in an issue of the organization's publication: "Never before has there been such an awareness that a well-developed system for discharge planning is essential for success in today's world of rapid change in the health care delivery system."

A headline in *Hospitals* proclaimed, "Case Management is Just the ticket for Home Care" (Traska 1986). The coordinator was likened to the conductor of an orchestra. While Halamandaris of NAHC was quoted as saying case management was a good idea, he did raise the issue of who manages the care. It was his opinion that it would be better not to have the hospital do so since there was a possibility of conflict of interest.

With the need for more community support services for patients who may be leaving the hospital earlier because of the new reimbursement scheme, homecare coordination will remain a top priority for any successful program endeavor.

Considering the levels of care, the elements of homecare, the specified services and the coordination, what type of individual benefits from a sound homecare program?

Persons Benefiting from Homecare

Homecare is particularly appropriate for the elderly, the rural, the poor, children, the handicapped, the chronically ill, the mentally ill, the terminally ill, and the disabled. Russell (1977) lists examples of people most likely to benefit from homecare:

- a middle-aged person with a cardiac disorder who requires a prolonged convalescence.

- a baby with diabetes, or a young mother with high blood pressure.

- a person who needs assistance in managing the home from a homemaker, nutritionist or family social service agency.

- an elderly person handicapped with arthritis in need of rehabilitation therapy.

- a child who needs assistance when the parent is hospitalized.

- persons under distress or disorganization who have no family available to help.

Common diagnoses for discharge to homecare services included the following, according to Nassif (1985,300): unstable diabetes, heart/circulatory conditions including unstable high blood pressure and pacemaker implant; stroke recovery; arthritis/joint problems; respiratory ailments; cancer; skin problems including bedsores and wounds; bowel and bladder conditions; nerve muscle disorders; digestive disorders including those requiring artificial feeding; postoperative recovery; and accident recovery.

Within this listing of people and problems, it becomes obvious that there may be a distinction between medical and social needs. If the World Health Organization (WHO 1947) definition of health is used as a baseline, health does not mean merely the absence of disease. Rather, health is broadbased and includes a "state of complete physical, mental, and social well-being." This unproductive trichotomy among medical, health, and social needs was analyzed by Blum and Minkler (1980). They concluded that there should be access to a variety of community-based caring alternatives to provide a continuum of care. Going back to the comments of Bluestone (1954) and Cherkasky (1949), there can be no doubt that their vision of the homecare program included adherence to the all-encompassing ideals of WHO's definition of health. There is no split in the services, but rather attention to the requirements of the patient and the family as a holistic unit.

Viewing the comprehensive range of conditions and services available to people in their own homes, consideration focuses upon the question of homecare as the alternative to institutionalization. That question has occupied the attention of numerous legislators, researchers, and consumer groups.

Is Homecare an Alternative?

Impassioned arguments have been made about he use of homecare as an alternative to institutional care. Even the business world got into the debate with the *Wall Street Journal* (Lubin 1975) proclaiming "Alternatives to Nursing Homes" in large, bold, black typeface. In the article, Dr. Robert Morris of Brandeis University raises a question and gives a possible answer:

> Why should anyone worry about alternatives? Public policy says, "Let's do things this one way, and we'll pay you for doing it."

Dr. Morris was alluding to the fact that health care providers and the others who pay for services have a bias toward the use of institutions to deliver the required care.

In response to the question of why anyone should worry about alternatives, we need to look at what happens to people placed in institutions. When individuals are put into institutions, there appears to be a speed-up in their physical and mental deterioration. "Transplantation shock" occurs when familiar surroundings and lifelong possessions are left behind. Patients often suffer severe depressions, with a speed-up in physical and mental deterioration, thereby shortening their lives. This takes place even in the well-run establishments and, of course, is compounded in the others. Furthermore, many people do not really need institutional care. Studies (Lowe 1976; Malafronte et al. 1977) estimate anywhere from 30 to 50 percent of nursing home residents could return home if adequate home health care services were available.

Despite these studies, there should be some caution. There are individuals who do require care in a facility of some type. This has been noted by Dr. Amitai Etzioni (Irwin 1978) of Columbia University:

> It is an illusion that most people currently in nursing homes could be sent home. Studies show that half of these people have no close relatives; a high proportion are mentally impaired and/or limited in physical mobility. A high proportion take potent drugs requiring medical supervision. Nevertheless, there are people presently in nursing homes who would prefer, and are physically well enough, to be cared for either in less costly facilities or at home on their own or with their family, if more and better in-home services were available.

Sylvia Porter (1978) wrote on the subject in her nationally syndicated column. In that article, "One Alternative Home Health Care," she quoted Walter J. McNerney, then president of Blue Cross and Blue Shield: "It may also be time to give serious considerations to homecare programs for the elderly as an alternative to nursing home care."

While the elderly appear to receive more attention in talking about alternatives, they are not the sole population at risk. Cang (1977), in his article, "An Alternative to Hospital," points out the desire for " . . . arrangements which are less expensive both in the narrow financial sense and in the sense of being simpler and less elaborate. The two currents thus merge in seeking less: less complexity, less remoteness, less expense, less red tape, less waste" (author's emphasis).

Cang and Clarke (1978) also delved into the problem of "social admissions" and the meaning of nursing vs. Nursing. Capital N nursing implies a higher and more professional level than lower case n nursing, indicating the type of care rendered at home. Social admission refers to placement in a facility when that level of care is not really needed. Thus, hospital care is not sacrosanct when considering alternatives. A General Accounting Office (1981) study made the blunt declarative that "Home health care is generally recognized as a beneficial and cost-effective alternative to prolonged hospital and nursing home care."

In an editorial discussion in the *American Journal of Public Health*, Callahan (1981) discussed long-term care. In founding a philosophy of care for those in need, Callahan stated, "In summary, what I am arguing for is a recognition that it is the institution which is the alternative. . ."

In an extensive review of home health services, Warhola (1980) filled in the gaps from Callahan's terse comment:

Homecare is the care of choice for many -- not all. Homecare is the care of choice at certain times -- not always. When home health services are used appropriately, they are not an alternative to institutional care, but rather the opposite. Homecare should be the first line of defense, and when no longer appropriate, its alternative is institutional care.

However, Lowenstein (1986) pointed out that the homecare alternative is not used because physicians are unaware of the state of the art. He reiterated the high technology list of services capable of being rendered at home and responded to a *New York Times* Op-Ed physician-author that homecare could have been used for the patient he described in the article.

If homecare is to be thought of as the prime location for care followed by other alternatives, it might be useful to examine some of the choices.

Alternative Choices

Alternatives to institutional care come in a variety of hues with labels such as extramural hospitals, hospitals without walls, hospital-at-home, comprehensive domiciliary patient care, domiciliary secondary care, nursing home without walls, home health care, home visiting and in France, hospitalisation-à-domicile. Cang (1976) remarks that the idea is far from new and operated in different forms in Australia, Canada, France, New Zealand, and the United States.

In the deliberations about homecare, Dr. E.M. Bluestone (1948) wrote about the extramural homecare function of the hospital. Despite the fact that these words were published in 1948, they still ring out loudly and boldly:

> ... the hospital that serves the public does not limit its superior scientific facilities to the patient within its walls. There is an area of expanding medical opportunity -- the patient's home ... which the hospital must take under its wing. Only by a combination of hospital and homecare under the same overall medical management can the hospital employ its unique facilities in the field of scientific medicine to best advantage.

Day Care, AFDP, and Group Living

Lubin (1975) described two additional alternatives in addition to homecare: day care centers and cash grants to families taking care of relatives at home.

Day care centers allow people to receive care during daytime hours when other family members may be at work or unavailable. Individuals going to the centers receive a comprehensive range of services Monday through Friday, including meals, transportation, baths, counseling, various therapies, recreation, and crafts. Families take care of the patient on weekends and evenings. Rafferty (1979) noted the improvement in the quality of life of adults in day care programs.

"Aid to Families with Dependent Parents" (AFDP) encourages families to care for their elderly parents at home. Similar to the long-standing governmental program called Aid to Families with Dependent Children (AFDC), the plan calls for families to receive a portion of the Medicaid allotment for care that would otherwise be required. Everybody would benefit from AFDP: government would save on high nursing home care; families who didn't have the financial resources would get some money; and elderly patients would regain family unity and dignity as well as an improved quality of life.

Congregate living arrangements also can be used as an alternative. These apartments or homes substitute for a family and provide all the same services (Irwin 1978,21). In a similar vein, foster homes can be used, as in the foster children programs. Families volunteer to take people into their homes and provide homecare, receiving reimbursement from the appropriate governmental agency (Manber 1980).

These homecare alternatives are only a sampling and other will be added as more experimentation and creativity take place in an expanding program. Innovations involving the use of home equity, new long-term care health insurance, and lifetime retirement communities are already under way.

In view of the attention to homecare as the primary choice for care, it should be useful to review the advantages and disadvantages of homecare and/or alternatives.

Advantages and Disadvantages of Homecare

Based upon 10 years of experience in the 1950s and 1960s with a hospital-based program in Pittsburgh, Odle (1967) identified the advantages and disadvantages of homecare for the physician and the patient/family. In his expert opinion, the positives far outnumber the negatives:

Advantages for Patient and Family

- They receive broad-based care.
- Long-term and terminal illnesses are better cared for at home.
- Family and friends provide closer care than does the hospital.
- Family is a part of the care team.
- Optimum recovery is expedited in those patients that can be rehabilitated.
- Physical rehabilitation can be carrier further.
- Patients with terminal illness get greater emotional support.
- Care is individually tailored.
- Patient's own food tastes can be met.
- Patient and family's sense of security is promoted.
- Prevents passive-dependency state engendered by long hospitalization.
- Patients seem happier in their own homes without the depression of long-term illness.
- Patients are not exposed to illness in hospitals.
- Patients retain their identities and sense of usefulness.
- More recordkeeping involved and attending clinical conferences.

Advantages for the Hospital

An *AMA Cost Containment Newsletter* (1981), "How Homecare Pays Off," cited significant cost benefits and the following reasons for hospitals to consider extending their services:

- Homecare is in keeping with the broad mission of the hospital to provide sound care at the most economical cost.

- Such programs improve continuity of care by giving hospitals control over the post-discharge care of their patients.

- Homecare programs enable the hospital, the patient, and the family to arrange for post-discharge care, including the acquisition and placement of equipment and the scheduling of personnel, well before the patient leaves.

- A homecare program can be a vehicle for providing hospice-type care to terminal patients in their own homes.

- Delivering patient care services to the home enhances the hospital's reputation in the local community.

Furthermore, hospitals have a built-in advantage because they already have the staff and back-up services to set up a homecare program. This is particularly true under the federal reimbursement scheme that presets allowances for specific diagnoses in the hospital.

In his book on the health care delivery system in the U.S., Jonas (1986,253) culled the following 12 advantages from a review of the literature:

- The company of one's family.

- A freer, more cheerful atmosphere.

- Comfort.

- The support and understanding of a visiting nurse.

- More personal freedom and dignity than in the hospital.

- Patient at home is not occupying a costly hospital bed.

- Patient may make more progress in activities of daily living and experience less deterioration in indices of social functioning.

- Hospital admissions may be reduced.

- Length of stay in the hospital for readmitted patients may be less.

- Patient learning and motivation may be better at home.

- Patient satisfaction with care may be at a higher level.

- Overall, homecare may be less expensive to patient and health care systems.

Cang's (1978) list contains many similar items but the wording is quite distinctive and adds a factor missing from other enumerations:

- A standard of care equivalent to that in hospital and perhaps even higher if the psychological benefit to those who dislike hospitals is counted.

- Implicit encouragement to renewed self-reliance in the patient and the family by allowing a greater degree of choice about where, and therefore, how to be ill and to be treated.

- Consequent reinforcement of family and local ties since caring aides would be hired from among local people.

- General de-mystification of illness, which is itself therapeutic.

- Protection of relatives from unreasonable strain, since homecare takes the effort into consideration.

- Flexibility and simplicity of organization and development.

- Provision of employment at low cost with implications for inner city problems.

- Cut in need for hospital beds.

Of particular concern as high technology comes into the fore, O'Donnell (1984) delineated the benefits of a hospital-based home IV therapy program. Advantages for patients, for physicians, for third-party payers, and for the hospital were listed. He concluded that "the availability of a multidisciplinary home IV therapy service may prove to be one of the most logical, and timely, extensions of hospital-level care."

These listings on the advantages of homecare are rather comprehensive in their exactness as well as in their possibilities for expansiveness.

Disadvantages for the Hospital

Every system has its drawbacks and homecare is no exception. Jonas (1986) again reviewed the literature to find the negatives:

- To be successful, the deep involvement of family members is required.

- Family functioning may be disrupted at the same time as homecare allows the family to remain intact.

- If the value of a family member's time is counted, the indirect costs may be high.

- Coordination may be lacking between physician, homecare agency, family, and patient.

- Quality of care may be problematic.

Even though Cang (1978) is speaking about the British National Health Service, his observations still contain that little extra about disadvantages:

- Homecare goes against the hospital-oriented outlook of some members of the public and the professionals alike.

- If implemented on any scale, modifications of the physician's pattern of work might be required.

- Administrative problems between a variety of health and homecare agencies would have to be sorted out.

While asking physicians if they were ready for the new homecare, Borders (1985b) synthesized the pro and con arguments. Exhibit 2-4 lists the major arguments for the patient, for the physician and for society.

Based on the numerous advantages for homecare, why do so many health care providers refer patients to institutional care instead of an alternative? There is some indication that the providers exercise poor risk assessment of the patient and that this results in inappropriate placement.

Inappropriate Institutionalization

A critical component in any homecare program is the ability to assess an individual's risk of institutionalization. What makes that task particularly onerous is that professionals frequently disagree in their conclusions about the same person. In a study of the appropriateness of long-term care placement in New Jersey, the Urban Health Institute (Malafronte, Moses, Bronson, et al. 1977,4) researchers reported that discharge recommendations from the eight offices studied ranged from 17 to 80 percent. Sager (1980, 24-26) investigated patient, family, and professional views of an alternative to institutionalization. Findings indicated that all three groups agreed on the average homecare needs, but disagreed in individual cases. Patients and families requested less paid help than professionals thought necessary. Professional agreement was strongest for technical care components and weaker for household and personal care services.

Exhibit 2-4

Where do you stand in the home care debate?

Few physicians question the benefits of home care in certain circumstances, but how much emphasis home care should receive is still a matter of great debate. Here's a summary of the major arguments, both pro and con.

	PRO	CON
For the patient	Patient has privacy, comfort, and dignity of remaining at home.	Other family members suffer inconvenience, especially when living quarters are crowded; they bear burden of out-of-pocket expenses.
	Patient feels better at home and avoids medical hazards of institutionalization.	Institutional care may be safer.
	Patient's functional status may improve more quickly at home.	Home care may not improve functional status in patients with relatively severe problems.
	Patient is attended by significant other(s).	Significant other(s) may be unwilling or poorly prepared to take care of patient or may suffer "burnout."
For the physician	Patient and family are usually more satisfied with care rendered by physician.	Patient or family may sue if "everything that could have been done" wasn't.
	House calls give physician important data about the patient at home and yield immense good will.	House calls are time-consuming and poorly reimbursed; they duplicate a service already well provided by visiting nurses anyway.
	Physician can efficiently provide high-quality care to patients who can't routinely come to the office.	Physician may find it difficult to manage the home care team, resulting in unnecessary services and expense; paper work and telephone calls may be a burden.
For society	Home care is cheaper than institutional care.	Home care can be more expensive than institutional care; institutional services subject to more scrutiny.
	Rate of avoidable admissions may be reduced.	Home care strengthens the trend started by DRGs: Patients with serious illness may be denied hospitalization; "social" admissions prohibited.
	Early discharge becomes more practical.	Patients with serious illness may be sent home too soon.
	Funds slated for expensive inpatient facilities may be diverted to other uses.	Hospitals now in financial difficulty may close; shortage of skilled nursing facilities may continue.

Source: Reproduced with permission from *Patient Care*, November 15, 1985. Copyright © 1985, Patient Care Communications, Inc., Darien, CT. All rights reserved.

Ham (1980) discusses the role of the family physician in preventing unnecessary institutionalization. He called for the physician to participate in a comprehensive medical, psychological, social, and financial assessment. In this case, "comprehensive" is open to interpretation and the time and ability of the practitioner.

Validation of professional judgment in a homecare agency was studied by Austin and Seidl (1981). Basically, they asked experts, "What information do you need to make a judgment as to whether an individual will be admitted into a nursing home?" Eventually, a list of 19 indicators in five general groupings evolved (see Exhibit 2-5). Then using those indicators,

---

Exhibit 2-5 Indicators for the Assessment of Institutionalization

1. Current general physical and emotional condition/disability, including past and present medical history with specific diagnosis.

   - Stability and/or severity of emotional condition(s).
   - Prognosis of diagnosed physical condition(s).
   - Ability/inability to cope with diagnosed condition(s).
   - Ambulation/mobility problems.

2. Amount of professional and nonprofessional (relatives) judgment needed in providing care.

   - Ability to follow/maintain dietary restrictions independently.
   - Type of medication(s) required and ability to self administer.
   - Supervisory/obaservation requirements--quantitative (hourly, daily) or qualitative (close, passive).

3. Availability of community resources and services.

   - Home-based supportive services.
   - Alternative living facilities (group homes, adult foster homes).
   - Nono-home-based supportive services.

4. Ability to cope physically and mentally with activities of daily living.

   - Ability to dress self.
   - Ability to prepare food and feed self.
   - Ability to deal with incontinence.
   - Ability to function socially.
   - Ability to program and to perform own activities.

5. Confusion/disorientation.

   - Time and place orientation.
   - Comprehension.
   - Reasoning.
   - Appropriateness of response.

Source: Austin, C.D., and Seidl, F.W. Validating professional judgment in a home care agency. *Health and Social Work.* 6(1): 50-56, 1981. Washington, D.C.: National Association of Social Workers, Inc. Reprinted with permission.

the experts were asked to evaluate 30 clients. Results showed that homecare agency managers tended to rate the clients at higher risk than a panel of outside experts. There was low agreement among panel members, but even that low level was higher than that between the panel members and the case managers. Homecare agency social workers had the same relationship with the social workers on the expert panel. In reviewing the disheartening data from this investigation, the researchers highlighted the low reliability of professional ability to predict risk assessment. Austin and Seidl (1981) concluded that, "The most immediate and compelling implication of the study is that professionals in long-term care must redouble their efforts to provide reliable, valid, comprehensive, and usable measurements to undergird our professional judgments." Coincidentally, the agency studied was established to prevent premature or continued institutionalization.

If experts are having that much difficulty making risk assessments, what is the average physician making a small number of referrals to alternative programs to do? Obviously, individuals at either end of the spectrum will be easier to classify. However, that leaves in the middle the bulk of the population, who may be inappropriately placed.

Typical Homecare Programs

Because of the rapid changes affecting the health care delivery system, the typical homecare programs will reflect those same changes. There has been an obvious increase in the use of high technology professional services along with an upsurge in the use of scientific equipment. However, before describing typical programs, it might be useful to consider generalizations about homecare agencies.

National Survey Data

In mid-1983, the House Subcommittee on Health and Long Term Care and the House Select Committee on Aging (1985) cooperated with the National Association for Home Care (NAHC) on the first survey to collect information about the operating characteristics of U.S. homecare agencies. A statistically valid sample of 673 agencies supplied data, although the vast majority of funding for those agencies came from the Medicare program.

An average home health agency employed a total of 45 full- and part-time people, a full-time equivalent (FTE) of 27.9 employees. An additional 7.7 FTEs were employed on a contract basis to provide direct services. Exhibit 2-6 shows the preponderance of RNs and Homemaker-Home Health Aides (H-HHAs) rendering services in the course of the 13,530 visits made by the average home health agency.

Exhibit 2-6 Average Home Health Agency Employees by FTEs, Contract FTEs, Home Visits, Visits per Employee and Percent of Agency Visits

Employ-ees	FTEs	Contract FTEs	Home Visits No.	%	Visits Per FTE	HHA* Visits No.	HHA** Visits	%	Zero*** Visits No.	%
RNs	11.2	1.15	7,025	52%	553	11%	218	33%	2	1%
H-HHAs	7.2	2.49	5,722	42	590	10	181	28	39	6
LPNs	1.1	.10	624	5	520	1	73	14	367	70
PTs	1.1	1.80	1,838	14	613	4	133	21	100	15
MSWs	.5	.20	253	2	361	1	98	16	295	49
OTs	.3	.58	319	2	363	1	107	18	304	51
STs	.3	.79	374	3	331	.2	159	25	206	33
MDs	.3	.09	14	0	3.6	.1	8	1.4	515	96
Agency Total			13,530							

* Based on HHA averaging 10,000-20,000 visits/year
** Based on largest number of reporting HHAs and their percentage of their total home visits.
*** Based on the number of agencies reporting zero visits and the percentage of the total number of reporting HHAs.

Source: House Subcommittee on Health and Long Term Care. 1985. *Building a long term care policy: homecare data and implications.* Washington, DC: Government Printing Office Comm. Pub. No. 98-484.

This average agency served 1,407 unduplicated clients with an average 9.6 visits per client. More than 75 percent of the clients were over 65; 35 percent 65-74; 29 percent 75-84; and 11 percent over 85. Women constituted the majority of the clients: 64 percent. To serve those clients, the average agency is open almost nine hours per day, six days a week, with 66 percent of the agencies providing 24-hour-per-day emergency services.

Average budget allocations increased 52 percent from 1980 to 1982 to a total of $740,931, with 67 percent of the total coming from Medicare; 9 percent came from Medicaid.

Agencies reported the "very common conditions" treated, in order, heart/circulatory conditions; high blood pressure; diabetes; carcinoma; and stroke recovery. "Common conditions," in order, were neuromuscular diseases; nutrition problems; skin problems; respiratory ailments; and bowel/bladder conditions.

Referrals usually come from hospitals (48 percent) and private physicians (26 percent). Self-referrals, community service agencies, government agencies, were all under 10 percent each.

As of January 1984, Williams, Gaumer, and Cella (1984,11) reported survey data regarding the 4,271 home health agencies and the services provided by their staff members. Skilled nursing was universal (100 percent) followed by H-HHA (96 percent) and physical therapy (83 percent). Other services included speech therapy (65 percent); medical social services (53 percent); occupational therapy (49 percent); nutrition guidance (24 percent); appliances and equipment (23 percent); pharmaceutical service (6 percent); and interns and resident (0.8 percent).

Ginzberg, Balinsky, and Ostow (1984,80-83) also add survey data about homecare clients. Medicaid's minor role in funding homecare for the elderly is noted, along with the fact that almost one-third of the patients had prior experience. Persons living with others were more likely to receive homecare services and were also probably pensioners. Results also suggested that home health care was not a substitute for most nursing home care. There was a spurt in hospital-based and proprietary homecare programs as well as variations in the existing agencies to meet demands and to resolve problems.

Hospital Homecare Programs

In an historic review, McNamara (1982) talked about the fact that hospitals were rediscovering comprehensive homecare. Lundberg (1984) later called homecare a logical extension of hospital services and discussed benefits, planning, organizing, and implementing a program. She also described a number of typical programs. Interestingly, a study by Balinsky and Rehman (1984) compared hospital and community-based homecare patients, and did find differences. Hospital-based patients were older, more limited in functional ability, received higher intensity care, and used more therapeutic services.

The Senior Care Network. Huntington Memorial Hospital in Pasadena, California, received a generous endowment to serve the community's older population. In partnership with the hospital medical staff, local community agencies and key area groups, the Senior Care Network was established to provide an integrated life care system with a complete range of medical, social, and personal services. Specific activities include a multipurpose senior services program, a linkage program to refer clients to appropriate sources, a community options effort to provide professional advice on alternatives to institutionalization, consultation on nursing homes, technical assistance to agencies, a consumer health education activity, professional education programs, development of Medicare alternatives, and a life services planning activity to take care of long-term needs. White (1985) reported on the program and called it a hospital-based coordinated community care system.

Hospital's Own Agency. Healthcorp Affiliates (*Profiles in Hospital Marketing* 1985), the forprofit division including Central DuPage Hospital in

Naperville, Illinois, set up its own homecare program using its own staff. All standard homecare services were provided using Healthcorp's own standards and guidelines. Using marketing techniques, Healthcorp promoted their homecare program and turned it into a successful venture -- so much so that Healthcorp packaged the activity, labeled it Harmony Home Care, and sold it to the other hospitals. "You can plug in (Harmony Care) as a basic system and then the hospital can plug in whatever else they wish to offer, such as their own physical therapy, occupational therapy, respiratory therapy -- that sort of thing."

In a more traditional vein, the nonprofit Huguley Memorial Medical Center in Fort Worth, Texas (Banfield 1985) licensed its own home health agency, which provides medical services, nursing care, medical social services, home health aides, homemaker chore services, physical, speech and occupational therapy services.

Hospital Contracts with Agency. Baptist Medical Center in Oklahoma City, Oklahoma, took another tack and contracted with an existing agency, Allied Nursing Care, to provide homecare. A hospital-employed coordinator works with the social services department and the physician referrals, while the existing agency rents space in the hospital and hires the hospital's marketing unit to promote the services. However, patients are not required to use the hospital's agency and can choose to go elsewhere. Baptist Medical Center (*Profiles in Hospital Marketing* 1985) believes, "We have more control over the quality of continuing care our patients are receiving and we maintain all the medical records right here."

Hospital Coalition Agency. More than 10 hospitals in the Minneapolis area formed Hospital Home Care, Inc. (Emerson 1985) to provide high technology services, specialized nursing care, hospice care and other homecare services to the seven-county metropolitan area. A staff of 40 full- and part-time personnel work for the free-standing homecare coalition that represents both religious and nonsectarian facilities. This arrangement allows smaller hospitals that otherwise could not afford it to expand care to their patients.

Disease/Condition Homecare Programs

Responding to the expressed needs of consumers as well as the needs of institutions and agencies, homecare activities have emerged that concentrate on specific healthcare aspects.

High Technology Homecare Teams. With the increased demand for highly technological services at home, the Dallas VNA established six specialty homecare teams: chronic pulmonary disorders, psychiatric, enterostomal therapy, IV therapy, diabetes, and cardiology (Weinstein 1984). Team members include a primary physician, nurse specialists, occupational therapists, nutritionists, and medical social workers. These teams seek to increase self-sufficiency, to reduce hospitalization, to maximize performance of activities of daily living, and to promote compliance with the medical regimen. "All high tech direct patient care is provided by nurses in our specialty program."

Bowyer (1986) describes a similar high tech program, the Complex Care Team (CCT) of the VNA of Morris County, New Jersey. A team consists of four staff nurses, a clinical coordinator responsible for daily functioning, and a clinical nurse specialist acting as liaison with administration. Team members use skills for IV therapy, ventilator utilization, wound drainage, and venous port medication. CCT members meet monthly to discuss cases and thus far problems have been minimal. "Patients and their families have expressed complete satisfaction and gratitude for the care and service offered them."

Acquired Immune Deficiency Syndrome (AIDS) Homecare Programs. Health professionals who care for Acquired Immune Deficiency Syndrome (AIDS) patients believe that homecare and hospice programs are effective and appropriate alternatives to inpatient care. However, few homecare services are generally available to help people who have AIDS. In fact, a Virginia law allows home health aides to refuse to care for Medicaid patients with contagious diseases. AIDS is being included in that grouping (Traska 1986). Nursing homes also generally avoid accepting AIDS patients. Successful efforts have been reported for homeless men with AIDS: the Shanti Project in San Francisco; AID Atlanta, operating a four-unit apartment house for those too ill to live alone; Chicago House and Social Service Agency with a residential program. San Francisco General Hospital also pays special attention to proper discharge planning for AIDS victims (Traska 1986).

Alzheimer's Disease Homecare Programs. By 1990, Perry (1984) estimates that one-third to one-half of the $75 billion institutional care bill will be for people with Alzheimer's Disease. She challenged nursing and the homecare system to do something about the lack of knowledge, the no-care gaps in funding mechanisms, the availability of services, and the mobilization of volunteers and support groups.

A December 1985 issue of *Caring* contained six articles relating to Alzheimer's Disease activities. Howell (1985) gave the medical background and identified the stages of this incurable condition. Possible casual nutritional factors were discussed by Martinez (1985) as a daily menu plan and mealtime hints for nutritional maintenance were elucidated. In Springfield,

Massachusetts, Skipper (1985) described the VNA's program of education and coordination. A coordinator services the area with information and referral services, educational seminars, a newsletter, and respite help. In cooperation with National Medical Enterprises, the John D. French Center for Alzheimer's Disease operates a 120-bed inpatient facility that focuses on an approach to this critical long-term care challenge. Laxton (1985) talks about the research center objectives, the workshops, and the educational activities. Finally, Stockton (1985) tells about how a wife lovingly coped with the illness of her husband, and a daughter tells a Congressional hearing about taking care of her mother (*Caring* 1985c).

Hospice Programs. Patients who are terminally ill can now choose to receive care at home. While not a new concept, the programs are relatively new in the United States with the early services beginning in the mid-1970s. McDonnell (1986) reviews the administration, organization, and models of hospice care with special attention to the quality of care. She compares models including the hospital-based, the homecare, freestanding facility, community-based and skilled nursing choices. In addition to the numerous references, McDonnell also covers patient grievance procedures, bereavement program resources, and patient care policies. Descriptions are given of the Continuing Care Team programs at Hospice of Pennsylvania, Inc., and a pain control program using morphine at Hospice of Northeastern Pennsylvania.

Diagnosis Specific Homecare. Enthusiastic physicians at Park Nicollet Medical Center (Roeder and Williams 1985) in Minneapolis developed four diagnosis specific homecare programs to meet changing demands in medical care. A Newborn-Family Care Program follows the family into the home within 48 hours of a routine vaginal delivery. At home the physical status of the baby and mother are evaluated, the family is educated about diet and care, and all questions are fully answered. Services include a prenatal visit, a postpartum hospital visit, and a home visit. A Bilirubin Phototherapy Program cares for infants with neonatal jaundice and usually lasts two to three days. Parents receive instructions in the use of phototherapy equipment, learn to take proper precautions and to record vital data on temperature and fluid input and output. There is close interaction with the hospital professionals as the program progresses. A Psoriasis Homecare Program treats patients with extensive plaques using a variation of the Goeckerman technique combining coal tar topical medication with ultraviolet exposure for six to 10 weeks. A Low Back Pain Program helps people who would otherwise be hospitalized for strict bed rest. Treatment includes traction, physical therapy, and medications as needed, with patients usually discharged after 10 days.

In setting up the four diagnosis specific homecare programs, the participants set up goals, identified outcomes, contained costs, trained personnel, selected patients, stimulated communication among all concerned, educated patients, and evaluated the activities.

Specific Population Groups Homecare Programs

While most all the homecare programs serve people of all ages, a number do specialize in particular groups. It is important to realize that homecare is not reserved only for the elderly, despite the fact that older people do actually use a great majority of the services.

Pediatric Homecare Programs.   An organization exists dedicated to children: Sick Kids need Involved People (SKIP). Shannon (1986; 1985) states that SKIP seeks "to foster and promote the feasibility of Specialized Pediatric Home Care for medically fragile children."

An entire issue of *Caring* detailed pediatric homecare programs. Perrum (1985) covered basic information about chronically ill children in America, Koop (1985) spoke to the commitment to the disabled child, and examples of homecare for fragile children were cited (*Caring* 1985d). A discussion of opportunities and obligations noted the denial of acute care at home for pediatric patients (Kohrman 1985) and Bock (1985) described the state of the art. Points were made about discharge planning (Kun and Brennan 1985), ventilator care (Goldberg 1985), hospice care (Dailey 1985), research (Moss 1985), helping organizations (*Caring* 1985e), funding strategies (Galten 1985), family stress (Feinberg 1985), transition from hospital to home (*Caring* 1985f), and a general appraisal of the situation (Halamandaris 1985b). In addition, ongoing pediatric homecare programs were described in Georgia (Halley 1985), Pennsylvania (Harris and McAllister 1985; Richardson 1985), Ohio (Houchen and Jones 1985), and New York City (Liota, Levene, Martin, et al. 1985).

From Hawaii, Sheridan (1985) told about home monitoring for apnea, or prolonged breathing pauses in infants. If an infant stops breathing or the heart rate falls too low, the machine goes "beep in the night," alerting the parents to take action.

Long-Term Home Health Care Program.   On January 18, 1973, St. Vincent's Hospital and Medical Center of New York initiated the Chelsea-Village Program that cares for a large number of very old people (Lipsman, Brickner, Sharer, et al. 1984). In the programs's more than 10 years of operation under the direction of Dr. Philip W. Brickner, the staff has striven to help patients "to remain in their own community, out of institutions, in adequate housing, in the best possible states of health, and at maximum attainable levels of independence" (Brickner 1985).

In an update on New York's Nursing Home Without Walls program, Lombardi (1986) commented that now there were 84 approved programs in 48 counties, with 53 operational in late 1985, serving 3,611 patients needing long-term care. Combining a full spectrum of homecare services available under Medicaid with a waiver to allow for community-based services, the programs provide a comprehensive 24-hour, 7-day-a-week effort.

Living at Home Program. A program funded by seven foundations aims to identify and support local organizations that will coordinate existing services and develop new ones to help frail elderly people remain home. Bogdonoff (1986) reported attention to housing, health care, and support services in the home, aiding family caregivers, ensuring a system for access to care, and help with financial planning. In the organizational stages a number of locations will be able to apply to be part of this innovative effort.

Rural Area Homecare Programs. Riffer (1985a) notes that cooperative arrangements are the key to providing home health care in rural areas. In Washington State, a two-hospital corporation and a nursing home in a rural area established just such a relationship. A hospital-based home health agency set up a branch office in the rural nursing home. Nurses, home health aides, homemakers, and secretarial staff are employed by the nursing home while the hospital employs the physical, occupational, and speech therapists, social workers, enterostomal therapists, and a branch office supervisor.

Foreign Homecare Programs

A special double issue of *Home Health Care Services Quarterly* (Reif and Trager 1985) gave international perspectives on long-term care. Homecare programs in Australia, Canada, France, Israel, Scotland, Sweden, the United Kingdom, and the United States were described. Conclusions urged that data be shared and that others adapt appropriate activities.

The *PRIDE Institute Journal of Long Term Health Care* (1984) also discussed international homecare programs in Canada, Denmark, France, and Hong Kong. Common threads in the programs dealt with serving the "old-old," the feminization of the elderly population, changing family life patterns, and the need to examine links between homecare and other community and institutional services.

Gunning-Schepers, Leroy, and DeWals (1984) related a case study in Belgium on using homecare as an alternative to institutionalization. In the semi-rural community of Braine Le Chateau, a coordinated homecare service was developed to provide medical and social services integrated horizontally and vertically, following the WHO concept of primary health care. Importantly, the investigators found that no extra services need be offered but that the commitment and enthusiasm of all staff members is critical to success.

In New Brunswick, Canada, an extra-mural hospital without walls serves 237,670 people with a wide range of homecare services (Steward 1985). Medical care comes from the physicians in the community while service delivery units serve as the foci for nursing care, physical and occupational therapy, dietic services, drugs, surgical and medical supplies, and the coordination of personal/social care services. About 100 staff members currently care for approximately 700 patients at seven delivery units. When fully operational, 20 service delivery units will be used. Technically, the New Brunswick Extra-Mural Hospital exists with a provincial board of trustees and administrative headquarters in the provincial capital, and is part of the national program under the Public Hospital Act. However, there are no inpatient beds and no usual facilities, except for the satellite unit delivery centers.

Homecare as a Business

A mere perusal of typical homecare activities leads to the immediate perception that there is a great deal of concern with the business of homecare. Various types of arrangements characterize the provision of homecare services as existing agencies reorganize or as new entities emerge. Kuntz (1983) reported on hospitals being offered a wide variety of partnership deals by home health care companies. Diversification opportunities and the relative safety of joint ventures was cited as a factor attracting hospitals by Mistarz (1984). In adjusting to the competing interest of hospitals, a new corporate structure was created for the Hospital Home Health Care Agency of California (Tatage 1984). That agency was founded by 10 Los Angeles area hospitals capable of forming partnerships with the agency and sharing in the profits. According to experts, more hospitals will use joint ventures to enter the homecare market (Anderson 1985). When deficits in public health agencies providing homecare mount up, hospitals, particularly in rural areas, join together to take over the service in a joint venture (Riffer 1985b). In a similar fashion, Pear (1986) commented on the growth of links between nursing homes and hospitals. A number of hospitals have nursing homes located on their own grounds. Logically, it could be expected that homecare services could also be located on the hospital or nursing home grounds to provide continuity of care. However, lawyers do issue a warning about antitrust laws regarding exclusive "downstream" referrals -- from hospital to nursing home or to homecare -- and "upstream" referrals -- from homecare and nursing home to the hospital (Shahoda 1986).

Hospital/Home Health Agency Relations

An entire issue of Caring (1984) concentrated upon the relations between the hospital and the home health agency, covering market considerations, legal aspects, financial factors, structural perspectives, delivery models, and hospital viewpoints. Most often the homecare services were set up in five variations (Andre 1984):

- hospital-based with all services supplied by the hospital;
- hospital-based with some services supplied and some under contract;
- hospital homecare department for continuity with contract for services from existing homecare agency;
- a joint venture with a home health agency;
- a contractual relation with a home health agency.

HMO and Homecare Relationship

Louden and Company surveyed health maintenance organizations (HMOs) and Preferred Provider Arrangements (PPAs) that represent about 25 percent of the enrollees in the nation (Firshein 1986). Results indicated that homecare was not the top priority, but was regarded as an important part of the total mix of services. Currently, the HMOs/PPAs spend about 1 to 3 percent of expenditures on homecare, with the projections of 5 to 10 percent in five years. While 17 percent of the HMOs/PPAs already operate home health care services, 60 percent indicate an interest in doing so. An HCFA official guessed that 20 percent of the 45 Medicare-certified risk contracts to provide care to beneficiaries under the aegis of an HMO or PPA will start their own home health agencies. A VNA administrator believes that the HMO/homecare relationship "should be a marriage made in heaven" (Firshein 1986).

Should the government relax the HMO regulations regarding home health certification, HMOs will be "able to beat the pants off any home health agency that has to be Medicare certified" (Firshein 1986).

With the innovative approaches to providing homecare service multiplying, it is obvious that attention has to be paid to the nuts and bolts of establishing and running the business of homecare.

Management Aspects of Homecare

New opportunities for out-of-hospital health services, including home health care, were cited in the *New England Journal of Medicine* by Moxley and Roeder (1984). This article reflected on the trends and radical changes in the health care delivery system.

However, Runner-Heidt (1985) detailed a business plan for assessing the feasibility of establishing a home health agency. That plan included five tasks: a market analysis; inquiry about licensing, accreditation, certificate-of-need and conditions of participation; consideration of status as profit, non-profit, joint venture, etc.; evaluation of the information; a report detailing recommendations. Holt (1985a and b) made a pitch for vertical integration in homecare, citing 11 advantages and six disadvantages, with a leaning toward integration. Vertical integration in homecare could result in groupings such as:

Facilities--hospital, hospice, rehabilitation unit, skilled nursing facility, intermediate care facility;

Housing--group home, foster home, congregate living, retirement village;

Homecare--hospice, long-term care, meals on wheels, pediatric care, intermittent acute care;

Community care--day care, mental health center, geriatric clinics, sheltered workshop, rehab center;

Equipment/Supplies--Infusion, respiratory, ambulatory aids, bedroom equipment, oxygen.

Vertical integration could take place in the manufacture and distribution of equipment and supplies, in the provision of services, in education and research activities, and even in all three areas.

Corporate Restructuring

Healthcare providers often dislike getting involved in the nitty gritty of the business of homecare.

Halamandaris (1985c) pinpoints the vital link between "corporate restructuring" and "diversification" and the healing arts and caring. He points out that health organizations need to insure their survival, and the acid test is whether or not the changes enhance the delivery of high quality services.

Reflecting the industry's concerns, *Caring* devoted an issue to corporate reorganization. Cabin (1985) presented an overview explaining terminology and diversification. He concluded that corporate reorganization was not a panacea. Opportunities for diversification included pharmacy, durable medical equipment, physical therapy, HMOs/PPOs, high technology care, joint ventures, and emergency alert systems (Windley 1985). Teplitsky and Hedlund (1985) explained how to set up combinations of profit and and nonprofit subsidiaries under a parent holding company.

Legal pitfalls in the conversion from nonprofit to forprofit was covered by Flanagan (1985a), as well as the problem of physician ownership of a home health agency (Flanagan 1985b). A legal checklist was compiled by Pyles (1985) to guide the choice of a structure. In a related area, Gardiner (1985) reviewed the tax problems encountered in reorganizing tax-exempt providers.

Accounting (Lorenz 1985a) and cost allocation (Simione 1985; Lorenz 1985b) material related to reimbursement under Medicare rules. HCFA's memo on cost finding for home health agencies gave the official word on that important area (Booth 1985).

Four key words highlighted DeVita's (1985) accounting perspective of corporate restructuring: identify, plan, evaluate, and implement. To identify and evaluate, an agency poses questions such as--should I restructure? Can I restructure? How do I restructure? To plan and implement, an agency must consider the why of restructuring in legal, tax, marketing, and reimbursement terms.

Variations of Corporate Restructuring. A number of examples of corporate restructuring illustrate the scope of the concept.

In Portland, Oregon, a VNA affiliated with a four-hospital chain to set up separate homecare and health services divisions (Elmslie 1985). Three separate entities evolved in Auburn, Massachusetts, connected via a parent holding company with overlapping governance. There was a Medicare certified home health agency, a private pay personal care unit, and a management services corporation (Perry 1985). VNA of Los Angeles established an intermittent care corporation, an extended care and a new business entity, and a Visiting Nurse Foundation to maintain continuity of sponsorship (Grigsby 1985). In Kansas City, Missouri, the VNA created four corporations including a VNA, a homecare services unit, a foundation, and a management corporation (Roberson 1985). In an affiliation with a medical center, a VNA in Illinois set up a governing body with three divisions: a homecare unit, a hospital center, and a foundation (Goodner 1985).

Creating a foundation unit allows that division to engage in research, to seek new ventures, and to assist the other entities.

Satisfaction with Restructuring. In a telephone survey of 108 freestanding home health agencies, Freishat, Gortmaker, O'Neill, et al. (1985) found that 85 percent were satisfied and thought the corporate restructuring was a wise decision--only 8 percent felt worse off and regretted the move. Geographically, 56 percent of the restructures were in the Northeast, 33 percent in the Midwest and Southeast, and 23 percent west of the Mississippi, with 46 percent in urban areas and 38 percent in suburban areas. In 83 percent of the cases, agencies had budgets of $3 to $10 million, and in 43 percent budgets of $1 to $3 million. Homemakers were added by 43 percent, and private pay nurses by 31 percent. As an aside, the agencies noted that the corporate restructure took longer than expected to accomplish.

Operational Management

A listing of 30 factors in management taking command were delineated by Bob (1985). While not an extraordinary listing, the factors included items such as taking credit, being prudent, repetition, meetings, communications, being prepared, planning, mastering facts, morale, and doing nothing. Logue and Garvey (1985) posed managerial dilemmas relating to eight primary values critical to the new era of business management: purpose, excellence, consensus, unity, performance, empiricism, intimacy, and integrity. In addition, the authors dealt with the dilemmas of financial management, maximization of employee potential, and patient's rights and responsibilities. The point was made that homecare is both a business and a profession, and perhaps values from each area can be combined for the benefit of all.

Developing managers for homecare expansion was Klane and Nestor's (1985) theme. It was suggested that agencies make a conscious effort to give priority to the development of management personnel. Career paths for in-house employees should be given top consideration.

VNA of Cleveland uses a system called Metroflex to manage agency resources. Gillaspy and Edwards (1985) describe mechanisms used to measure productivity, to award incentives and bonuses, to identify equipment needs, to improve cash flow, to review utilization, and to use the non-profit division effectively. In addition, staff can be scheduled by level of care required, by skills needed, by type of services, for maximum use of each caregiver, and for allocations of indigent care.

Financial Aspects of Management. Fields (1985) comprehensively examines financial planning for the home health agency. He covers the benefits of formal financial planning, long range and annual planning, potential problems, the need for financial ratios, and the four types of ratios: liquidity, activity, leverage, and profitability. Obviously, an agency needs to manage its funds to succeed. With prospective payment on the horizon for homecare, Cushman (1984) argues for greater attention to program budgeting in agencies.

A major operational financial function of any agency is billing, credit and collection to obtain "full, prompt payment of all amounts owed" (Gleeson, Riddell, Yuncza, et al. 1984). To do this the homecare agency pays attention to the four Ps: philosophy, policy, procedures, performance. Despite the humanitarian outlook, staff must be aware of the agency's philosophy of a realistic approach to billing and collection. Policy positions must link the agency's collection efforts to the ability to provide services in the future. Procedures and performance combine to actually secure funds from clients.

Productivity. Why is productivity important in homecare? Bonstein and Mueller (1985) illustrate that an increase in nursing visits from 5 to 5.5 to 6 per day results in profits rising from -4 to 5 to 13 percent. However, obstacles to even these small increases in productivity are linked to values placed on high quality care, rigidity in productivity standards, and a misunderstanding of the standards by managers. Elements to be reported for productivity control include total time visit, non-visit time, visits per day per worker, average visit time, average visits per client, and utilization rates. An algebraic model (Oni 1984) calculates productivity using recorded time and activity factors. "With minor local adaptations, this model can evaluate current programs and study the influence which any proposed adjustments will have upon cost, time, and quality without disturbing existing arrangements unnecessarily." Rozelle (1985) also illustrates a related productivity method, while Borden (1985) suggests that administrators make house calls to gain an understanding of what staff is being asked to produce in terms of productivity.

Critics contend that attention to productivity negates the altruistic goals of the agencies and results in employee stress. Walsh (1985) explains a stress management program for home attendants using two-hour weekly seminars for staff and management. A noticeable change in behavior was noted in the evaluation leading to a reduction in the stress level. An article by Riddell (1981) said that productivity was a dirty word in the voluntary nonprofit agency. Yet, his message was that homecare agencies should adopt more of the business ethic in their daily operations.

Marketing Homecare. Competition is the key to organizational positioning and posturing today, according to Pappas (1985a). To position themselves in the market, agencies must concentrate on target segments, identify their rank in service offerings, and select a service position attractive to a relevant market. Factors to evaluate in arriving at a position base include service attributes, benefits usage situation, user classifications, competition, and types of services. Pappas (1985b) states that strategy options could be in specialization, services diversity, and in consumer satisfaction. Growth could be stimulated via market penetration by promoting more referrals, by adding new services, by marketing to new population groups, and through diversification. Pitfalls detailed by Pappas included not anticipating competitive responses or negative reactions by consumers and/or professionals, attempting too much too soon, and mismatching staff resources and strategies. Shaw (1985) notes that marketing must meet the needs and perspectives of the patients. "Listen to their needs."

Computers. In these times, it would be an obvious omission to leave a discussion of operational management without mentioning computers. Leafing through any of the homecare trade journals, we see numerous advertisements for computer programs to manage homecare agencies.

These software applications aim to produce all types of data and to maintain records vital to reimbursement, quality control, productivity, and assorted information. Harris and McAllister (1985) elucidate microcomputer applications for home health care services. Starting with the selection of hardware and software, they proceed to illustrate the use of menu screens for therapy applications, inventory management, billing, work calendars, report generation, patient monitoring, and linkages to other computers elsewhere.

Management Survival Strategies

Governmental policies stimulating utilization while increasing the gap between patient needs and reimbursement threaten the survival of homecare agencies. Reif (1984) outlines six strategies for survival that reflect much of the management guidelines for homecare agencies:

1. Reduce expenditures on overhead and administration.

2. Use service staff efficiently.

3. Diversify programming.

4. Implement financial planning procedures.

5. Maximize reimbursement.

6. Retain old and develop new funding sources for services.

Reviewing the business aspects of the homecare industry and the direct application to the daily operation of agencies, malpractice becomes a critical issue. Of course, this issue is also part of the entire health care delivery system.

Malpractice and Homecare

In 1980, an AMA official (Schwartz) made a strong statement about medical malpractice in homecare:

> Physicians should not fear an increased exposure to medical liability as a result of involvement with homecare services.

> The *AMA Guide* notes that no cases of alleged injury to patients who received services that were ordered by their attending physicians and were provided by employees or agents of home health care agencies or organizations have been reported to date.

Schwartz commented that the physician is not a guarantor of home health care services. Separately incorporated agencies can be held legally responsible for negligence by their employees.

After interviewing expert consultants on homecare liability, Borders (1986) concluded that "the medical risk you face managing patients in the home may actually be less than that for patients in the hospital." Basically, inpatients are probably sicker and the outcome may be poorer and result in a lawsuit " with or without errors in judgment." These consultants offered specific guidelines to reduce liability risk:

Discharge patients on solid medical grounds and not in reaction to financial pressure.

- Make sure there's good continuity of care.

- Be sure to obtain adequate information by phone.

- Know the patient/family and develop a good relationship.

- Get the patient/family involved in the care regimen.

- Obtain informed consent for specific procedures done in the home.

A possible danger in homecare is that the physician may give undue weight to the convenience of the patient when the medical situation clearly calls for transfer to a higher level of care.

Liability risks in homecare are not fully known because the area is relatively new and changing rapidly. However, the experts agree that the courts will not make allowances for the physician just because the patient is at home. It is anticipated that the courts will expect the same high standards of care regardless of the setting.

Greenberg (1986) discusses the legal implications of home health care by nonprofit hospitals and covers liability issues. He points out the need for the hospital to ensure that the homecare staff is well trained, and that services meet appropriate standards of care. In addition, there must be suitable criteria for patient selection and training for the homecare program. While Greenberg states that "there is a greater risk of provider and professional negligence in home health care," he does raise the aspect of contributory or comparative negligence by the patient or family members. Contributory negligence seeks to prove that the patient's actions contributed to the injury. Comparative negligence tries to compare the actions of the provider and the patient to show that the patient's negligence exceeded that of the provider.

Expert consultants (Borders 1986) also commented on the physician's lack of knowledge of noncompliance with instructions by the homecare patient when injury resulted. To avoid liability, providers will need good documentation to support their contention that the patient was instructed.

The combination of the business ethic and the financial pressures burgeoning in the homecare industry is causing people to become concerned about the ethics of the situation.

Ethics and Homecare

Bayer (1984) reflected about the ethical challenges of the movement for homecare. Beginning with the premise that the current emphasis concentrates on containing costs and not on extending care to those in need, several questions arise. "What does social justice demand in terms of the provision of homecare services? How much of the burden of paying for such care should be borne by those of diminished capacity and in ill health? How much by their families? How much by the government?" Quoting the President's Commission for the Study of Ethical Problems in Medicine and Biomedical and Behavioral Research, Bayer notes that "society has an ethical obligation to ensure equitable access to an adequate level of health care without excessive burden." Social planners appear to be frightened by the potential population group that might use homecare and thereby enormously increase expenditures. A moral obligation exists to resolve this situation so that future generations will not be saddled with the abandonment of the ethical challenge presented earlier.

Home birthing was questioned by Hoff and Schneiderman (1985), from the viewpoint of both safety and ethics. Their position was that the morality of home births should be based on these priorities: safety of the mother; safety of the fetus; benefit to the fetus; potential benefit to the mother. Contending that risks existed in either setting, the authors advised physicians to "honor the personal ethics and choices of parents" while determining risks, and while making both procedures as safe as possible.

It is apparent that the ethical issues are not confined to homecare alone. These dilemmas are inherent in the entire health care delivery system. Specifically, the cost containment crush has increased the intensity of the ethical decisions as pressures are brought to bear upon a variety of health care providers. Basically, the critics maintain that health care is becoming more of a business than a humane professional calling.

References

Anderson, H.J. 1985. More hospitals will use joint ventures to enter home care market--experts. *Modern Healthcare* 15 (23): 51-52.

Andre, J, and L.D. Bella. 1984. United Western Medical Centers/VNA home care. *Caring* 3 (7): 86-88.

Austin, C.D. and F.W. Seidl. 1981. Validating professional judgment in a home care agency. *Health and Social Work* 6 (2): 50-56.

Balinsky, W., and S. Rehman. 1984. Home health care: a comparative analysis of hospital-based and community-based aging patients. *Home Health Care Services Quarterly* 5 (1): 45-60.

Banfield, S.K. 1985. Huguley home health agency--a look at how and why it works. *Texas Hospitals* 40 (11): 16-20.

Bayer, R. 1984. Ethical challenges of the movement for home care. *Caring* 3 (10): 57-62.

Blue Cross Association. 1978. Home health care. *Model benefit program and related guidelines.* Chicago, IL (June).

Bluestone, E.M. 1948. Homecare: an extramural hospital function. *Survey Mid-monthly* 84:99.

Bluestone, E.M. 1954. The principles and practice of home care. *Journal of the American Medical Association* 155:1379-1382 (14 Aug.).

Blum, S.R., and M. Minkler. 1980. Toward a continuum of caring alternatives: community-based care for the elderly. *Journal of Social Issues* 36:133-152.

Bob, M.L. 1985. Take command. *Caring* 4 (11):14-15.

Bock, R.H. 1985. State of the art--pediatric homecare in 1985. *Caring* 4 (5):26-28.

Bogdonoff, M.D. 1986. Letter to author. Cornell University Medical College, New York.

Bonstein, Jr., R.G., and J. Mueller. 1985. Improving agency productivity. *Caring* 4 (11):4-9.

Booth, C.R. 1985. Memo on cost funding for home health agencies. *Caring* 4 (7):72-73.

Borden, R. 1985. House calls for administrators. *Caring* 4 (11):6.

Borders, C.R. 1985a. Preparing for posthospital homecare. *Patient Care* 19(20):27-62.

Borders, C.R. 1985b. Are you ready for the new homecare? *Patient Care* 19(19):20-46.

Borders, C.R. 1986. Reducing liability risk in homecare. *Patient Care* 20(5):57-67.

Bowyer, C.K. 1986. The complex care team: meeting the needs of high-technology nursing at home. *Home Health Care Nurse* 4(1):24-29.

Brickner, P.W. 1985. Annual report. Department of Community Medicine, St. Vincent's Hospital and Medical Center of New York.

Brody, J.E. 1986. Personal health column. *New York Times* (22 Jan.).

Cabin, W. 1985. Corporate reorganization overview. *Caring* 4 (7):4-7.

Callahan, Jr. J.J. 1981. How much, for what, and for whom? *American Journal of Public Health* 71:987-988.

Cang, S. 1976/77. Why not a hospital at home here? *Age Concern Today* No. 20:9-11 (Winter).

Cang, S. 1977. An alternative to hospital. *Lancet* 1 (8014);742-743.

Cang, S., and F. Clarke, 1978. Homecare of the sick -- an emerging general analysis based on schemes in France. *Community Health* 9 (3):167-172.

Caring. 1984. Special issue on hospitals/HHA relations. 3(7):1-92.

Caring. 1985a. National Health Care Week. 4:37.

Caring. 1985b. Case studies. 4 (8):27-56.

Caring. 1985c. Congress acts on Alzheimer's disease: two statements from the 1983 congressional hearing. 4 (12):26-29.

Caring. 1985d. Fragile children. 4 (5):8-10.

Caring. 1985e. Organizations providing help. 4 (5):58-62.

Caring. 1985f. Providing a transition setting between hospital and homecare. 4 (5):69-70.

Cetron, M. 1985. The public opinion of homecare. A survey report executive summary. *Caring* 4 (10):12-15, 1985.

Cherkasky, M. 1949. The Montefiore hospital homecare program. *American Journal of Public Health* 39:163-166.

Coleman, B. 1985. *A consumer guide to home health care.* Washington, D.C.: National Consumers League (June).

Congressional Record. H.J. res. 319, 99th Cong., 1st Sess., 131 Cong. Rec. (1985).

Connecticut Community Care, Inc. 1985. *Annual Report.* Bristol, CT. pp. 8, 10.

Cost Containment Newsletter. 1981. How homecare programs pay off. 3 (11):3,6.

Cushman, M.J. 1984. Program budgeting in homecare agencies. *Nursing Economics* 2 (6):409-412.

Coyle 1984. Pain program helps cancer patients. *Hospitals* 58 (5):56,60 (1 March).

Dailey, A. 1985. Hospice care and the role of children's hospice international. *Caring* 4 (5):66-67.

Daniels, K. 1985. Hospital Home Health Agency of California. *Caring* 4 (7):16-18.

Department of Health, Education and Welfare. 1976. *Home health care. A discussion paper by the Intra-Departmental HHC Policy Working Group.* Washington, DC, unpublished (December).

DeVita, R., and D. Elwell, 1985. Corporate restructuring. *Caring* 4 (7):60-62.

Elmslie, J. 1985. VNA Health Resources, Inc. of Portland, Oregon. *Caring* 4 (7):19-21.

Emerson, D. 1985. Hospital's home health coalition improves care, cuts costs. *Health Progress* 66 (5):26.

Feinberg, E.A. 1985. Family stress in pediatric homecare. *Caring* 4 (5):38-41.

Fields, M.A. 1985. Financial planning in the home health agency. *Family and Community Health* 8 (2):33-45.

Firshein, J. 1986. Prepaid use of home health services booming. *Hospitals* 60 (8):66-67.

Flanagan, E.M. 1985a. Conversion from non-profit to profit: legal and practical consideration. *Caring* 4 (7):52-54.

Flanagan, E. M. 1985b. Home health agency physician ownership: legal considerations. *Caring* 4(7):56-59.

Flashenberg, L. 1985. Celebrate home care week: A hypothetical agency celebrates national home care week. *Caring* 4 (8):8-26.

Forum. 1978. Supermarket of services allows dependent adults to avoid institutions. 2 (4):16-21.

Frasca, C. 1981. Home health care program offers comprehensive services. *Hospitals* 55 (6):39-42.

Freishat, H., S. Gortmaker, E. O'Neill, et al. 1985. The corporate reorganization survey: Management indicates satisfaction. *Caring* 4 (11):40-45.

Freidman, J. 1986. *Home health care: A complete guide for patients and their families.* New York: W.W. Norton.

Friedman, S.R., and L.W. Kaye. 1979. Homecaring for the frail elderly: implications for an international relationship. *Journal of Gerontological Social Work* 2:109-123 (Winter).

Galten, R. 1985. Funding strategies: advice to parents. *Caring* 4 (5):54-57.

Gardiner, N.B. 1985. Tax problems in corporate reorganization of tax-exempt providers. *Caring* 4 (7):49-51.

General Accounting Office. 1981. *VA's home care programs is a cost-beneficial alternative to institutional care and should be expanded, but program management needs improvement.* Washington, DC: Government Printing Office. Pub. no. HRD-81-72 (27 April).

Gillaspy, J.L., and J. Edwards, 1985. Metroflex: home health agency resource management. *Caring* 4 (11):10-13.

Ginzberg, E., W. Balinky, and M. Ostow. 1984. *Home health care: It's role in the changing health services market.* Totowa, NJ: Rowman & Allanheld Pub.

Gleeson, S.V., A.J. Riddell, J.W. Yuncza, et al. 1984. The four Ps of billing, credit and collection for home health care agencies. *Nursing Administration Quarterly* 8 (2):74-81.

Goldberg, A.I. 1985. Homecare for the ventilator-dependent person in England and France. *Caring* 4 (5):34-36.

Goodner, L. 1985. VNA of Sangamon County, Illinois. *Caring* 4 (7):34-37.

Greenberg, R.B. 1986. Legal implications of home health care by nonprofit hospitals. *American Journal of Hospital Pharmacy* 43:386-390.

Grigsby, S. 1985. VNA of Louisiana. *Caring* 4(7):26-28.

Gunning-Schepers, L. X. Leroy, and P. DeWals. 1984. Homecare as an alternative to hospitalization: a case study in Belgium. *Social Science Medicine* 18 (6):531-537.

Halamandaris, V.J. 1985a. Caring thoughts. *Caring* 4 (8):72.

Halamandaris, V.J. 1985b. Caring thoughts. *Caring* 4 (5):96.

Halamandaris, V.J. 1985c. Caring thoughts. *Caring* 4 (7):80.

Halley, N.I. 1985. Ogeeche home health agency of Statesboro, Georgia. *Caring* 4 (5):80-81.

Ham, R. 1980. Alternatives to institutionalization. *American Family Physician* 22 (1):95-100.

Hansen, R., and R.J. Gallentine. 1985. The organization review: health care management. *Caring* 4 (4):44-48.

Harris, M., M. Nyman, and L. Harmer. 1985. VNA of Eastern Montgomery County, Abington, Pennsylvania *Caring* 4 (5):82-83.

Harris, Jr., W.L. and J.C. McAllister, III. 1985. Microcomputer applications for home health care services. *American Journal of Hospital Pharmacy* 42:2702-2708.

Hayslip, Jr., B., M.L. Ritter, R.M. Oltman, et al. 1980. Homecare services and the rural elderly. *Gerontologist* 20:192-199.

Heritage Foundation. 1984. *Mandate for Leadership II*. Washington, DC (7 Dec.).

Hennessey, M.J. and B. Greenberg. 1980. The significance and impact of the home care of an older adult. *Nursing Clinics of North America* 15 (2):349-369.

Hoff, G.A., and L.J. Schneiderman. 1985. Having babies at home: is it safe? is it ethical? *Hastings Center Report* :19-27 (Dec.).

Holt, S.W. 1985a. Vertical integration in home care -- Part I. *Caring* 4 (3):54-57.

Holt, S.W. 1985b. Vertical integration in home care -- Part II. *Caring* 4 (4):50-52.

Houchen, B., and K. Jones. 1985. City of Columbus home health services of Columbus, Ohio. *Caring* 4 (5):88-91.

House Subcommittee on Health and Long Term Care. 1985. *Building a long-term care policy: homecare data and implications.* Washington, DC: Government Printing Office. Comm. Pub. No. 98-484.

Howell, M. 1985. The diagnosis and treatment of Alzheimer's disease. *Caring* 4 (12):12-16, 64.

Irwin, T. 1978. *Home health care: when a patient leaves the hospital.* New York: Public Affairs Committee, Inc (July).

Jonas, S. 1986. *Health care delivery in the United States.* New York: Springer Publishing Co.

Klane, E.M., and O.W. Nestor. 1985. Management development: the critical element in homecare expansion. *Caring* 4 (11):28-31.

Kohrman, A.F. 1985. Pediatric homecare opportunity and obligation. *Caring* 4 (5):42-46.

Koop, E. 1985. Our commitment to the disabled child. *Caring* 4 (5):8-23-25,95.

Kun, S., and K. Brennan. 1985. Pediatric discharge planning: challenges and rewards. *Caring* 4 (5):37.

Kuntz, E.F. 1983. Hospitals move into homecare by striking partnership deals. *Modern Healthcare* 13 (12):116,118.

Lancaster, J. 1985. From the editor. *Family and Community Health* 8 (2):VI-VII.

Laxton, C.E. 1985. The John D. French center for Alzheimer's disease. *Caring* 4 (12):22-24.

Lee, J.T., and M.A Stein, 1980.. Eliminating duplication in home health care for the elderly: the Guale project. *Health and Social Work* 5 (3):29-36.

Liota, M., M.H. Levene, L. Martin, et al. 1985. VNS of New York, New York. *Caring* 4 (5):76-79.

Lipsman, R., P.W. Brickner, L.K. Scharer, et al. 1984. The Chelsea-Village program in *Hospitals and the aged. The new old market* edited by S.J. Brody and N.A. Persily. Rockville, MD: Aspen Systems Corp., pp. 191-201.

Logue, J.H. 1984. Patient education challenges in home health care. *Patient Education Newsletter* 7 (5):3-4.

Logue, J.H., and E. Garvey. 1985. Managerial dilemmas in home health care. *Family and Community Health* 8 (2):46-53.

Lombardi, Jr., T. 1986. Nursing home without walls--An update. *Health Bulletin #75-F.* Albany, New York (1 Jan.).

Long Term Care Management. 1985. News. 14 (22):2.

Lorenz, B. 1985a. Corporate reorganization: the accounting perspective. *Caring* 4 (7):62-65.

Lorenz, B. 1985b. More sophisticated cost finding. *Caring* 4 (7):75-78.

Lowe, J. 1976. The alternative to hospitals. *Modern Maturity.* 19 (2):29-31.

Lowenstein, H. 1986. Home-care alternative. *New York Times* (6, Feb.).

Lubin, J.S. April 4, 1975. Alternatives to nursing homes. *Wall Street Journal.*

Lundberg, C.J. Spring 1984. Home health care: a logical extension of hospital services. *Topics in Health Care Financing* 10 (3):22-23.

Malafronte, D., H.H. Moses, R.M. Bronson, et al. 1977. *Appropriateness of long-term care placement.* East Orange, NJ: Urban Health Institute.

Manber, M.M. 1980. Patients with no place to go. *Medical World News* 21 (16):57-63.

Martinez, C.K. 1985. Dietary management of Alzheimer's disease. *Caring* 4 (12):18-20.

McBroom, A.C. 1985. President's message. *Access* 3 (2):1.

McDonnell, A. 1986. *Quality hospice care. Administration, organization, and models.* Owings Mills, MD: Rynd Communications.

McNamara, E. 1982. Homecare. Hospitals rediscover comprehensive home care. *Hospitals* 56 (21):60-66 (1 Nov.)

Mistarz, J.E. 1984. Safety of joint ventures may attract hospitals. *Hospitals* 58 (5):42,44.

Moss, F. 1985. Foundation for hospice and homecare sets research on pediatric homecare as top priority. *Caring* 4 (5):72-73.

Moxley, J.H., and P.C. Roeder. 1984. New opportunities for out-of-hospital health services. *New England Journal of Medicine* 319:193-197.

Murphy, L.B. 1982. *The home hospital.* New York: Basic Books.

Nassif, J.Z. 1985. *The home health care solution.* New York: Harper & Row.

National HomeCaring Council. 1983. *All about home care: A consumer's guide.* New York.

National League for Nursing. 1978. *Prospectus for a national homecare policy.* New York.

Odle, S.G. 1967. *What are the advantages and disadvantages of hospital homecare for the patient and family in The physician speaks on homecare.* Washington, DC: Government Printing Office Pub. No. (PHS) 1654 (June).

O'Donnell, K.P. 1984. Hospital-based home health care: Gaining a competitive advantage where everyone benefits. American Journal of Hospital Pharmacy 41:147-148.

Oni, A. 1984. Measuring productivity in home health care. Nursing Management 15 (3):14-16.

Pappas, J.P. 1985a. Marketing homecare: Organizational posture and positioning. *Caring* 4 (11):48-50.

Pappas, J.P. 1985b. The marketing audit and communications. *Caring* 4 (12):54-59.

Pear, R. 1986. Change in Medicare prompts hospital - nursing home ties. New York Times (16 April).

Perrin, J.M. 1985. Chronically ill children in America. *Caring* 4 (5):16-22.

Perry, B.J. 1984. Alzheimer's disease. A challenge to nursing and the homecare system. The Maine Nurse 70 (1):5-7.

Perry, B. 1985. Great Falls Corporation, Auburn, Maine. *Caring* 4 (7):22-25.

Porter, S. 1978. One alternative home health care. *N.Y. Daily News* (13 Feb.).

Pride Institute Journal of Long Term Home Health Care. Summer 1984. International perspectives on home health care. 3 (3):8-44.

Profiles in Hospital Marketing. 1985. Home health services. Two approaches to doing it yourself. 17:50-60 (Jan.).

Pyles, J.C. 1985. The legal checklist for home care ventures. *Caring* 4 (7):38-40.

Rafferty, L.J. 1979. Adult day care: Its effect upon the psycological quality of life of otherwise homebound older persons in an urban setting. *Long Term Care and Health Services Administration Quarterly* 3 (3):119-221.

Reif, L. Fall 1980. Expansion and merger of home care agencies: Optimizing existing resources through organizational redesign. *Home Health Care Services Quarterly* 1 (3):3-36.

Reif, L. 1984. Making dollars and sense of home health policy. *Nursing Economics* 2 (6):382-388.

Reif, L., and B. Trager. Winter 1985. International perspectives on long-term care. *Home Health Care Services Quarterly.* 5:(314).

Richardson, K. 1985. Home nursing agency of Altoona, Pennsylvania. *Caring* 4 (5):84-86.

Riddell, A.J. 1981. Productivity: a dirty word in the voluntary nonprofit agency. *Home Health Review* 4 (1):13-20.

Riffer, J. May 16, 1985a. Cooperative arrangements are key for home health care in rural areas. *Hospitals* 59 (10):81.

Riffer, J. May 16, 1985b. Public health deficits spur hospital joint ventures. *Hospitals* 59 (10):70.

Roberson, R.G. 1985. VNA home health services of Greater Kansas City, Missouri. *Caring* 4 (7):30-33.

Roberts, I. 1978. Planning care at home. *Nursing Times* 74 (4):154-156.

Roeder, B.J., and D.N. Williams. 1985. Diagnosis-specific home care: the Park Nicollet model. *Postgraduate Medicine* 77 (2):79-88.

Rozelle, G.J. 1985. Calculation of productivity. *Caring* 4 (11):7.

Runner-Heidt, C.M. 1985. Initiating hospital-based home care. *Home Healthcare Nurse* 3 (4):33-36.

Russell, D.L. 1977. Home health care - another way to reduce costs? *Pennsylvania Medicine* 80:19-22.

Ryder, C.F. 1967. *Changing patterns in home care.* Washington, DC: Government Printing Office. PHS Pub. No. 1657.

Sager, A. 1980. *Who should control long term care planning for the elderly?* Waltham, MA: Brandeis University, Heller School.

Schwartz, G.B. 1980. Physicians support home health care. *Hospitals* 54 (4):52,56,65.

Seidl, F.W., R. Applebaum, C.D. Austin, et al. 1981. Delivering in-home services to the aged and disabled: The Wisconsin experiment. Report. University of Wisconsin-Madison.

Shahoda, T. 1986. Clustering services? Consider antitrust laws. *Hospitals* 60 (8):38,42.

Shannon, K.A. 1985. Sick kids need involved people. *Caring* 4 (5):65-67.

Shannon, K.A. April 22, 1986. Letter to Author. Severna Park, Maryland.

Shaw, S. 1985. The changing marketplace. *Caring* 4 (7):8-9,79.

Sheridan, M.S. 1985. Things that go beep in the night: Home monitoring for apnea. *Health and Social Work* 10 (1):63-70.

Simione, Jr., W.J., and D. Elwell 1985. Cost allocation: The problem and the solutions. *Caring* 4 (7):67-70.

Skipper, M. 1985. Alzheimer's disease touches home--and a VNA responds. *Caring* 4 (12):5-11,64.

Steward, J. 1985. Hospitals without walls. The New Brunswick extra-mural hospital. *International Nursing Review* 32 (6):181-184.

Stewart, J.E. 1979. *Home health care.* St. Louis: C.V. Mosby Co.

Stitt, P.G. 1985. Home health care innovations in health care delivery. *Hawaii Medical Journal* 44:166-169.

Stockton, M. 1985. Book review of For Sasha, with Love. *Caring* 4 (12):31.

Tamme, P. 1985. Abuse of the adult client in home care. *Family and Community Health* 8 (2):54-65.

Tatage, M. 1984. Homecare agency adjusts to competing interests of hospitals. *Modern Healthcare* 14 (11):32-34, 38.

Teplitsky, S.V., and C.T. Hedlund. 1985. HHA restructuring opportunity for the future? *Caring* 4 (7):42-44.

Tolkoff-Rubin, N.E., S.L. Fisher, J.T. O'Brien, et al. 1978. Coordinated homecare. The Massachusetts General Hospital experience. *Medical Care* 16:453-464.

Trager, B. 1972. *Home health services in the U.S.A. Report to the U.S. Senate Special Committee on Aging.* Washington, DC: Government Printing Office (April).

Trager, B. 1980. Home health care and national health policy. *Home Health Care Services Quarterly* 1 (2):1-103.

Traska, M.R. Jan. 5, 1986. No home means no home care for AIDS patients. *Hospitals* 60(1):69-70.

Traska, M.R. 1986. Case management is just the ticket for home care. *Hospitals* 60 (6):80-81.

Walsh, M. 1985. Stress management: A case oriented program for a home attendant agency. *Caring* 4 (11):18-22.

Warhola, C.F. Ryder. 1980. *Planning for home health services: a resource handbook.* Washington, DC: Government Printing Office. Pub. No. HRA 80-14017, p. 41 (Aug.).

Weinstein, S.M. 1984. Specialty teams in home care. *American Journal of Nursing* 84:342-345.

Weller, C. 1978. Home health care. *New York State Journal of Medicine* 78:1957-1961.

White, M. Nov. 1985. A hospital based coordinated community care system: The promise, the problems, the strategies for solving them. Presentation at annual meeting of American Public Health Association, Washington, DC.

Williams, J.L., G. Gaumer, and M.A. Cella. 1984. *Home health services: An industry in transition.* Cambridge, MA: Abt Associates, Inc (3May).

Windley, R. 1985. Diversification opportunities in the 1980s. *Caring* 4 (7):10-14.

World Health Organization 1947. The constitution of the WHO. *WHO Chronicle* 1:29.

Chapter 3

DRGs Stimulate High Technology and DME Services

Revolutionary changes are taking place in the home health care field because of the emphasis upon cost containment to control the runaway inflationary spiral upward. Using a prospective payment system (PPS), the federal government employs diagnosis related groups (DRGs) to place a cap on expenditures. This regulatory combination of PPS/DRGs has led to a surge in the use of high technology homecare services, along with a concomitant increase in the use of durable medical equipment (DME). Although the boundaries between high technology and DME are somewhat blurred due to reimbursement criteria, developments in both areas are worth noting, along with a brief explanation of the PPS/DRG methodology.

PPS/DRGs

On October 1, 1983, the federal government initiated a new reimbursement methodology for individuals receiving inpatient hospital care when they are covered by the Medicare program. Under the new program the hospital will be reimbursed based upon preset allowances (PPS) for the services rendered to the patient. Each patient is classified into one of the 467 diagnosis related categories (DRGs), which are also grouped into 23 major diagnostic categories (MDCs). Each of the 467 DRGs also has indicators determining the length of stay (LOS) for that particular condition. If the patient stays beyond the indicated LOS, the hospital has to explain the "outlier" and request additional reimbursement. Thus, the hospital receives the same reimbursement allowance regardless of the services rendered or the number of days in the hospital within the LOS range. There are many additional complexities to the PPS/DRG scheme dealing with exempted facilities, stipends for teaching hospitals, variances for comorbidities, complications, surgery and/or medical procedures and age. However, the heart of the method revolves around the predetermined prices set for all inpatient services rendered by the hospital. This PPS/DRG methodology has turned hospital administrators into management people concerned with the "winners and losers" among their inpatient census (Spiegel and Kavaler 1986).

Quicker and Sicker

In 1980, the State of New Jersey instituted an experimental DRG scheme and Livengood, Smith, and Hallstead reported on the impact of DRGs on home health care toward the end of 1983 (Livengood, Smith, and Hallstead 1983). These investigators inquired about the quality of care, the discharge of patients in more acute stages of illness, the change in the type of patients seen in home health agencies, and the overall impact on home health services.

Utilization review, quality assurance, and discharge planning programs all monitor the quality of care in New Jersey hospitals. Readmissions and premature discharge were indicated as evidence of lowered quality of care. There was no data to reflect an increase in the number of readmissions over the three years that DRGs were operational in New Jersey. However, the consideration of premature discharge did raise the issue of sicker patients being discharged to home health care services.

While not using the actual words, "quicker and sicker," at that time the New Jersey researchers did report that noticeable trend. There was an increased need for daily homecare visits and for longer LOS nursing visits. This was not a universal trend among the hospitals, however.

Emphasis was noted in attention to discharge planning by a variety of hospital staff members as patients were identified early for potential homecare services after discharge. Home health agencies increased their relations with hospitals and some even arranged for the placement of Home Care Intake Coordinators within hospitals.

Advances in medical technology also intervened during the 1980 to 1983 time period, and the new technology allowed patients to be discharged to homecare earlier. Of course, the technology also intermingled with the concept of avoiding overstepping the LOS range. Therefore, patients were able to make use of insulin pumps, apnea monitors, enteral nutrition, and ventilators at home without detriment.

In concluding their investigation, the authors advised home health agencies to improve relations with hospital administrators and discharge planners, to develop the requisite skilled professional capability to use the new technology, to expand services, and to create alternatives to institutionalization (Livengood, Smith, and Hallstead 1983).

On April 28, 1983, a symposium discussed the potential impact of DRGs on long-term care. More than 30 long-term care professionals gathered to talk about the financial issues, the placement of patients, and the ethical dilemmas raised by the conflict between the needs of human beings and the needs of the institutions. Points raised were similar to those already noted in the New Jersey article regarding the quality of care, premature discharge, discharge planning, and the use of medical technology. Representatives of the Connecticut and Massachusetts hospital associations, the Visiting Nurse Service of New York, and the Yale-New Haven Hospital made presentations, while Dr. Philip W. Brickner of St. Vincent's Hospital moderated (*PRIDE Institute Journal of Long Term Home Health Care* 1983). Livengood commended the symposium convenors and reiterated her observations about experiences in New Jersey under DRGs in a letter to the editor (Livengood 1984a). Another New Jersey nurse, Mitchell, also commented on the symposium but pointedly observed the opportunities for creativity in home health care offered under the new reimbursement system (Mitchell 1984).

Concepts of "quicker and sicker" discharges under the new Medicare reimbursement system received reinforcement in studies by the Senate Special Committee on Aging, the Inspector General of HHS, the General Accounting Officer (GAO), an AMA survey, and an editorial in *American Medical News* (Cancila 1986).

In fact a Hospitals issue (1986b) noted that the "quicker and sicker" controversy began one year earlier, when the GAO report released by Senator John Heinz quoted the study (*Hospitals* March 5, 1986, 9). This GAO study found that "patients are being discharged from hospitals after shorter lengths of stay and in a poorer state of health than prior to PPS." In addition, the GAO noted that "PPS may increase the effective demand for post-hospital nursing and home health services covered by Medicare." The GAO also commented that "PPS creates a strong incentive for hospitals to shorten patients' lengths of stay" (General Accounting Office 1985a).

Two reports from the Senate Committee on Aging, in September and October of 1985, repeated the earlier GAO findings and added case studies to dramatize the impact. These studies concluded that, "Seriously ill Medicare patients are inappropriately and prematurely discharged from hospitals" (Senate Special Committee 1985 a & b). Another study by a University of California researcher found that hospitals are forced to move older patients out "quicker and sicker" due to DRGs (Perlman 1986). Reporting in his local medical society journal, Herrington spoke to the increased pressure to discharge patients to homecare (Herrington 1985).

Consumer groups call the incentives the "dumping" of patients by the hospital to save or make money (Pear 1986). Tehan et al. even created an euphemistic phrase to describe the phenomena: Planned Accelerated Discharge (PAD). Under the PAD Program, hospitals pay the homecare agency to provide more intensive homecare than available under Medicare for a maximum of four days using a descending charge schedule (Tehan, Daniels, and Daniels 1985). Whether it is called "dumping" or "planned accelerated discharge," the federal government requires hospitals to tell Medicare patients that they have a right to challenge the discharge if they think they are being sent home prematurely (Pear 1986).

Differing Views of Quicker and Sicker

A research arm of the Hospital Association of Pennsylvania examined 4.5 million discharges from 244 community hospitals in that state between 1982 and 1985. While the report noted a 20.7 percent decrease in length of stay for Medicare patients and increasing transfers to home health care, there was no support for the allegation that PPS results in "quicker and sicker" discharges (*Hospitals* 1986d). An interview with former HCFA Deputy Administrator Paul Willging found him admitting evidence of quicker discharges--but not necessarily prematurely. He reminded the interviewer that a shorter length of stay was the intent of Congress (*Hospitals* 1986b).

Paul Kerschner, President of the National Foundation for Long Term Care, conceded that DRGs may be responsible for 60 to 70 percent of the blame for the "quicker and sicker" discharges. However, "sicker" discharges are related to the previously unidentified villain, the "demographic connection." Individuals over 75 to 85 would be showing up in the long-term care facilities regardless of whether or not the DRG system had come into being (Kerschner 1986).

Despite some differences about the "quicker and sicker" syndrome, a recent survey of 2,000+ home health agencies by the National Association for Home Care (NAHC) found that 92 percent reported a sharp increase in the number of sicker patients seeking care (*Home Health Journal* 1986c). U.S. Representative Matthew J. Rinaldo (R-NJ) repeated the cry in 1986: "There is widespread concern that changes in Medicare's payment system have resulted in the elderly being sent home from the hospital sooner and sicker than they used to be" (*The News Tribune* 1986).

Enter Home Health Care

Coleman and Smith (1984) posited that the economics of DRGs would drive hospitals and physicians to seek out home health agencies for monetary relief from the low PPS allowances. In exploring opportunities as a result of the PPS, Johnson (1985) suggested that home health agencies assist hospitals to identify the DRGs where homecare services can reduce the length of stay. In a review of health care delivery trends, Riffer (1985) concluded that "Medicare's prospective pricing system continued to be one of the major forces driving hospitals' interest in establishing homecare programs during 1985."

Almost an entire issue of *Caring*, the official publication of the NAHC, was devoted to the impact of DRGs on home health care. More than 24 articles discussed the DRG system, the Peer Review Organizations (PROs), the Prospective Payment Assessment Commission, the opportunities and the problems, planning for DRGs for home health care, experiences in waivered states, referrals, and future trends (Caring 1984).

DRGs as a Reason for Discharge

In testimony before Congress, Donald F. Reilly, Deputy Executive Director of the National Council on the Aging, Inc., summed up the critical consequences resulting from the implementation of the PPS. Generally, Reilly seconded the comments already made, but did add another point about the early discharge factor. He said that families were being told that their Medicare benefits had run out and that Medicare would not pay for any more hospital days (Reilly 1985). The American Medical Peer Review Association had also reviewed medical records and found physician notes saying "since the DRG reimbursement had run out" as the reason for discharge (Garner 1986).

Studies Supporting Increased Homecare

Meiners and Coffey (1985) studied 103,635 patients over 65 who were discharged from Maryland hospitals in 1980. Nearly 2 percent were discharged to home health care. Data from 18 random for-profit hospitals in San Diego, California, was also reviewed. About 37 percent of the patients referred to home health care came from the following 10 DRGs: heart failure and shock; specific cerebrovascular disorders; chronic obstructive pulmonary disease; atherosclerosis; unrelated operating room procedure; diabetes; esophagitis, gastroenteritis, and miscellaneous digestive disorders; respiratory neoplasms; major small and large bowel procedures; hip and femur procedures. These investigators concluded that home health care patients were more likely to require long-term care but were not necessarily debilitated. In addition, they predicted that hospitals and home health agencies would do more in long-term care and change their patient mix as the need grew (Meiners and Coffey 1985).

A survey of 100 home health agencies in 1983 revealed that 57 percent increased their full-time staff and 70 percent reported an increase in clients due to the PPS. Homecare clients were 75 or older and required multiple services (Wood and Estes 1984).

Investigations in New Jersey (Livengood 1984b; Sweeney-Stanhope 1984) and Maryland (McCleary and Driscoll 1984) studied care, the former using DRGs and the latter a state rate-setting commission. Each showed increases in the use of home health care services to patients more acutely ill, requiring more intensive and sophisticated services.

Area Agencies on Aging were surveyed in 1985 by the Southwest Long Term Care Gerontology Center in cooperation with the National Association of Area Agencies on Aging. Data on pre- and post-DRG programs were compared for evidence of changes that could be linked to DRGs. Comparisons revealed major program shifts: a 365 percent increase in case management services, a 196 percent increase in skilled nursing in the home, a 69 percent increase in housekeeping, and a 63 percent increase in personal care services. Length of service and services per client increased for most agencies and particularly so for agencies where DRGs had been in effect for the longest time. Researchers concluded that, "The cost containment policy utilizing prospective reimbursement and DRGs appears to be shifting a major portion of the burden of health care away from acute care hospitals to the community-based care system" (Harlow, Wilson, and Gorshe 1986). A study by the Eastern Washington Area Agency on Aging reported a 46 percent increase in home health visits in urban areas when comparing the first six months of 1983 with those in 1984 (*Hospitals* 1985b).

Another pre- and post-DRG study also confirms sharp increases in home health care utilization. A county health department reported a 43 percent rise in new home health care patients, and a 44 percent increase in those considered seriously ill (Senate Select Committee on Aging 1985a, 7).

Northwest Oregon Health Systems Agency researchers in Portland compared an 18-month period before and after DRGs, looking at patient dependency at discharge, using six activity scales: activity and mobility, bathing and hygiene, number of medications, procedures, signs and symptoms, and age. Activity rating ranged from 0 to 6 and fell into 4 classes from least to most dependent. A total of 3,200 medical record charts from four hospitals were reviewed, concentrating on three medical and two surgical DRGs. Initial results show a significantly shortened LOS with no apparent dependency increase for DRG 14-stroke. However, DRG 89 and DRG 127, pneumonia and heart failure, both showed a shortened LOS associated with an increase in dependency (Coe, Wilkinson, and Patterson 1986).

If the information is accurate, it is probable that the PPS/DRG scheme is referring patients to home health care or other alternatives in a physical condition necessitating more care. This would obviously raise the issue of the hospital's role in discharge planning.

Discharge Planning, DRGs, and Homecare

In review of legislative and regulatory aspects of discharge planning, Hall (1985) states that, "Generally speaking, discharge planning is in its infancy in terms of laws and regulations." Noting that services follow dollars and regulators are currently inhibiting expenditures for home health care, Hall posits that discharge planners will have limited options to avoid overutilization of institutionalization.

Seven New Jersey discharge planning professionals gathered to discuss the impact of DRGs on May 24, 1983, after about three years of experience with the system in that state. These professionals agreed that DRG impact was minimal in their institutions because effective discharge planning programs already existed. However, there was a consensus that there could be potential difficulties if an appropriate discharge system did not exist.

The existing programs integrated staff involvement, identification of referrals, coordinated services, documentation, and links to the community (Stonerock 1983).

Advising homecare agencies to take the initiative in improving relations with hospitals, Feather and Nichols (1985) report on a two-year study of discharge planners at 200 hospitals. They cite discharge planners noting a 24 percent increase in caseload as a result of DRGs and a 54 percent increase in contacts with home health care agencies. On the negative side, planners commented that "the hospital administrator is likely to bring at least subtle pressure" to make use of the hospital's homecare agency, if one exists.

Pressure on the entire process of discharge planning involves not only the professional planner but physicians, nurses, patients, and their families (Zimmerman-Cathcart 1983). According to an active community nurse (Krup 1985), ". . . DRG coordinators, discharge planners and social workers are pressured to move patients through the system as fast as possible."

In speaking to the adoption of discharge planning to PPS, Rossen (1984) identifies these elements of discharge planning: screening, assessment, planning, and follow-up. "Discharge planning is essential for a hospital's successful adaptation to prospective pricing." Since discharge activities effectively transfer patients out of the hospital, the hospital has a strong incentive to upgrade the quality of that particular service (Newcomer, Wood, and Sankar 1985). Austin (1986) agrees with this position, and calls discharge planning a currently pivotal service. That view is reflected in the AHA's *Introduction to Discharge Planning for Hospitals* (1983). According to the AHA, the volume is a practical blueprint for establishing, implementing, and maintaining a coordinated, interdisciplinary planning program.

A staff report for the Senate Special Committee on Aging (1985b) reported on the problem of discharge planning. Noting the inadequate service in 1975, the report states, "At most hospitals, however, the quality and professionalism of discharge planning has not improved significantly. . . the absence of Federal requirements in this area is remarkable." Recommendations suggested federal rules for predischarge consultation between all involved professionals, and that patients be informed of post-hospital benefits and appeal rights. Local agencies should be available for consultation about continued care.

PPS/DRGs for Home Health Care

With the "quicker and sicker" syndrome, the documented increase in referrals, the rising number of visits, and the attention to discharge planning, it is reasonable to consider the future application of PPS/DRGs to the home health care field.

In April of 1983, John D. Thompson, one of the DRG developers from Yale University, wrote, "In homecare I do not feel at this time that we know enough about the kinds of patients, the treatment they receive, or the resources they use to design a DRG-type system" (House Select Committee on Aging 1985, 48). In 1986, Bishop and Stassen (1986) considered prospective reimbursement for home health care from the perspective of the growth of expenditures necessitating payment changes, the specific components of a reimbursement system, and the broad context of a national health policy. Reimbursement components included timing (retrospective or prospective), payment unit (per visit, per case, per unit time or capitation), rate method (individual cost, group cost or fee schedule), and payment adjustments (wage index, transportation cost, patient mix, agency size and agency auspices). In a counter-to-the-cost-containment-at-all-costs philosophy, the authors declared, "cost containment, however, is not the sole objective of reimbursement policy." Grimaldi (1985) adds another consideration as he notes that the DRGs generally do not take into account functional impairments and the inability to perform activities of daily living. Kornblatt, Fisher, MacMillian, et al. (1985) call attention to the required emphasis on care rather than diagnosis, and the possible distinctions between public and private agencies.

Advising home health care agencies on preparing for DRGs, Bridges (1984) suggests a base year strategy: avoid blatant base year cost loading; prudently make reasonable expenditures; avoid costs that may not be recoverable; make properly financed capital expenditures in technology such as computer systems.

On a request from Representative Claude Pepper, the GAO (1985c) conducted simulations of a Medicare prospective payment system for home health care. Methodology provided for national payment rates set at the 75th percentile, with visit rates for skilled nursing, physical therapy, combined speech therapy, occupational therapy and medical social services, and rates for home health aides. Consideration for urban/rural differences, geographical wage differences, and integration of management costs into a total per visit cost was included in the simulation. Conclusions indicated that the basic methodology would increase total Medicare costs for home health care services--at the 75th percentile costs would be 15 percent higher. To achieve budget neutrality (no increase in current costs), the payment rates would have to be set at the 45th percentile. Modifications simulated showed a 9 percent increase (about $133 million) when visits were weighted, and a 2 percent decrease (about $26 million) when separate payment rates were established for each of the nation's nine census regions. Regionalization showed "significant potential promise for reducing total program costs" in this GAO simulation.

At the end of 1983, ABT Associates (1985) began a three-year HCFA-funded investigation of home health agency prospective payment alternatives. This project involves 120 home health agencies in 10 states, with 40 agencies following each one of the alternative payment methods: either per visit by discipline, per patient month of care, or per episode of care. Each of the three payment methods includes variables regarding the actual dollar rates, the treatment of long stays, a risk cap, rate adjustments for casemix, and utilization control rates. However, a report in Hospitals indicated that the study was put on hold in July 1985, when HCFA initiated per visit cost caps (Riffer 1985).

An accounting consultant discussed planning for the future of prospective payment in home health agencies and came up with the following recommendations: collect all required information; fine tune the budgeting process; monitor the budget monthly; summarize costs into variable and fixed categories; install new management systems now; analyze cost and revenue by diagnosis, by age and other variables; plan for other payers following Medicare's PPS model; explore the need for new services; analyze hospital computer printouts on discharged patients; educate the staff about PPS; consider purchasing equipment, especially under $500, now rather than waiting (Lorenz 1985).

DRG Impact Summary

There appears to be almost universal agreement that the PPS/DRG scheme has resulted in creating revolutionary changes in the home health care industry. "Quicker and sicker" appears frequently in the literature as shorthand for indicating that patients are being discharged earlier and still needing a higher level of care. Studies of pre- and post-DRG data conclude that the number of clients referred to home health care and the number of visits per client have increased. A new emphasis envelops the discharge planning program as the staff becomes pivotal in arranging for shorter lengths of stay. Walker (1985) commented on the particularly heavy impact of DRGs on home health care of the elderly at a Congressional hearing on cost containment and protection of the elderly.

Since the data is also evident to the government, there are a number of efforts to develop a prospective payment methodology to apply to home health care services. RUGs (Resources Utilization Groups), RIMSs (Relative Intensity Measures), and AVGs (Ambulatory Visit Groups) are a few of the new initials appearing in connection with prospective payment for home health care.

DRGs Spur High Technology Use in Home Health Care

With patients being released from the hospital requiring more intensive and sophisticated care, it is obvious that greater use will be made of high technology services, equipment, and supplies. Whether the services are classified as a high tech or durable medical equipment may be a quirk of the reimbursement criteria, although the actual category may be a mixture of both high tech and DME. Regardless of the categorization, it is becoming "virtually possible to create a minihospital for each homebound patient, complete with equipment and the necessary technical staff" (Brickner 1985).

What is High Tech?

"High technology homecare is nothing more than therapeutic pharmacy services formerly offered only in the hospital," according to Michael Popper, M.D., of Metro Foster Home Care in Berkeley, Illinois (Anderson 1986). Krup (1985) a community nurse, agrees, and says that, "Procedures once performed only in the hospital now are taught to patients and their families" to use in their own homes. Specifically, Epstein and Johnstone (1985) state that "high tech services generally refer to total parenteral and enteral nutrition (TPN and EN) services, intravenous (IV) chemotherapy and antibiotic therapy, and to a lesser degree, other areas of homecare such as insulin therapies and ventilator-dependent services." Noting the migration of technology from the hospital to the doctor's office to the home, Haffner (1985) adds blood glucose testing, in vitro tests, oxygen therapy, and transcutaneous electrical nerve stimulation (TENS) for pain management to the list.

There appears to be agreement that the major components of high tech fall into the following infusion groupings, even though the label is applied to a number of different therapies:

- *Total parenteral nutrition*--intravenous infusion of nutrients to patients who are unable to digest food

- *Enteral nutrition*--infusion of nutritional formula to the functioning portion of a patient's digestive tract

- *Intravenous antibiotic therapy*--the administration of antibiotics through the vein for treatment of infections

- *Continuous intravenous chemotherapy*--the intravenous infusion of drugs to fight cancer.

- *Other infusions*--includes pain-relieving drugs after surgery and fluids for dehydrated patients (Anderson 1986).

Hoffman (1985) accurately labeled high technology nursing at home a "silent revolution."

A PRIDE Institute (1984) conference on December 8, 1983, devoted the entire day to a discussion of high technology and home health care. Technology applications reported upon included respiratory care (oxygen therapy and mechanical ventilation); home dialysis (continuous ambulatory peritoneal dialysis (CAPD); and parenteral technology (enteral nutrition, chemotherapy, insulin therapy). Consequences of high technology, reimbursement, regulatory issues, future research and development were also on the agenda.

In speaking to the future, Scheinberg (*PRIDE Institute Journal of Long Term Health Care* 1984, 54) cited two research goals for high tech homecare; interactive computerized television, and an automated, mechanical defibrillating and pacing apparatus to be used in cardiopulmonary resuscitation. In addition to the telemetry and automatic external defibrillator, Haffner (1985) added the following list of homecare devices likely to be marketed in the near future: automated cardiopulmonary resuscitation devices; electrical stimulation for scoliosis; electromedicine therapy for a variety of conditions; in vitro testing of saliva, urine, and blood to monitor antibodies and drug levels; and liquid crystal thermography to detect heat-related disease changes in the body. "Because of continuing advances in both science and engineering, the possibilities of new and improved devices for the home patients are limitless."

Interestingly, participants at the 1983 PRIDE Institute (1984, 3) Conference commented on the fact that the "high tech" of flashing lights, tubes, and machines also brought with it the "high touch" of maximizing an individual's lifestyle.

Issues Common to High Tech at Home

Factors common to the management of a patient at home appear to be similar regardless of the high technology involved. Bishop (1984) identified the following six considerations:

1. *Patient Screening and Selection*--Interest and willingness to learn is the most important factor along with prognosis, patient stability, family support, access to medical care, reimbursement coverage, type of high tech, and logistics.

2. *Patient and Family Education and Training*--There must be a thorough and flexible educational program, including demonstrations, audiovisual aids, and written materials to insure comprehension and ability to undertake the tasks involved.

3. *Equipment and Supplies*--Considerations involve the setting-up and maintenance of equipment, storage of supplies, and safety precautions in the home for family and caregivers.

4. *Psychological and Sociological Concerns*--Emotional support from home health care providers is needed to alleviate anxiety, fear, hostility, and powerlessness in the patient and the family. Personal

and/or telephone reassurance and empathy is vital to assure that family caregivers realize that they are meeting expectations. Referrals to community support groups of people in similar situations can do much to help people cope with psychological and sociological situations.

5. *Clinical Management*--Coordination and communication through a single homecare professional is basic to efficient clinical management, especially when many caregivers may be rendering service. Attention should be given to the adjustment period, 24-hour on-call system, therapeutic monitoring, untoward effects of monitoring and documentation.

6. *Quality Assurance*--There should be qualified staff with written policies and procedures, medical records reviews, audits of emergency procedures, safety checks, evaluation of collaborative agreements, and reinforcement of education and training programs.

These factors have also been thoroughly examined and elaborated upon by Grizzard (1985), Harris (1984), and Schneider (1984).

Reimbursement Commonalities

Medicare reimbursement for parenteral and/or enteral nutrition is limited and deemed inadequate by most providers. Antibiotic therapy payment from Medicare is problematic at best. Insurance companies do better at reimbursement for high tech. A recent report of the national Blue Cross and Blue Shield plans (1986) indicate that 95 percent pay for antibiotic therapy; 91 percent cover parenteral nutrition; and 93 percent pay for chemotherapy. Out-of-pocket payments are still a major concern of individuals opting for high tech care at home.

High Tech Growth Factors

Cost containment efforts, an increasing elderly population, and new developments in science and engineering have already been mentioned as growth factors in high tech usage. Hoffman (1985) adds the improved educational level of the population, attitudes toward deinstitutionalization, and willingness of third-party insurers to cover the services. From a business viewpoint, Arlotta and Steele (1984) comment on home infusion therapy as a "rapid growth, high-profit margin, low-barrier-to-entry market."

Elements cited in the decision process include considerations of time and financial resources, reimbursement, patient potential, and collaborative ventures. Adding deliberations about applicable regulations, taxes, joint ventures, and legal liability, Epstein and Johnstone (1985) discuss the necessity of corporate restructuring to enter the high tech homecare market. Citing both competition and partnership opportunities for hospitals and other companies, an article in *Hospitals* (1984a) described the high tech business activities of Baxter Travenol Laboratories, Upjohn Healthcare Services, Abbott Laboratories, and American Hospital Supply's Continue-Care Division. Rucker and Holmstedt (1984) added Healthdyne, Omnicare, and Home Health Care of America to the major companies dominating the home infusion therapy market.

Relating to the growth, a June-July 1985 survey of 168 hospitals by the brokerage firm of Dean Witter Reynolds revealed that about 28 percent are planning to offer home respiratory and home IV therapy in the future. About 22 percent plan to do so in a joint venture of some type (*Hospitals* 1985c).

Marketing Analysis

In an analysis of the home infusion therapy market, the firm of Hambrech and Quist, Inc. of San Fancisco, California, identified the following four intertwining overall growth factors:

1. Home infusion therapy offers a cost effective system to the patient.

2. High margins are in store for industry participants who compete effectively.

3. Total parenteral nutrition revenue per patient will decline, but the patient base will grow.

4. Newer therapies will come to the fore (Rucker and Holmstedt 1984).

Comparative revenues and percentage of market from 1983 to 1988 reveal why the marketing firm advised clients to develop an investment strategy for home infusion therapy:

Therapy & Typical Indicators	Revenues (in millions)		% of Market	
	1983	1988	1983	1988
Total parenteral nutrition Chrohn's disease Head/neck cancer Stroke Inflamatory bowel disease	$170	$400	65%	37%
Enteral Nutrition Head/neck cancer Stroke Inflammatory bowel disease	$ 75	$250	28%	23%
Antibiotic Therapy Endocarditis Osteomyelitis Septic arthritis Deep Wound infections	$ 15	$359	6%	23%
Chemotherapy Cancer	$ 5	$ 85	2%	8%
Total infusion market to 1988	$265	$1 billion	33% annual growth	

Source: B.B. Rucker, and K. Holmstedt, 1984. *Home Infusion Therapy Market*. San Francisco: Hambrecht and Quist, Inc.

While TPN is currently the dominant therapy, antibiotic therapy is projected to be the fastest growing, at an estimated annual rate of 80 percent. Another market research firm, FIND/SVP (1985), also reported on Home Care Products and Services and forecast the high technology grouping as having the largest growth potential, adding oxygen therapy, renal dialysis, electromagnetic bone growth stimulators, and inhome infant apnea monitors to the home infusion categories. This study noted that high tech accounted for 20 to 25 percent of the total home health care market sales because of the use of costly drugs, equipment, and skilled labor. However, only 5 percent of the patient volume received such services (*Hospitals* 1985a). "Growth in the industry will stem from an increasing patient base, not increasing prices," according to the Hambrecht and Quist report (Rucker and Holmstedt 1984).

Safety and Training

Barstow (1985) called attention to the safe handling of cytotoxic agents in home health care activities. Risks in the home can be reduced by experts mixing the agents, washing before and after usage, wearing latex gloves when cleaning up, proper disposal of leftover materials, no clipping of needles, and reduction of exposure. Obviously, similar safety precautions apply to many of the components used in home health care therapies. Related to the safety emphasis is the need for better trained nurses and other home health care personnel to monitor the risk aspects of the technical and sophisticated care (Hospitals 1984c).

Standards for High Tech

Standards for nutrition support have been prepared by the American Society for Parenteral and Enteral Nutrition (ASPEN 1985). These standards begin with definitions and elaborate on organization providers, patient selection, the therapeutic plan, implementation, patient monitoring, and termination of therapy. Using clinical examples, Chrystal (1985) discusses the use of the National Intravenous Therapy Association (NITA) standards for home IV therapy. She lists 22 points to consider in initiating therapy, many guidelines relating to the use of cannulas, criteria for intermittent IV therapy, points about micron air eliminating filters, and communication norms. Abbott Laboratories' Home Care Division follows an IV therapy protocol of patient assessment, patient training, and follow-up care to assure quality standards for their services (*Hospitals* 1984b). Bender and Faubion (1985) relate their recommendations to the pediatric patient and call for a nursing checklist including physical, technical, and psychological assessment. A nutrition support team including pharmacists, a dietitian, a social worker, a nurse, and physicians was evaluated, with particular attention given to the hours of input required of each professional in a home parenteral nutrition program. Their average of 16 hours of care per patient per year can be considered relative to input required of professionals in similar programs (Dzierba, Mirtallo, Grauer, et al. 1984).

In an issue of *Drug Intelligence and Clinical Pharmacy* (1985), a symposium of six articles was published dealing with antibiotic therapy at home. Presenters spoke about cost containment, the role of the pharmacist, development and implementation of programs, and evaluation of activities. Special attention was given to assuring the high quality of the services delivered to patients.

A commercial home health care provider publishes *The Home Health Care Professional* for its employees. Typical issues cover computerized medication reporting systems, with sample print-outs illustrating the quality assurance aspects (Klotz, Chamallas, Benson, et al. 1985) as well as a warning that "intravenous Dextran 40 for the prevention of postoperative thromboembolism is not recommended for homecare use" (Andrusko 1985).

High Tech Impact Summary

DRGs are directly linked to the growth of high technology, since patients need sophisticated care when discharged sicker from the hospital. Home infusion therapies appear to be the major portion of required services, although there are common issues for all the high tech modalities. Market analysis reveals considerable projected growth in volume of patients as well as in anticipated revenues. A number of quality standards have been developed and attention has been called to the potential danger of noxious agents improperly being used in the home by professionals and family caregivers.

Durable Medical Equipment (DME): Keeping Pace in Home Health Care

In an editorial in *Rx Home Care,* a journal devoted mainly to DME interests, Garnett Jones (1985) began by saying, "It is no secret that DME supply is considered to be one of the most profitable businesses in the health care industry." She expanded on that point by stating that the degree of knowledge and expertise of DME dealers was not as well known. In fact, the upswing in the DME supply business is directly linked to the PPS/DRGs and the quicker and sicker syndrome that utilizes high technology services and the necessary medical devices and supplies to care for people in their own homes.

DME Defined

HCFA instructions, regulation 405.514, define DME as equipment that can withstand repeated use, is primarily and customarily medical in nature, is generally not useful to a person who does not have an illness or injury, and is appropriate for use in the home. To be covered by Medicare under HHS regulations, the equipment must be used in the patient's home and be considered medically necessary and reasonable for the treatment of the patient's illness or injury. Items such as canes, hospital beds, wheelchairs, respirators, oxygen regulators, crutches, commodes, walkers, and traction equipment are considered to be DME. A power-operated vehicle may be used as a wheelchair on the basis of the individual's medical and physical condition and the meeting of safety requirements set by HHS.

DME Historical Overview

Since its inception in 1965, Medicare has included a DME rental benefit. While Congress legislatively authorized the HEW Secretary to experiment developing alternative reimbursement methods for DME under Medicare in 1972, no action ensued. In 1977, Congress enacted legislation allowing HHS to reimburse for purchase rather than rental of DME when purchase is less costly. Pointedly, a National Association of Medical Equipment Suppliers (NAMES 1985) report comments that Congress had scant data to use in setting guidelines because HEW did not undertake the earlier experimentation. Final regulations were published in June 1980, implementing the 1977 law. Critics expressed concern about the regulations being costly and burdensome, and not having an analysis of those factors in the implementation of the guidelines. In response to the critics, a new HEW Secretary stayed implementation of the regulations. Researchers at Williams College, Massachusetts, received a $600,000 contract to conduct a cost benefit study that same year and the GAO also examined the costs of DME. Differing conclusions were reached by the two investigations. According to the GAO (1982), the DME Medicare payments were higher than necessary, while the William College group claimed that the HCFA regulations would not save money and recommended not implementing the 1977 law (Over, Bradburd, Williams, et al. 1983). In June 1983, the Senate Finance Committee asked the GAO to reconcile the differences between the two reports with no action to be taken on the 1980 regulations until the completion of the new GAO study. Despite the fact that the GAO study was still not completed, HCFA issued Transmittal 1067 on December 13, 1984, scheduling a February 1, 1985 date for the implementation of the 1980 regulations regarding lease or purchase of DME.

To the dismay of Medicare carriers, the DME industry, political leaders and consumers, numerous implementation difficulties arose relative to claims processing, computer reprogramming, orientation/informational meetings, and cash flow problems. Reacting to the critics, HCFA officials met with NAMES representatives and did make some changes. However, HCFA did not delay the regulations. Additional meetings between HCFA and the DME industry representatives have taken place without a resolution.

On July 30, 1985, the GAO report was published. It was recommended that Medicare payment procedures for DME be modified relative to the 1980 regulation. With the ups and downs of the legislation, the regulations, the guidelines, and the critics, the DME controversy is still unsettled.

In March 1986, a group of trade associations urged HHS to declare a "moratorium on further substantial changes in the DME benefit under Medicare" (*Home Health Journal* 1986a). NAMES led the group that included the American Association for Respiratory Therapists, the Health Industry Distributors Association, the Health Care Contractors Association, and the National Association of Retail Druggists. These critics argued that too many changes were taking place at one time, making it extremely difficult for Medicare carriers and suppliers to keep up with events. HHS was asked to wait for an analysis of the impact of prior changes on DME before proceeding with additional changes. HHS Secretary Bowen was told that "Carriers and industry cannot turn on a dime repeatedly in the course of a few months" (*Home Health Journal* 1986a).

A press release from the Health Industry Manufacturers Association (1986c) announced the formation of a new Home Care Products Committee "to address critical issues confronting this dynamic industry, particularly issues of Medicare reimbursement for homecare products and services."

A portion of the rationale for the intense concern by the federal government and the DME industry can be understood by looking at the growth and potential for DME.

DME Growth and Potential

A publication by the market research firm of FIND/SVP (1985) discussed the standard medical products portion of the homecare industry. Three major products in that category were identified as durable medical equipment, ostomy products, and disposable incontinence products. In 1984, those three products accounted for $730 million in sales with an additional $88 million from specialized pressure sore products and TENS equipment. Furthermore, the market is expected to grow at a compounded annual rate of 12.1 percent through 1990. Frost & Sullivan (1983), another market research firm, noted a $219 million DME market in 1982 with predicted jumps to $318 in 1985 and $385 in 1987, with similar growth rates at 10 to 13 percent compounded annually. Incontinence products were estimated to have a 20 percent growth, moving from $458 million in 1982 to $1.1 billion in 1985 and $1.5 billion in 1987.

Another Frost & Sullivan (1984) analysis of rehabilitation products and services identified mobility aids (wheelchairs), walking aids (canes, crutches, walkers), activities of daily living aids (dressing aids, bibs, reachers), and nerve and muscle stimulators as major DME products used in rehabilitation.

Comparative market revenues reveal the extensive growth potential:

Revenue in millions

Products	1983	1990
Mobility aids	$154.4	$362.4
Walking aids	33.4	54.4
ADL aids	37.0	100.6
TENS	60.01	21.6
Wheelchair, manual	108.0	213.0
Wheelchair, powered	26.0	87.0
Carts/Scooters	20.4	62.4

Impressive compounded annual growth rates were also noted for many of the specific categories.

International growth is another potential as HIMA (1986a) held a seminar on changes affecting trade barriers that prevented easy access of American medical equipment to the market in Japan. Seminar topics dealt with the extent of the Japanese market, business strategies for success there, promotion and assistance programs, Japanese regulatory and reimbursement approval, and existing U.S.-Japan agreements.

DME's broadening scope can be illustrated by *Rx Home Care's* (1984) efforts to provide "up-to-date coverage of relevant issues ranging from industry expansion and regulatory developments to technologic advancements and new products." Journal articles are indexed into ambulatory aids, business operations, profiles and perspectives, rehabilitation and respiratory aids and issues. In addition, special issues have been devoted to wheelchairs, ostomy, hospital beds, respiratory therapy, family education, sports injuries and DME, and to nonprofit competition.

However, in testimony before a House appropriations committee, Samuel (1986) noted that the Food and Drug Administration (FDA) required a premarket approval for many medical devices similar to that required for new drugs. Representing HIMA, Samuel complained that the time lag was close to 16 months, citing patient care, innovation, cost effectiveness, and global competitiveness. HIMA favored an additional $5 million for the FDA Center for Devices and Radiological Health to allow staff to "arrest a growing device lag."

DME is growing in dollar terms, in volume of customers, and in the ranging scope of services. An obvious collateral to the growth of DME is the effort to market the services.

Marketing DME

In a general article on health care marketing, Franklin (1985) points out six mistakes as guidelines for developing a sound approach avoiding those pitfalls

1. A marketing mix consists of four basic elements: product, place (distribution mechanisms), price, and promotion. Advertising is part of an integrated whole and should not be equated with marketing in toto.

2. Following the leader can lead to disaster. Marketing requires direction, and farsightedness to keep ahead of the competition.

3. Don't let the marketing message become obscured by overattention to the graphics. Approaches should be developed in concise, factual, meaningful, and descriptive writing.

4. Failing to balance the marketing effort among radio, TV, flyers, direct mailings, telephone calls, and other media can result in poor marketing. Nothing works all the time and different audiences need different appeals.

5. Measurable objectives can and should be used to evaluate the marketing effort.

6. Fresh perspectives from unprejudiced critical sources should be welcomed as opportunities to rethink your marketing concepts. At times, market professionals may be too close to the activity to really see what is happening.

At a meeting on home health care competition sponsored by NARD, a number of experts spoke about marketing. It was pointed out that healthcare providers, such as hospitals, HMOs and PPOs are logically moving into marketing DME, stimulated by the PPS/DRG push to seek new revenue sources. Since hospitals already stock DME for their own use, administrators consider DME as a rational extension of their services. Furthermore, the hospital could consider the DME service as a patient acquisition tool, in that the patient will have a relationship with the hospital should the inpatient need arise (*National Association of Retail Druggists Journal* 1985b). A related type of facility is the medicenter, or free standing diagnostic/treatment center. The Nelsons (1985) claim that "DME dealers in large and small firms are eyeing the growing medicenter market figuring out how they can participate."

Pathmark Supermarkets entered into an arrangement with Professional Care Equipment Corporation to provide space for DME kiosks adjacent to pharmacy centers in return for a commission on the business generated.

Shoppers can stop at the DME information kiosk, view transparencies of 20 products on a screen, discuss the purchase with the pharmacist, and then use the kiosk's direct phone line to complete the transaction and pay for the DME by credit (Rondeau 1985). Videotex marketing is an interactive mass communications medium enabling people to access information electronically and to conduct transactions at a variety of locations (Udeleff 1985). In a similar vein, Peoples Drug Stores, Inc. opened a chain a freestanding total capability DME centers, mainly in the Maryland, Virginia and D.C. area. Marketing includes emphasis on information, choice of equipment on hand for immediate delivery, and follow-up on all details (Henry 1986).

Referrals and Marketing. Part of a marketing campaign involves the development of an awareness program that encourages health care providers to refer people needing DME to your company. Logical sources would be hospitals, nursing homes, prepaid health plans, and individual professionals such as physicians, nurses, social workers, and rehabilitation personnel. However, the increasing appearance of wholly-owned DME subsidiaries affiliated with health care facilities has raised the issue of "captive referrals." Bigman (1985) advices DME dealers to cultivate loyalty in customers to deter the competition. "Unfair advantage" and "antitrust" law violations are also entering the heated conversations.

Physicians came in for special mention at a marketing conference on home health care. Audience members were reminded that the physician starts the process and is often overlooked in the home health care field. Physicians want their share of the pie, too. Louden, a home health care consultant, said, "When they refer them to homecare--if they don't get a piece of it--they lose in the end" (*National Association of Retail Druggists Journal* 1985b). In fact, some physicians raise the issue of being reimbursed for services performed in coordinating home health care services and preparing treatment plans.

Despite the "captive referral" situation and the real dependence upon solid health professional/DME dealer relationships, an 1985 survey bolstered the satisfied consumer self-referral as a major consideration in choice. A marketing telephone survey of almost 400 DME consumers, names supplied by the *National Association of Retail Druggists*, sought data about the behavior of home health care customers. Results indicated that a majority of the respondents felt that their pharmacy provided better or much better service than other outlets. It was also found that 80 percent purchase all their products at the same place. Small price differences were not as important as the trusting relationship and the availability of the desired product. Factors critical to marketing DME included professionalism, service, knowledge of home health care, concern for the customer as a person, giving time/information in person or on the phone, operating hours, and delivery of products (National Association of Retail

Druggists Journal 1985b). These variables should generate ideas for marketing activities to stimulate referrals and to boost business.

DME Wheeling and Dealing

Within six months of the initiation of the PPS/DRG reimbursement methodology, the official journal of the Health Industry Distributors Association, *Medical Products Sales* (1984), had a major headline on page one: "Hospitals Eye Potential for DME Dealer Alliances." In general, the article alerted DME dealers to the fact that they should be calling on hospitals to cement their referral relationships, "perhaps under some form of shared revenue partnership." In addition, the article talked about hospitals setting up their own DME units and trade association efforts to discourage that movement through legislative lobbying. On the other hand, there was also information about collaborative arrangements---joint ventures. In a similar journal for materials management professionals, *Hospital Purchasing News*, Albertson (1984a) describes the hospital inroads into DME. Luther General Hospital, Park Ridge, Illinois, purchased an existing DME distributor "seeking to profit from potential synergetic efforts . . . The affiliation has reportedly proved highly profitable."

Toward the end of 1984, a two-day conference on "Home Care . . . The Hospital's Business?" attracted almost 200 participants, about equally divided between hospital executives and vendors seeking homecare alliances. One consulting firm estimated that "many hospitals could earn about $800,000 in net profit after five years in DME" (Albertson 1984b). Another example involved a DME alliance between Foster Medical Corporation and Philadelphia's Grandview Hospital to form the jointly-owned Grandview Home Care. "Financial projections showed Grandview earning $3.5 million, with $1 million in pretax profits after five years." Benchmarks for that estimate are based on about 71 homecare patients per month with charges of around $66 per patient per month with a 10 percent annual growth rate (Albertson 1984b).

In reaction to the hospital/DME alliances, a Georgia DME supplier took the county hospital authority to court in February 1985 to prevent the public hospital from selling homecare DME. In prohibiting the hospital from selling DME, the court found that the venture fell outside of the Georgia Hospital Authority Law and such activity was not specifically written into the existing law. Arguments were made that the public hospitals didn't pay taxes and received interest rate breaks, and thereby created an unfair advantage for the nonprofit entity (*NAMES Washington Report* 1985). Whether or not the decision holds up under appeal, the issues raised are not fading away and other jurisdictions are reviewing their laws to see if similar situations prevail.

Case (1984) also explored the legal considerations of DME contracting with hospitals. He asked, "Is this new competition illegal or unfair or simply tougher?" The realities of the situation are:

1. Under restraint of trade laws, hospitals have as much right to enter the DME business as DME dealers have to enter other medical fields. However, the hospital must not abuse its unique relationship with the patient.

2. Reimbursement to hospitals for DME sales or rentals to home care outpatients under Part A or Part B are not at 100 percent unless the hospital owns a home health agency.

3. DRGs will force hospitals to be more businesslike and to seek new revenues sources, including DME.

4. High capital investment and lack of expertise is moving hospitals to enter into contractual relations rather than setting up their own DME units.

5. Some of the hospitals/DME dealer relationships could violate federal Medicare/Medicaid anti-kickback laws. Hospitals must perform services for which they receive compensation, patients remain customers of the DME supplier, and the transactions must be consistent with traditional business practice.

6. Despite restraint of trade lawsuits, Congressional activities, FTC rulemaking, changes in Medicare guides, and state legal actions, the DME supplier still has to adapt to the changing marketplace with sound business practices.

Evidently, there is still more to come regarding the legal ramifications of the issues. Citing the 1984 U.S. Supreme Court decision in Copperweld Corp. et al. v. Independence Tube Corp., a *Hospitals* article (Shahoda 1986) warned about violation of antitrust laws when multihealth care companies cluster services under one umbrella.

In May 1986, the nation's largest nonprofit home healthcare agency, Visiting Nurse Service of New York (VNSNY), entered into a joint venture with the nation's second largest health care services company, National Medical Enterprises (NME), to market medical equipment and home health care supplies. This new firm, VNS Med-Equip, will sell bedroom and bathroom accessories, ambulatory aids, respiratory therapy devices, and enternal nutritional equipment. Based on the 105,000 patients currently served in Manhattan, Queens, and the Bronx, it is projected that $6 million worth of medical supplies will be sold annually. However, there are plans to expand to other markets in the near future, as VNSNY seeks to replace the losses from declining federal aid (*American Medical News* 1986).

As with other aspects of the home health care industry, DME cannot escape the commercial concerns encompassed within the "wheeling and dealing" concept. Even if an organization is engaged in rendering services for the public good, that agency still has to survive economically. Of course, ethical issues arise when financial considerations overwhelm all others. The reimbursement issue in DME may be the root of all evil.

Reimbursement--The Root of It All

In 1976, prior to the start of PPS/DRGs, HCFA awarded a three-year contract to Exotech Research and Analysis, Inc., to provide a first-time-ever large-scale primary date analysis relating to Medicare DME reimbursement. Data from five Medicare carriers provided information about the DME experiences of 403,818 beneficiaries for analysis. Variations had a relatively large number of Medicare beneficiaries using a relatively small amount of DME (as in California) and vice versa (as in Florida). Medicare payed for about 73 percent of the allowed charges after the denials, the reasonable charge reductions, the deductibles, and the coinsurance, Over 1976 and 1977, the distribution of reimbursement for given categories of equipment was fairly stable, although the vast array of equipment clearly revealed the complexity of the DME field. An important finding revealed that about 50 percent of DME reimbursement involved oxygen gas and related delivery of therapy equipment. DME rentals of one year or less explained 85 percent of the expenditures and 92 percent of the episodes. Conversely, longer term DME rentals accounted for 15 percent of payments and 8 percent of the episodes. Regarding rental/purchase, this study found a nearly 50/50 split in 1976 and almost 60 percent spent on purchases in 1977.

In view of the exploratory nature of the study, Janssen and Saffran (1981) conclude that their data should provide benchmarks for further research and policy investigations. An earlier 1972 GAO study had similar conclusions with the exception of rental/purchase ratios. That GAO investigation found 82 percent rentals and 18 percent purchases.

Rent or Purchase Agreements. Through hearings and reports Congress learned of excessive rental abuses of DME. In one case a hospital bed and wheelchair was rented for four years and Medicare paid $3,234 when the purchase was $900. Stories about the "golden commode" were in a similar vein. Understandably the members of Congress were outraged at the possible fraud and abuse in the DME Medicare program.

Passage of the Medicare and Medicaid Anti-Fraud and Abuse Amendments in 1977 aimed to resolve the problem of uneconomical long-term DME rentals. Legislation required that after October 1, 1977, the HHS Secretary, acting through the Medicare carrier, would determine whether the expected need for the DME warranted purchase or rental. That decision would be based upon the medical necessity information supplied to the carrier by the attending physician. Based on the carrier's decision, reimbursement would be made to the supplier or beneficiary, with payment in a lump sum or installments through a lease-purchase arrangement. When more economical, suppliers were encouraged to develop lease-purchase agreements. Provisions also allowed for HCFA to permit rental if the beneficiary experienced financial hardship in paying the coinsurance.

Regulations planned to implement that 1977 legislation beginning in December 1980. For a variety of reasons, not the least of which was the intense criticism by the DME industry, the implementation was delayed. In the interim, two additional studies took place.

A GAO report (1982) claimed that Medicare payments for DME are higher than necessary. GAO investigators estimated excess DME rental payments after October 1, 1977 at $2 million, about 21 percent of the total 1979 DME payments. Had the 1977 law been implemented in 1977, the GAO estimated that one-third of the excess payments could have been avoided. That GAO study recommended that HCFA require reimbursement on a purchase basis on items costing $100 or less and the purchase of items costing more than $100 when more economical than rental, based upon the anticipated period of need.

In April 1983, researchers from Williams College published their report on the determinants of current and future Medicare DME expenditures and the impact upon beneficiaries. Based upon 1976 and 1977 data secured from Exotech Research and Data Analysis, Over, Bradburd, Williams, et al. (1983) analyzed 21,658 rental episodes occurring in seven states. A rental episode was defined as a beneficiary renting a single item for one or more months. Costs were simulated using HCFA's new regulations. This study concluded that the new HCFA regulations should not be implemented because program costs would increase.

According to a reviewer reflecting upon the conflicting GAO and Williams College studies, the "William College report sent tremors through HCFA, much to the glee of NAMES and HIDA (Health Industry Distributors Association)" (Brown 1985). Three important differences were identified between the two investigations:

1. GAO estimated excess rental payments at about 35 percent, while Williams College put the excess figure at only 14 percent of rental payments.

2. GAO estimated that reimbursing for purchases under $100 would increase cost effectiveness since two-thirds of rental items were under that figure and resulted in excess rentals. Williams College estimated that implementing such a policy would increase costs by about 15 percent.

3. GAO assumed that Medicare carriers could make appropriate rent/purchase decisions based upon the estimated duration of need gleaned from improved data from physicians' medical necessity forms. Williams College disagreed on the assumption that incorrect purchase decisions and the carriers costs of administering the provision would offset any potential savings (General Accounting Office 1985b, 14-15).

"A major reason for the different findings and conclusions involved the distribution of DME rental episode lengths." William College had about 64 percent of the rental episodes for one or two months and 8 percent for more than a year. GAO (1985b, 18) found 22 percent for the shorter period and 33 percent for the longer time period.

In response to a request from the Chairman of the Senate Finance Committee, the GAO investigated to find out if implementing HCFA's rental/purchase instructions would save money. In addition, the GAO was asked to address the differences between the William College study and the GAO report of July 1982. That Congressional request resulted in the July 30, 1985 GAO publication, *Procedures for Avoiding Excessive Rental Payments for Durable Medical Equipment Under Medicare Should Be Modified*.

This 1985 GAO report still differed from the Williams College study. Overall, the GAO found that excess rentals represented about 54 percent of the amounts allowed for lower cost items ($120 or less) and about 34 percent for higher cost items (more than $120).

Regarding excessive DME low cost rentals, a major part of both earlier studies, the GAO recommended to the HHS that the HCFA December 1984 instructions be modified based on findings at three of the four locations in the 1985 investigation. At those three sites, the GAO found that HCFA could increase savings from excessive rentals from 21 to 30 percent if they allowed beneficiaries one month's rental to see if they really needed to purchase the equipment. That additional month's rental would be more than offset by the savings achieved when the beneficiary only required the equipment for one month and did not purchase the item. HHS did not agree with the GAO recommendation and noted that the HCFA instructions did not mandate the purchase of low cost DME. In fact, HHS said that beneficiaries were encouraged to rent DME if needed for only short periods. Adding a one-month waiting period would complicate claims procedures and reduce savings, according to the HHS (General Accounting Office, 1985b, 75).

On high cost DME items ($120 or more), the GAO did not make any recommendation about implementing HCFA's July 1982 and December 1984 instructions that carriers make decisions no later than the 5th month regarding the most economical choice. That conclusion was based upon the uncertainty of avoiding excessive rental allowances due to the unreliability of the medical necessity forms, and the subsequent potential for errors by the carriers in their rental/purchase decisions. HHS disagreed and argued that carriers would be able to properly administer the instructions and achieve savings. HCFA is to carry out various activities to assure improvements in the completion of medical necessity forms through physician education, improved carrier processing, and monitoring by HHS personnel (General Accounting Office 1985b, 75-76).

Nevertheless, GAO did suggest that the Senate Finance Committee consider a legislative change to limit rental allowances for high cost DME items to a specific percentage of the purchase price. That change would provide that Medicare rental payments for DME be made only on the basis of an assignment where the supplier agrees to accept the Medicare allowance and related limitations. HHS felt the cap idea was similar to existing policy, but agreed to study the issue as legislative proposals were developed by HHS (General Accounting Office 1985b, 76).

Alternative rental/purchase arrangements were also discussed by the 1985 GAO report (1985b, 51, 54, 56). A NAMES proposal suggested a 24-month cap on rentals for non-oxygen related DME items with an ensuing monthly maintenance fee. Under a New York Blue Shield proposal, a non-oxygen DME item would be rented until the payments equaled the purchase price, and then the item would be purchased. A New Jersey plan limits rental payments to 120 percent of the purchase allowance, at which time the item is deemed purchased. Massachusetts has a plan that calculates a credit percentage to be applied to purchase that results in a cap of about 130 percent of the purchase price.

NAMES comments (General Accounting Office 1985b, 78-87) concluded that the document was a valuable resource. "The analysis demands that HCFA proceed with implementation of the provision for inexpensive items and withdraw the guideline provisions for expensive items." In addition, NAMES offered the GAO and their own cap proposals for the withdrawn provision. Finally, NAMES asked for a comparison chart to show anticipated savings and additional expenses.

HIDA (General Accounting Office 1985b, 88-90) also agreed that the GAO conclusions paralleled many of their own regarding purchase of low cost DME, decisions on high cost items, and consideration of a cost cap concept. An issue relative to the dealer supplying the same warranty on used as on new equipment was labeled as unrealistic. Generally, the GAO was praised for doing an excellent job in outlining the uncertainties and difficulties. In addition to their comments on the one-month wait for low cost items and the high cost legislative proposal, HHS (General Accounting Office 1985b, 77) also spoke to two other items in the GAO report. HHS agreed that requiring the same warranty for used and new equipment was unrealistic and actions would be taken to change that regulation. On lease/purchase agreements as a cost saving mechanism, HHS said that they will work with industry representatives to foster such arrangements, including regulatory changes.

No Way to Avoid Excess Rentals? Noting the outrage of the DME industry, the *National Association of Retail Druggists Journal* (April 1985a, 36-37) detailed the HCFA rent/purchase guidelines under fire in Transmittal 1067. HCFA initiatives regarding the under and over $120 cost of DME, the options for rent/purchase decisions and "reasonable charge" for DME were labeled as "inconsistent and vague." Although the outcry did result in some changes by HCFA, there are still many clarifications required, according to the DME industry representatives.

In testimony before the House Select Committee on Aging in mid-July 1985, Stephen G. Yovanovich (1985, 201-203), President of the American Federation of Home Health Agencies, Inc., addressed the issue of co-payment for DME as well as the rent/purchase problem. He said that the requirement that home health agencies bill beneficiaries a 20 percent coinsurance for DME will inhibit the elderly from using DME when needed. Furthermore, the HCFA lease/purchase regulations simply did not permit adequate reimbursement. "Recent changes in federal policy have made it less likely that the elderly will gain access to needed DME items."

In response to the question, "Could excess rental allowances be avoided?" the GAO (1985b, 30) replied as follows:

In the absence of a policy which would provide that Medicare rental payments would stop when the rental allowance equaled the purchase allowance on an item-by-item or episode-by-episode basis, there is no practical way that all excess rentals can be avoided.

Federal Budget Activity and DME. Cost containment continued to play a dominant role in trying to save federal monies, including a number of actions affecting DME. Beginning February 1, 1985, the HHS Secretary implemented three methods for reimbursing DME under Medicare: lease/purchase, lump sum purchase, or rental charges. In early 1986, Curtiss (1986) reviewed recent developments in federal reimbursement for home health care. He covered the lease/purchase rules for DME with the more economical decision coming no later than the fifth rental month; the moratorium on lease/purchase rules for oxygen concentrators, regulators, ventilators, and liquid oxygen systems; the less restrictive rules on home oxygen therapy; changes in the coverage of parenteral and enternal nutrition programs; coverage of morphine infusion; coverage of infusion pumps; coverage of blood clotting factors; and a policy to delay Medicare payments that was later retracted. In addition, Curtiss cited the basis for the collection of a 20 percent coinsurance charge from Medicare beneficiaries by the agency supplying DME to the customer.

O'Sullivan (1985) analyzed the federal FY 1986 Medicare budget for members of Congress. Regarding DME, she noted the administration's proposal to freeze customary and prevailing charges for DME and related items for one year, beginning in FY 1986. Beginning in 1987, prevailing charges would be indexed to the consumer price index (CPI). That proposal would change the payments previously made on the basis of reasonable charges. Outlays would be reduced by $50 million in FY 1986 and $750 million over the FY 1986-FY 1990 period. A House Ways and Means Committee proposal would limit the increase in reasonable charges for rented DME to 1 percent in FY 1986. Thereafter, reasonable charges for both rented and purchased DME could rise no faster than the CPI. Payment could only be made on the basis of mandatory assignment. Suppliers would be required to accept Medicare's determination of the reasonable charge and could bill the beneficiary no more than the applicable deductible and coinsurance (O'Sullivan 1985).

According to federal budget documents, "Evidence indicates that Medicare is paying excessive amounts for these services (DME) . . . Under this initiative, reasonable charge levels will be reviewed, and payments will be revised where appropriate to reduce overpriced charges" (*Home Health Journal* 1986b). There was an immediate response from the DME industry regarding the proposals to cut reimbursements along with foreboding of the anticipated impact upon beneficiaries and suppliers.

Testifying before the House Subcommittee on Health on the 1986 Medicare budget, Linden (1985a) represented the 1,400+ members of the National Association of Medical Equipment Suppliers (NAMES). He was joined by the Health Industry Distributors Association (HIDA) in his comments. While the trade associations expressed support for the proposal to freeze and index DME rental charges, issues were raised relative to recent HCFA initiatives on oxygen coverage guidelines, oxygen reimbursement guidelines, and rent/purchase payment procedures. Specifically, the contention was made that "there are very few customary or prevailing purchase charges for new and used equipment" with significant errors and hopelessly outdated source material. Linden predicted lower quality products, decreased service on the equipment, and a lower rate of assignment. Four recommendations were made to the Committee:

1. Consider the significant changes affecting beneficiaries receiving DME that have resulted from the policy changes recently implemented by HCFA.

2. Consider the need to establish fair and reasonable purchase charges for DME before freezing those charges.

3. Consider the savings to be achieved by withdrawing the HCFA rent/purchase payment instructions for expensive equipment and substituting the NAMES alternative payment proposal.

4. Consider the need for Congress to provide review and appeal for Medicare Part B beneficiaries and providers.

In a statement before the Senate Finance Committee on the 1986 budget, Linden (1985b), expanded a bit on the earlier positions. He asked that CPI indexing for purchase of DME begin in 1988 and rental in 1987; reiterated support for rental limitation in 1986 but not for purchase in 1986; opposed mandatory assignment and linked consideration to HCFA's issuing formal regulations defining "inherently reasonable" charges and to legislation granting new appeal rights; supported legislation requiring HHS to study alternative reimbursement methodologies for DME and to report the findings to Congress.

Reasonable Charges for DME. Proposed rules on reasonable charge limitations for Part B under Medicare were published in the *Federal Register* (1986). Reasonable charge was defined as the lowest of the actual charge, the customary charge by a supplier, or the 75th percentile of customary charges in a locality. It was noted that unreasonable charges can occur when the market is not competitive; when Medicare and Medicaid are the primary payment sources; when new technology is used without a history of charges; when technology use changes as skills required are reduced; when charges are out of line with other localities; and when charges are grossly in excess of acquisition or production costs. Factors to be considered in limit setting included price markup, utilization, cost of providing service, charges in other areas, a comparison of charges to non-Medicare and Medicare patients, and other appropriate factors. This proposed rule also provided for public participation in setting limits and exemptions. HCFA intended the rule to protect Medicare from excessive outlays and adverse effects on beneficiaries.

Using strong language, HIMA (1986b) sent a letter to HCFA commenting on the February 18, 1986 proposed rule on reasonable charge limitations. HCFA was accused of trying to "end-run" Congress by exceeding the legal authority authorized by the Medicare statute. HIMA said that the rule was a substantial departure from Part B and that restructuring should be accomplished by joint legislative/executive branch planning, not piecemeal efforts by HCFA. Even assuming HCFA's statutory authority, HIMA pointed out that the rule needed to clarify vague and ambiguous provisions regarding specific criteria to protect Medicare beneficiaries, the special circumstances, the specific charge calculation methods, and the distinctions between costs and charges. "HCFA is in a backdoor fashion ratcheting down a program that seriously affects the safety, quality and access of healthcare for the elderly."

With the piling up of actions aimed at doing something about the DME reimbursements in HCFA policies, in budget cost cutting, and in Congressional initiatives, consideration of alternative methods is a logical next move.

Alternative Reimbursement Methods. A number of suggestions for alternative DME reimbursement methods were noted in the 1985 GAO report including variations on percentage cap on purchase, a one month rental waiting period before making a purchase decision, and a fixed time period for rentals, However, NAMES (1985) did come forward with a six-point legislative and regulatory plan to control Medicare costs, while preserving both the DME benefit and the rental nature of the industry. Recommendations included retaining the present method for low cost DME; establishing three categories for expansive DME depending upon the high risk intensive service, an 18-20 month cap on rentals of all other DME with maintenance service follow-up to be resolved later, and the last category of exceptions where purchase is appropriate; setting up a national pricing system; reducing the number of Medicare carriers; establishing an advisory committee similar to the Prospective Payment Assessment Commission in the PPS/DRG scheme; and uniform policy regarding the enforcement of the collection of coinsurance and deductibles. NAMES noted that the six point reimbursement proposal must be viewed as a package.

Competitive bidding on supplying DME to Medicare patients will be tried by HCFA in late 1986 as part of a five-year demonstration project by multiple winning bidders in six cities to be selected. Bids will be made on either a per capita basis, episodes-of-care or unite-of-service basis with the most likely to be the latter with payment per wheelchair, per cane, etc. "I wouldn't be surprised if competitive bidding could drive down reimbursement by as much as 25 percent," said Jeff McCombs of HCFA's Office of Research and Demonstrations. McCombs also was of the certain opinion that DME reimbursement based on usual, customary, and reasonable charges is on the way out (*Hospitals* 1986a).

DME Impact Summary

While the ferment continues and the arguments become heated on both sides, DME appears to be heading toward a path consistent with other federal actions to contain costs in the provision of health care services to Medicare beneficiaries. Coverage of capital costs already exists in the PPS/DRG provisions and the discussions have addressed classifications such a movable equipment versus bricks and mortar facilities. These divisions could be compared to low and high cost DME and a similar type of resolution could be applied in DME reimbursements. Competitive bidding is the latest effort to supplant the usual, customary, and reasonable basis as reimbursement of DME.

It is apparent that the growth potential of the DME industry is seen as an opportunity for the expansion of health care delivery services by hospitals, nursing homes, proprietary organizations, and others seeking to broaden their financial bases. Joint ventures are even being suggested by the DME trade associations as a way of forestalling cutthroat competition. DME dealers are encouraged to be creative in their marketing, even to selling DME in a food chain supermarket via a video/telephone hook-up.

Even though the legislation to change DME reimbursement methods was passed in 1977, it is obvious that the impact of the PPS/DRG implementation in 1983 accelerated the agitation for change. As the federal government is buoyed up by the successful PPS/DRG results, it can be anticipated that DME will feel the impact in increased efforts to contain the DME costs in the Medicare program.

DRGs, High Tech, and DME--An Overview

Evidence is mounting that DRGs are directly linked to patients being discharged from the hospital "quicker and sicker." In a chain reaction, high technology home health care services and DME suppliers responded to the real needs of an ailing population for those specific components of care. In fact, the success of the federal government in controlling Medicare inpatient costs is apt to foster initiatives in applying DRG-like techniques to ambulatory and home health care services.

High tech care is the movement of activities formerly done only inside the sterile hospital walls into the home. Modern science and engineering combined to develop and deliver the newest and best mechanical marvels to the doorstep. Prognosticators expect a bright future for high tech at home in terms of the volume of patients and dollar growth. While governmental programs are not reimbursing adequately at the moment, private insurers do better in the interests of saving on hospital costs. Although the case can be made for savings, those savings are achieved without loss of quality, as standards for high tech services exist in a number of professional association documents.

While the dividing line between high tech and DME is sometimes vague, DME essentially deals with equipment and maintenance rather than professional services. At times, the reimbursement criteria make the determination. Again, analysts predict a rosy future for DME in customer volume and dollar growth. However, there does seem to be more commercial acumen applied to DME as marketing, referrals and joint business ventures come into play. With the federal government claiming that excessive payments are the norm, HCFA has taken the lead in promoting a morass of regulations and policies. This situation has prompted the DME industry to call for a moratorium until all the pieces of the puzzle can be fit into place.

At the base of all this activity in high technology services and DME supplies is the PPS/DRG scheme. It behooves individuals and organizations in high tech and DME to study the workings and unfoldings of PPS/DRG for a preview of their own future.

References

Abt Associates Inc. 1985. *Summary of payment methods. National home health agency prospective payment demonstration.* Cambridge, MA (20 Feb).

Albertson, D. 1984a. Homecare involvements. A new horizon for buyers. *Hospital Purchasing News* 8 (3):1, 10, 49.

Albertson, D. 1984b. Hospitals review options for homecare involvement. *Medical Products Sales* 15 (11):86-87.

American Hospital Association 1983. *Introduction to discharge planning for hospitals.* Chicago, IL.

*American Medical News*1986. Nursing service, firm to market supplies. 29 (17):36.

American Society for Parenteral and Enteral Nutrition. 1985. *Standards for nutrition support.* Silver Spring, MD (January).

Anderson, H.J. 1986. High-technology services help cut lengths of stay, save money. *Modern Healthcare* 16 (4):90,92.

Andrusko, K. 1985. Prevention of postoperative thromboembolism: Dextran 40 in the home. *The Home Health Care Professional* 2 (4):6-8.

Arlotta, J., and S.L. Steele 1984. Analysis of the home health care market: the vendor's perspective. *Topics in Hospital Pharmacy Management* 4 (3):72-79.

Austin, C.D. 1986. DRGs and the elderly. Positive potential. *Health and Social Work* 11 (1):69-70.

Barstown, J. 1985. Safe handling of cytotoxic agents in the home. *Home Healthcare Nurse* 3 (5):46-47.

Bender, J.H., and W.C. Faubion 1985. Parenteral nutrition for the pediatric

patient. *Home Healthcare Nurse* 3 (6):3239.

Bigman, D. 1985. Captivating referrals. *Rx Home Care* 7 (8):7.

Bishop, C.T. 1984. Home parental chemotherapy. *Topics in Hospital Pharmacy Management* 4 (3):35-42.

Bishop, C.E., and M. Stassen. 1986. Prospective reimbursement for home health care: context for an evolving policy. *PRIDE Institute Journal of Long Term Health Care* 5 (1):17-26.

Blue Cross and Blue Shield Association. 1986. *Home health care survey report.* Chicago, Illinois.

Brickner, P.W. 1985. Long-term home health care. Undated draft of manuscript. Letter to author.

Bridges, R. 1984. Planning ahead for homecare DRGs. *Caring* 3 (2):29-30.

Brown, R.E. 1985. HCFA's rent/purchase guidelines. *Rx Home Care* 7 (4):21-27.

Cancila, C. 1986. Medicare's policies blamed for premature discharge. *American Medical News* 29 (16):2,9.

Caring. 1984. Special issue on DRGs. 3 (2):13-58.

Case, F.H., III. 1984. DME contracting with hospitals. *Caring* 3 (7):27-28.

Chrystal, C. 1985. Making NITA standards work for you. *National Intravenous Therapy Association* 8:363-365.

Coe, M.F., A. Wilkinson, and P. Patterson, 1986. *Dependency at discharge study. Impact of DRGs. Final report.* Beaverton, OR: Northwest Oregon Health Systems (May).

Coleman, J.R., and D.B. Smith. 1984. DRGs and the growth of home health care. *Nursing Economics* 2:391-395, 408.

Curtiss, F.R., 1986. Recent developments in federal reimbursement for home health care. *American Journal of Hospital Pharmacy* 43 (1):132-139.

Drug Intelligence and Clinical Pharmacy. 1985. Antibiotic cost-containment in the home health care environment. 19:278-296 (April).

Dzierba, S.H., J.M. Mirtallo, D.W. Grauer, et al. 1984. Fiscal and clinical evaluation of home parenteral nutrition. *American Journal of Hospital Pharmacy* 41:285-291.

Epstein, J.D., and D. M. Johnston. 1985. The necessity of corporate restructuring to enter the high tech home care market. *Caring* 4 (7):46-48.

Feather, J., and L.O. Nichols. 1985. Working with discharge planners in a post-DRG world. *Caring* 4 (11):52-54.

Federal Register. Feb. 18, 1986. Medicare program: reasonable charge limitations. Proposed rule. 51(32):5725-5728.

FIND/SVP. January 1985. *Home care products and services.* Firm Report. New York.

Franklin, D.P. 1985. Health care marketing: An emerging discipline. *Rx Home Care* 7 (12):65-72.

Frost & Sullivan. August 1983. *Home healthcare products and services in the U.S. New York.*

Frost & Sullivan. 1984. *Rehabilitation products and services.* Company Report. New York.

Garner, J.D. 1986. Social Darwinism to the fore? *Health and Social Work* 11:70-72 (Winter).

General Accounting Office. 1972. *Need for legislation to authorize more economical ways of providing DME under Medicare.* Washington, DC: Government Printing Office.

General Accounting Office. 1982. *Medicare payments for DME are higher than necessary.* Washington, DC: Government Printing Office. Pub. no. HRD-82-61 (July).

General Accounting Office. 1985a. *Information requirements for evaluating the impacts of Medicare prospective payment on post-hospital long-term care services: preliminary report.* Washington, DC: Government Printing Office. Pub. no. GAO/PEMD-85-8 (21 Feb.).

General Accounting Office. 1985b. *Procedures for avoiding excessive rental payments for DME under Medicare should be modified.* Washington, DC: Government Printing Office. Pub. no. GAO/HRD 85-35 (30 July).

General Accounting Office. 1985c. *Simulations of a Medicare prospective payment system for home health care.* Washington, DC: Government Printing Office. Pub. no. GAO/HRD-85-110 (30 Sept.).

Grimaldi, P.L. 1985. DRGs and long-term care. *American Health Care Association Journal* 11 (1):6-9.

Grizzard, M.B. 1985. Home intravenous antibiotic therapy. *Postgraduate Medicine* 78 (6):187-195.

Haffner, M.E. 1985. New horizons in home medical devices. *Rx Home Care* 7 (12):59-62.

Hall, H.D. 1985. *Historical perspective: Legislative and regulatory aspects of discharge planning in Continuity of Care* edited by E. McClelland, K. Kelly, and K.C. Buckwalter. New York: Grune and Stratton, pp. 11-19.

Harlow, K.S., L.B. Wilson, and N. Gorshe. 1986. PRIDE Institute Journal 5 (1):29-31.

Harris, W.L., Jr. 1984. Home parenteral antibiotic therapy. *Topics in Hospital Pharmacy Management* 4 (3):43-55.

Health Industry Manufacturers Association. 1986a. Changes in Japanese approval system to highlight upcoming HIMA seminar. Press Release. Washington, DC (6 Feb.).

Health Industry Manufacturers Association. 1986b. Comments on the Medicare program: reasonable charges and limitations. Washington, DC (29 March).

Health Industry Manufacturers Association. 1986c. Health Industry Manufacturers Association forms homecare committee. Press release. Washington, DC (1 May).

Henry, T. 1986. Drug firm opens total capability centers. *Home Health Journal* 7 (2):8,10.

Herrington, K.B. 1985. Three MDs discuss DRGs and the changing practice climate. *Michigan Medicine* 84:332, 334.

Hoffman, J.R. 1985. High-technology nursing at home. *Home Health Journal* 5 (10):19.

Home Health Journal. 1986a. Moratorium on DME. 7(3):1.

Home Health Journal. 1986b. 87 federal budget proposes cutback on homecare services. 7 (3):8-9.

Home Health Journal. 1986b. National association says Reagan out to dismantle Medicare home benefit. 7 (4):5,8.

Hospitals. 1984a. Suppliers' sophisticated options demonstrate their market interest. 58 (5):49,52.

Hospitals. 1984b. IV protocol a result of high tech service. 58 (5):52.

Hospitals. 1984c. Nursing skills require more sophistication. 58 (5):65 (1 March).

Hospitals. 1985a. High tech homecare market has greatest growth. 59 (7):45 (1 April).

Hospitals. 1985b. Homecare bears brunt of DRG system. 59 (12):70-71 (16 June).

Hospitals. 1985c. Hospital home IV, RT will see growth spurt. 59 (17):44,47.

Hospitals. 1986a. Competitive bidding coming for DME. 60 (4):92.

Hospitals. 1986b. Interview with Paul Willging. 60 (5):88-89.

Hospitals. 1986c. 60 (5):9.

Hospitals. 1986d. News at deadline. 60 (6):15.

House Select Committee on Aging. 1985. *Building a long-term care policy: homecare data and implications.* Washington, DC: Government Printing Office.

Janssen, T.J., and G.T. Saffran. 1981. Reimbursement for durable medical equipment. *Health Care Financing Review* 2 (3): 85-96.

Johnson, K.A. 1985. Exploring home health care opportunities as a result of the prospective payment system. *Caring* 4 (4): 54-60.

Jones, G. 1985. The best kept secret in home health care. *Rx Home Care* 7 (5):9.

Kerschner, P. 1986. Quicker and sicker syndrome: the unidentified villain. *Provider* 12 (4):28-29.

Klotz, R., S.N. Chamallas, T. Benson, et al. 1985. New HHCA computerized medication system (benefits patients, physicians, nurses and pharmacists). *The Home Health Care Professional* 2 (3):1-7.

Kornblatt, E.S., M.E. Fisher, D.J. MacMillian, et al. 1985. *DRG ripple: the shifting burden of nursing care in the community.* Presentation at the annual meeting of the American Public Health Association, Washington, DC (20 Nov.).

Krup, C. 1985. PPS, DRGs and elder care. Comment by a community nurse. *Geriatric Nurse* 6 (5):273.

Linden, S.J. 1985a. NAMES statement on 1986 Medicare budget. Washington, DC: House Subcommittee on Health (17 July).

Linden, S.J. 1985b. NAMES statement on 1986 Medicare budget. Washington, DC: Senate Finance Committee (12 Sept.).

Livengood, W.S. Winter 1984a. Letter to Editor. *PRIDE Institute Journal* 3 (1):25.

Livengood, W.S. 1984b. DRG system in New Jersey. Impact on reimbursement. Caring 3 (2):48-49.

Livengood, W.S., C. Smith, and S. Hallstead. 1983. The impact of DRGs on home health care. *Home Healthcare Nurse* 1:29-31, 34.

Lorenz, B. 1985. Prospective reimbursement: planning for the future. *Caring* 4 (10):47-54.

McCleary, M., and R.R. Driscoll. 1984. Health services cost review: the impact on home health services in Maryland. *Caring* 3 (2):46-47.

Medical Products Sales. 1984. Hospitals eye potential for dealer alliances. 15 (2):1, 16, 18.

Meiners, M.R., and R.M. Coffey. 1985. Hospital DRGs and the need for long-term care analysis: an empirical analysis. *Health Services Research* 20:359-384.

Mitchell, R.D. 1984. Letter to Editor. *PRIDE Institute Journal* 3 (1):25-36.

National Association of Medical Equipment Suppliers. 1985. Alternative reimbursement program for DME under Medicare. Washington, DC (July).

NAMES Washington Report. 1985. Georgia hospital prohibited from selling DME. 3 (8):2.

National Association of Retail Druggists Journal. 1985a. HCFA rent-purchase guidelines under fire. 107(4): 36-37.

National Association of Retail Druggists Journal. 1985b. Home health care competition intensifies: pharmacists can beat "em . . . or join em." 107 (6):32-33.

Nelson, J., and M. Nelson. 1985. Marketing to medicenters. *Rx Home Care* 7 (12): 105-108.

Newcomer, R., J. Wood, and A. Sankar. Summer 1985. Medicare prospective payment: anticipated effect on hospitals, other community agencies, and families. *Journal of Health Politics, Policy and Law* 10 (2): 275-282.

O'Sullivan, J. 1985. *Medicare: FY 86 Budget.* Washington, DC: Congressional Research Service, Library of Congress (8 Nov.).

Over, A.M., Jr., R.M. Bradburd, R.C. Williams, Jr., et al. 1983. *Determinants of current and future expenditures on DME by Medicare and its program beneficiaries.* Springfield, VA: National Technical Information Services (April).

Pear, R. 1986. Medicare extends patients' rights. *New York Times* (9 Jan.).

Perlman, D. 1986. Study finds elderly in cruel health dilemma. *San Francisco Chronicle* (16 Feb.).

PRIDE Institute Journal of Long Term Home Health Care. Fall 1983. Symposium: the potential impact of diagnosis-related groups on long term care. 2 (4):3-9.

PRIDE Institute Journal of Long Term Home Health Care. Spring 1984. High technology and home health care. 3 (2):1-58.

Reilly, D.F. 1985. Testimony before U.S. House of Representatives on the Medicare PPS, Washington, DC (21 Oct.).

Riffer, J. 1985. PPS, diversification push home care rise. *Hospitals* 59 (24):52, 54.

Rondeau, J. 1985. DME kiosks: the next best thing to being there. *Rx Home Care* 7 (12):76.

Rossen, S. 1984. Adapting discharge planning to prospective pricing. *Hospitals* 58 (5):71, 75, 79.

Rucker, B.B., and K. Holmstedt. 1984. Trends in the home infusion therapy market. *Caring* 3 (11):65-70.

Rx Home Care. 1984 Index. 7 (11):111-118.

Samuel, F.E., Jr. 1986. Testimony before House Committee on Appropriations re

FDA budget. Health Industry Manufacturers Association, Washington, DC (16 April).

Schneider, P.J. 1984. Home parenteral nutrition. *Topics in Hospital Pharmacy Management* 4 (3):26-34.

Senate Special Committee on Aging. 1985a. *Impact of Medicare's prospective payment system on the quality of care received by Medicare beneficiaries.* Washington, DC: Government Printing Office (26 Sept.).

Senate Special Committee on Aging. 1985b. Impact report as above (24 Oct.).

Shahoda, T. 1986. Clustering services? Consider antitrust laws. *Hospitals* 60 (8): 38,42.

Spiegel, A.D., and F. Kavaler. 1986. *Cost Containment and DRGs: A guide to prospective payment.* Owings Mills, MD: National Health Publishing.

Stonerock, C. 1983. The impact of DRGs on discharge planning to home care: the New Jersey perspective. Kalamazoo, Michigan: Upjohn Healthcare Services (24 May).

Sweeney-Stanhope, N. 1984. MCOSS nursing services--one agency's experience with DRGs. *Caring* 3 (2): 51-53.

Tehan, J., K. Daniels, and W. Daniels. 1985. Planned accelerated discharge: home care's response to DRGs. Presentation at American Public Health Association annual meeting, Washington, DC (20 Nov.).

The News Tribune. April 24, 1986. Rinaldo seeking Medicare changes.

Udeleff, M. 1985. Videotex: tomorrow's retailing technology. *Rx Home Care* 7 (12):75-79.

Walker, G. 1985. Testimony before House Select Committee on Aging in *Health care cost containment: Are America's aged protected?* Washington, DC: Government Printing Office; pp. 81-87 (9 July).

Wood, J.B., and C.L. Estes. 1984. Home health care under the policies of the new federalism. *Caring* 3 (6):58-61.

Yovanovich, S.G. 1985. Testimony before House Select Committee on Aging in *Health care cost containment: Are*

America's aged protected? Washington, DC: Government Printing Office, pp. 201-203 (9 July).

Zimmerman-Cathcart, B. 1983. What's DRG's impact on home health? *Pennsylvania Nurse* 38 (10): 6,8.

Chapter 4

Need Assessment in Homecare

Determination of the need for homecare is not strictly a statistical task. There are many areas where data may not be readily available and assumptions are made to justify the need. In a study of homecare use in New York City, Revenson and Bell (1985, 27) found that "limited and non-integrated information available about current utilization and costs prevents us from projecting unmet and future needs." However, a number of variables are usually considered, including retrospective and anecdotal approaches, as well as formulas for mathematical projections of need assessment. A number of federal legislators champion the cause of homecare, outstanding among them Congressman Claude Pepper, with his long-time support as Chairman of the Subcommittee on Health and Long-Term Care. In a report of that Committee on homecare data and implications (House Select Committee on Aging 1985, iii), Congressman Pepper noted that "in excess of 5 million people are going without the homecare services that they need. . . We are spending billions of dollars to place individuals in nursing homes and only a few million to take care of them at home."

Measuring the Need

Aging of the nation's population dramatically shows the potential need for long-term care services. In 1900, only 4 percent of the U.S. population was 65 or older. By 1980, the percentage was 11.3, more than 25 million people. Projections to 2020 estimate 17.3 percent, more than 51 million elderly. To compound the problem, the portion of "old-old" will increase faster. In 1980, those over 85 constituted 1.0 percent of the population, about 2 million people. By 2020 that percentage will rise to 2.4 percent, more than 7 million "old-old" people. Currently, the 85+ population is the fastest growing age group in the nation; by 2020, that group will make up 14 percent of the 65+ population. Futhermore, the aged support ratio (that is, the ratio of the 65+ population to the working population age 19-64 years) increased from 7.6 in 1900 to 18.6 in 1980 and will be an estimated 29.3 by 2020 (O'Shaughnessy, Price, and Griffith 1985, 4-5).

Given that the elderly do require more health care services, both in and out of institutions, the demographic projections forcibly support the necessity of reevaluating the needs assessment methodologies used by the health care delivery system.

Approximately 1.3 million Americans over 65 reside in nursing homes, about 5 percent of the total elderly population (Pear 1986). Assuming a declining mortality rate, nursing home residents could increase by 115 percent around the year 2000. There could be 2.8 million individuals institutionalized, with half of that group 85 or older. In addition, ". . . for every person 65 years of age and over residing in a nursing home, there are twice as many persons living in the community requiring the various kinds of care provided in an institution" (O'Shaughnessy, Price, and Griffith 1985, ix).

Yet, despite the huge number of elderly in institutions, it is estimated that at least 70 percent of the elderly receive homecare from family or friends rather than in nursing homes (Liu and Manton 1985, 22). "By far, the majority of long-term care services are provided by family members" (O'Shaughnessy, Price, and Griffith, viii). Liu and Manton (1985) calculate that 27 million days of informal care are delivered weekly in comparison to 4 million days weekly by formal caregivers. Obviously, the elderly being cared for at home do not easily accumulate in the statistical data since mechanisms for collecting that data are not readily available. Dr. Philip W. Brickner stated it bluntly many years ago in an article in the *Journal of the American Medical Association*: "The medical community is not reaching the isolated, homebound aged" (1973).

While the aged are usually thought of when homecare is discussed, there are many children and adults who also need such services. A National Health Interview Survey in the U.S. in 1980 reported that 31.4 million people had some activity limitation and 23.8 million people were restricted in relation to their major activity (Department of Health and Human Services 1981a, 24). Exhibit 4-1 shows the age distribution for those with activity and major activity limitations.

Weissert (1985) uses 1979 and 1980 National Health Interview Surveys data and the following four types of dependency for another analysis:

- *Personal care* included assistance in eating, continence, transferring, toileting, bathing, and dressing.

- *Household activities* included meal preparation, shopping, chores other than yard work, and financial management.

- *Mobility* included assistance in walking and going outside.

- *Health services* included injections, changing sterile dressings, and specific therapies.

Personal care can be equated with activities of daily living (ADL) and household activities can be equated with instrumental activities of daily living (IADL) (Liu, Manton, and Liu 1985).

Exhibit 4-1 Limitation of Activity Due to Chronic Conditions by Degree of Limitation and Selected Age Groups, 1981

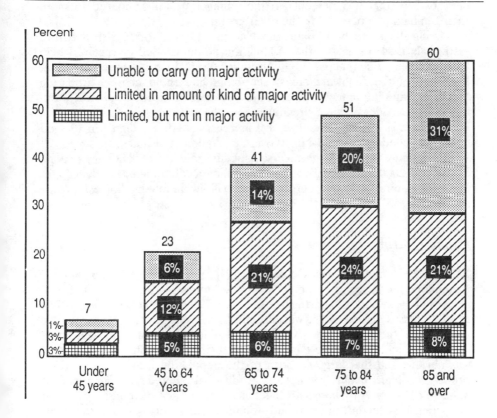

Source: Department of Health and Human Services. National Center for Health Statistics. Sept. 14, 1983. *Americans needing help to function at home.* Washington, DC: Government Printing Office. Pub. No. 99.

  Based on the four dependency classifications, Weissert arrives at a total of almost 5.5 million noninstitutionalized dependent people--about 2.6 million under 65 and nearly 3 million over 65. Those under 65 constitute 1.4 percent of the total noninstitutionalized population compared to 7.1 for those 65-74 and 20.6 for those 75 and over. Overall, this dependent population makes up 2.6 percent for all age groups. For all age groups, those in the personal care grouping (most severe dependency) and in the household activity classification (less severe dependency) are the largest categories: 1.9

million (0.9 percent) and 2.0 million (0.9 percent) respectively. Under 65 there were 820,000 people (0.5 percent) needing personal care, compared to more than 1 million over 65 (4.4 percent). Household activity dependency had 937,000 (0.5 percent) in the younger group compared to more than 1 million (4.3 percent) in the older group.

Using the same basic data, the National Center for Health Statistics (Hospitals 1984) estimated that 4.1 million adults needed or received help from another person, about 2 million under 65. Help could have been in at least one of the following areas: shopping, household chores, preparing meals, or handling money. An estimated 3.4 million needed aid with walking, going outside, bathing, dressing, using the toilet, getting in or out of a bed or chair, or eating. Of course, age increases need: less than 1 in 10 aged 65 to 74 needed help, while 4 in 10 over 85 required assistance.

"Assuming the same age-race-sex specific rates of dependency prevail, by the year 2000, the dependent aged population will number nearly 6.5 million people, more than one-third of whom will live in nursing homes" (Weissert 1985).

Public Hearings on Need

Between September 20 and October 1, 1976, the federal government held regional public hearings on homecare in Atlanta, Chicago, Dallas, Los Angeles, and New York (Department of Health, Education and Welfare 1977). Most witnesses agreed that it was difficult to measure precisely the need for homecare in the community. Even in the absence of adequate measurement instruments and incomplete data, those testifying commented that the need was obvious and that large sections of the population lack access to comprehensive high quality homecare. Individuals noted the numbers of patients discharged by homecare agencies due to lack of funds, the length of waiting lists for institutional and noninstitutional services, and the number of homebound in the community not receiving care.

In determining the need for homecare, individuals cited a lack of adequate standardized patient assessment tools and the frequency with which the level of need changes. In addition, it was noted that need determinations should be a joint endeavor undertaken by consumers and their families, health planners familiar with short-and long-range health requirements, and social service planners knowledgeable about personal care needs. Witnesses emphasized the need to consider resources for families with developmentally disabled, physically handicapped and chronically ill infants, children and adults under 65. Planners often assume that the nonelderly will be taken care of by family members. Evidence suggests that that assumption may not be valid, particularly for independent adults.

Factors in Need Determination

Accurate estimates of the potential demand for homecare services are sketchy, although most third-party payers, including the government, fear that the demand will be overwhelming. Studies examine various aspects related to need determinations and possible homecare requisites: functional assessment (Morris, Sherwood, and Mor 1984; Fortinsky, Granger, and Seltzer 1981; Baker 1980) utilization of homecare services (Wolock et al. 1985; Revenson; and Bell 1985; Liu, Manton, and Liu 1985; Trager 1972; Lemon and Welches 1967); long-term care needs (Weissert 1985; O'Shaughnessy, Price, and Griffith 1985; House Select Committee on Aging 1985; Sager 1979; Department of Health and Human Services 1981b); disability and limitations (Liu and Manton 1985; Weissert 1985). These studies have been going on for some time and critics contend that the results have been inconclusive.

A Congressional Budget Office report (General Accounting Office 1979) showed the tremendous differences between actual utilization and estimated use of homecare services for 1975-1976 and projected use for 1985 as follows:

	1975-76 Utilization	1975-76 Estimates	1985 Projections
Adults receiving homecare services	200,000-4000,000	3.0-4.4 million	3.5-5.2 million
Percent increase over 1975-1976		1,000-2,100%	1,650-2,500%

GAO calculations were made using governmental data, mainly Medicare statistics, with an orientation toward episodic illnesses. Obviously, the numbers are conservative based on the excluded population.

An array of perhaps confusing and perhaps conflicting numbers on need determination have been presented. It may be worthwhile to also examine methods and techniques, including various formulas, for calculating need assessment for homecare services.

Homecare Need Assessment Methods and Techniques

Most of the formulas rely upon a common denominator that estimates the incidence rate for persons requiring homecare over a one-year period. Nine diverse approaches use factors relative to the under 65, 65+ and 75+ age of the population at risk, hospital discharges, and the nursing home population (Griff 1984; Lundberg 1984; Warhola 1980, 21). Exhibit 4-2 compares the nine techniques and applies the method to a hypothetical community to illustrate the outcomes of need assessment. A brief description of each of the statistical approaches follows:

- *Department of Health Education and Welfare* (1972) -- Of obscure origin, only individuals over 65 are considered the high risk population with an estimate that 6.7 percent will need homecare services. That arbitrary division obviously misses a sizeable group under age 65 needing care.

- *Portland Kaiser-Permanente Group* -- This health maintenance organization based its formula on the assumption that seven percent of people treated for acute illness in a hospital will need homecare upon discharge. Nonhospitalized people and those already at home are ignored in this formula.

- *Health Systems Agency of Southwestern Pennsylvania, Inc.* -- Based on a 1973 study of acute care hospital discharges, this method estimates that 4 percent of acute discharges will need homecare services. An equal number is added on the assumption that there will be referrals from other sources. Of course, the calculation is rooted in retrospective information that may date itself quickly.

- *Southern Piedmont (North Carolina) Health Systems Agency* -- Age comes into play in this formula with estimates being 7 percent for those over 65 and 0.5 percent for those under 65 who require homecare.

- *National League for Nursing* -- This organization has developed a number of methods for calculating need. All are population-based, coupled with varying probabilities for degrees of physical disability or limitation by age to estimate hospital discharges and/or need for homecare. Exhibit 4-2 illustrates a method that uses 2.6 percent of the 65 + group and 1.3 percent of those under 65.

- *Ohio Department of Health and Batelle Laboratories* -- Using 1972 vital and health statistics, a formula emerged taking 0.2 percent of those under 14; 1.15 percent of those 15-64; and 11.8 percent of those over 65.

- *Georgia Department of Human Resources* -- Using data from a homemaker/home health aide training program, this method estimates 25 percent of the 75 + age group and 14 percent of the 65-74 group. Here, the formula takes note of the higher risk in the "old-old" age group.

- *New York/Pennsylvania Health Systems Agency* -- Using a
  Philadelphia Blue Cross study and National Health Survey data, this
  formula was developed by the Home Health Council of New York
  State. It is estimated that 6 percent of those over 65, plus 8 percent
  of hospital medical and surgical discharges, plus 50 percent of those
  discharged from nursing homes and intermediate care facilities will
  need homecare services.

- *University of California at Berkeley* -- Three factors are considered in
  this formula: age, nursing home residency, and acute care discharges
  from the hospital. Based on earlier studies, a range of from 11.8 to
  16 percent is predicted for the 65+ group. Nursing home residents
  produce a 15 to 30 percent estimate. From 3 to 9 percent of acute
  hospital discharges are estimated to need homecare services.

Application of the Nine Formulas

Dependent upon the size and characteristics of the total population, the patterns of hospital care and the nursing home situation, variations will occur
when any of the nine formulas are used for need assessment. Taking a
hypothetical community with the data given below, each of the nine formulas are applied in turn to show the differences:

Hypothetical Community

Population	Number	Percent
14 and under	109,272	26.2
15-64	260,442	62.5
Total under 64	369,714	88.7
65-74	28,500	6.8
75 and over	18,600	4.5
Total 65 and over	47,100	11.3
Total Population	416,814	100.0

Hospital discharge rate = 141 per 1000 persons

Long-term care institutional population = 5 percent of 65+ group

Results of the calculations are in the last column in Exhibit 4-2 (Number in Need of Homecare). Note that the need ranges from 3,156 to 10,556,

Exhibit 4-2 Comparison of Formulas Used for Need Determination

Source	Age of Population at Risk Under 65 / Factor A	65+ / Factor B	75+ / Factor C	Hospital Discharge D[1]	Nursing Home Population E[2]	Factors Used	Number In Need of Home Care[3]
1. DHEW (1972)	-	.067	-	-	-	B	3,156
2. Portland Kaiser Permanente Group	-	-	-	.07	-	D	4,114
3. HSA of Southwestern Pennsylvania, Inc.	-	-	-	.04x2	-	D[4]	4,702
4. Southern Piedmont HSA	.005	.07	-	-	-	AB	5,146
5. NLN	.013	.026	-	-	-	AB	6,031
6. Ohio Dept. of Health Batelle Laboratories	14-.002 15-64-.0115	.118	-	-	-	AB	8,772
7. Georgia Dept. of Human Resources	-	.140 (65-74)	.25	-	-	BC	8,640
8. New York/Pennsylvania, HSA	-	.080	-	.06	.50	BDE	8,472
9. Univ. of California at Berkeley	-	.118-.160 m̄ - .138	-	.03 to .09 m̄ - .06	.15 to .30 m̄ - .225	BDE5	10,556
m̄ values	.009	.09	.25	.058	.320		

[1] Assumes hospitalization rate of .141
[2] Assumes .05 of population over 65 in long-term care facilities
[3] Using hypothetical community data
[4] Assumes equal number of patients from community referrals
[5] Mean values of rates used

Source: Warhola, C.F.R. *Planning for Home Health Services: A Resource Handbook.* Washington, DC: Department of Health and Human Services. Pub. No. (HRA) 80-14017, August 1980, p. 22.

despite the fact that the same hypothetical population was used for the calculations.

Half of the methods use only the factor of age in determinations. However, all but one of the formulas considered different rates for different age groups. Hospital discharge was used in four methods, either by itself or in combination with age groupings. Only the last two formulas used three factors: age, hospital discharge, and inappropriate nursing home placement.

Basically, the use of a formula to calculate need has three disadvantages: retrospective data is used; there may be a geographic bias in the data not applicable to other areas; and most of the formulas reflect pre-DRG information bases (Griff 1984).

Consensus Patterns in Need Determination

Reviewing all nine formulas results in the identification of the following five major variables, in priority order, with the ranges and the means for each factor:

Factor	Range	Median
65-74 population	2.1 to 16%	9.0%
Under 65	0.5 to 1.3%	0.9%
75 and older		25.0%*
Hospital discharge	3.0 to 9.0%	5.8%
Inappropriate placement in long-term care	15.0 to 30.0%	32.0%

*Only one formula estimates a rate for this high risk group.

It would appear that the inclusion of the five common variables in need determinations should yield a reasonable figure for planning for homecare. Warhola (1980, 25) suggests a technique to arrive at an appropriate calculation by applying the common factors, in order of priority, using the hypothetical community data:

Factor	Calculation	Additive Need
Over 65	47,100 X 9% = 4,239	4,239
Under 65	369,714 X .9% = 3,327	7,566
Over 75	18,600 X 25% = 4,650*	10,566
Hospital Discharges	58,711 X 5.8% = 3,409	13,965
Inappropriate Placements	2,355 X 32% = 754	14,819

*Adjusted for duplication in over 65 group.

Thus, the hypothetical community would need services for 14,819 individuals. Starting with the group in greatest need and moving forward, planners could reasonably consider the expansion of homecare services.

Another consensus pattern for continuing care was identified by Hamill and Ryan (1985). They found that the best predictors of future need were the following data items: descriptors of functional status; living arrangements in the community; family and other supports; number of times in the hospital in the past 12 months; and prior use of community services. These predictor data items were quite similar to those enumerated by an earlier GAO report (1977, 124).

When considering consensus, the opposite poles of need and demand arise. Demand may be based upon expressed wishes of the population for a particular service. A recent survey indicated that 68 percent of consumers agree that "hospitals should provide health care services to the elderly in their homes" (Inguanzo and Harju 1985). Need commonly uses concepts of determinations using data and professional expertise. Consumers may be unaware of needs and therefore the demand could be nonexistent. On the other hand, consumers could reject the expressed needs as seen by the professionals.

Another factor under the veneer of humane civility is the feelings of family members called upon to render care. One study (Sharma 1980) identified the following three reasons for families not to accept the patient home again, regardless of whether more extensive homecare services were available:

- They had already cared for the patient at home as long as they were able.

- Family caregivers themselves were too old and chronically ill to provide the necessary physical care.

- Adult children had been burdened with the care of their patients throughout their adult lives and now, at age 67 or 70, felt they deserved some freedom to enjoy life before they, too, became debilitated.

Availability of homecare services alone cannot resolve the need/demand dilemma. Accurate, reliable needs assessment measures can supply the data but not the changes in attitude to go along with the programs.

Hospital-based Need Determinations

With DRGs spurring hospitals, the facilities have stressed discharge planning and screening to determine the need for aftercare in the community. While there can be no denying of the economical motive behind the move, it is clear that the hospital requires an ability to determine needs. Consideration is given to care at home including follow-up care, rehabilitation, terminal care, and maintenance care.

Berry (1980) reported on projecting demand for home health care among more than 2,600 patients discharged from medical and surgical services over a five-month period. A nurse screened the patients for appropriate homecare. For the most part, her judgments agreed with the staff of the hospital's homecare service. Only patients meeting the following nine criteria were assessed as proper referrals to homecare:

1. The patient is homebound, nonambulatory, or has many medical problems.

2. The patient requires more professional care than can be rendered in outpatient clinic visits.

3. The patient has a caregiver at home who is available when needed.

4. The caregiver is willing to be of assistance.

5. The patient's physical home environment is such that daily care can be rendered.

6. The patient and caregiver require instruction and support to sustain the patient at home.

7. The patient's and caregiver's behavior and emotional status are stable.

8. The patient's use of alcohol and/or illicit drugs does not interfere with his/her ability to function.

9. The patient will do better with homecare than with other options for post-hospital care.

Comparisons of nurse and homecare staff referrals showed that the neurology service tended to over-refer. Other services, especially general surgery, neurosurgery, and rehabilitative medicine, tended to under-refer.

Data from another hospital need assessment study (Inui, Stevenson, Plorde, et al. 1980) revealed a substantial unmet need for homecare services. "By study estimates, 64 percent of the patients who qualify do not receive services. This percentage is a minimum estimate of unmet need."

If facilities are discharging patients "quicker and sicker" under DRGs, need assessment techniques may merely reflect the economic incentive above all other criteria and/or factors.

Need Determination by Attending Physicians

Physicians evaluate their patients and decide on whether or not to discharge them. In the past, patients were allowed to stay a day or two more if there was no readily available community placement or for extra rest--a social stay (Department of Health, Education and Welfare 1978, 81). Now, with the cost containment emphasis, the social stay is open to severe criticism as well as causing economic loss to the hospital.

Early identification of post-hospital needs is the watchword for the attending physician. Inui et al. (1981) describe the application of a simple and objective clinical index found to be useful for such purposes. Patients are evaluated within 48 hours of admission to discover those who require discharge planning to arrange for special care. A CAAST method (Glass and Weiner 1976) rates a patient in five areas and correlates each area with a disposition difficulty rating:

Continence -- fully continent/ incontinent for two days to one month/ incontinent for more than one month;

Ambulation -- fully ambulatory/ unable to move independently more than 20 feet two days to one month/ unable for more than one month;

Age -- younger than 65/ 65-79/ older than 79;

Social background -- admitted from home and likely to return home/ admitted from an extended care facility (ECF) and likely to return to the same ECF/ admitted from home and likely to be discharged to an ECF/ admitted from one ECF and likely to be discharged to another; and

Thought processes -- fully oriented/ disoriented for more than one month.

Each of the items in the CAAST index is scored from 0 to 2, based on severity and weighted for chronicity. When the total score for the patient is added, a higher score indicates a higher degree of difficulty with posthospital arrangements.

Screening nurses using the CAAST technique were able to pinpoint at least 63 percent of the patients who later required special arrangements at discharge. Those patients were identified during the first two days of their hospital stay.

This technique for need determination is reiterated from a family physician viewpoint by Ham (1980) and is similar to CAAST. However, Ham believes that social assessment is often overlooked by the physician. This includes an evaluation of the patient's home situation, the help available if the patient becomes ill (or requires urgent aid), the patient's social life, hobbies, access to transportation, financial status, and the patient's feelings about living at home. Because many physicians do not know about community services, Ham includes a "laundry list" of things such as meals-on-wheels, congregate housing, home health aides, and day hospitals.

Physicians, nurses, social workers, discharge planners, and others involved in the referral process also use their anecdotal experiences to document the need for homecare. Sometimes, the information is collected during interviews and translated into a needs assessment technique with numbers projected on to a total population. Obviously, the method could be biased based upon the subjective analysis by those contributing the anecdotal material.

Patient Assessment/Classification for Need Determination

Related to the individual physician's evaluation are the methods of individual patient assessment/classification techniques for continuing and long-term care. These methods collect data at admission that is predictive of post-hospital needs. During hospitalization, the information is given to patients, family and staff to make post-hospital decisions. At discharge, information is shared to help meet post-hospital needs (Hamill and Ryan 1985). A computer-assisted assessment procedure (Lloyd, Bowling, and Kozlowski 1985) analyzes 20 sociodemographic items, 13 medical status factors, 14 functioning status items, and 7 service-related variables. All that data is translated into service needs and eventually into physician orders for follow-up care.

Eisenberg and Amerman (1985) believe that the use of assessment instruments results in the likelihood that all relevant variables are fed into the decision; that a common language is produced for professional use; that potential assessor bias is reduced; and that a basis for problem identification and care planning is established. They review four assessment instruments: In-Home Assessment (IHA) of the Philadelphia Corporation for the Aging; Social Adjustment Assessment Form (SAAF) of the Philadelphia Geriatric Center; Baseline Assessment Instrument (BAI) of Mathematica Policy Research; and the Pre-Admission Assessment Form (PAAF) of the Temple University Institution on Aging. Five commonalities emerge in all the assessment instruments: all collect multidimensional data; all emphasize current functioning and prognosis; all are designed to record data from the patient but use a proxy if needed; all are administered by social workers;

and all take 50 minutes to one hour to complete the interview. In their review of the assessment instruments, the authors also commented on the importance of the order of the content, the need to be terse and to the point in the questions, the design for synthesis of the data, and the page format and physical size of the instrument.

Morris, Sherwood, and Mor (1984) detailed the use of the HRCA Vulnerability Index for use in identifying functionally vulnerable people in the community. Developed by the Hebrew Rehabilitation Center for the Aged in Boston, key measures of mobility, personal and instrumental ADL, orientation and activities are addressed. Data comes from self-reporting or from a proxy respondent. This instrument provides "a logical and clinically validated system for simultaneously weighing a complex set of functional deficits and determining whether a person is or is not restricted."

Specific patient classification systems for home health care patients have been developed by Hardy (1984), Harris, Santoferraro and Silva (1985), and Buchanan (1985). All seek to discover functioning ability of the patients and to classify individuals based on their dependency requirements.

Inappropriate Placements in Need Calculations

A number of studies reveal a long history of inappropriate placement of individuals in institutional settings. People end up in facilities because they have no family, because they are waiting to be transferred elsewhere, or for a so-called social stay. Tidewater Regional Health Planning Council (1974) in Norfolk, Virginia, surveyed and studied home health care services; Beattie and Jordan (1975) reported on hospitalized patients in Massachusetts who were ready for discharge but awaiting placements; a Massachusetts Department of Public Health (1975) study looked at discharge summaries of home health agency clients; Malafronte, Moses, Bronson, et al. (1977) looked at appropriateness of long-term care placement in the New Jersey Medicaid program. Exhibit 4-3 shows the assessment form service checklist used by the evaluation team of a physician, nurse and social worker to indicate the help required to allow the patient to live in the community.

Medicaid assessment procedures for long-term care were listed as one of three causes of avoidable admissions in Congressional hearings (House Subcommittee on Health and the Environment 1980). Testifying for the GAO, Harry S. Havens stated that Medicaid's ". . . present system of financing and delivering long-term care creates strong incentives to use nursing care services." Exhibit 4-4 graphically presents the institutional bias of Medicaid procedures. Havens further noted that most chronically impaired elderly were placed in a nursing home without comprehensive needs assessment. While the physician alone was the typical professional to examine the individual, it was noted that the medical exam was not sufficient for a deter-

Exhibit 4-3 Service Checklist in Assessment Form

If the patient could be maintained in a non-institutional setting, the team's judgement is requested about the patient's service needs in two categories: (1) licensed nursing and (2) homemaker/home health aid services.

Please check the specific services and amount of time these services would be required in an alternative care setting.

LICENSED NURSING SERVICES

Hours per day _____
Hours per night _____
Times per week _____
Other (explain) _____

__ Assessment of total needs at intervals
__ Supervision of home health aide
__ Ambulatory/transfer teaching
__ Catherization/Catheter Care
__ Colostomy care
__ Change dressings
__ Determination of fluid balance
__ Diet Management
__ Enemas
__ Exercises (not phys. therapy)
__ Follow-up of special therapies
__ Fracture care
__ IPPB
__ Irrigations (lesions, etc.)
__ Monitor vital signs (TPR)
__ Preventive health instruction
__ Prothesis assistance
__ Special mouth care
__ Special skin care
__ Supervise & administer medications
__ Utilize suction machine
__ Other (Specify)

HOMEMAKER/HOME HEALTH AIDE SERVICES

Hours per day _____
Hours per night _____
Times per week _____
Other (explain) _____

__ Assist with ambulation
__ Assist with appliances incl. wheelchairs, binders, walkers, etc.
__ Assist with colostomy care
__ Assist with enemas
__ Assist in & out of bed
__ Assist with medications
__ Assist with prothesis
__ Baths
__ Care of catheters
__ Change dressings
__ Clean room
__ Exercises
__ Laundry
__ Meal preparation
__ Measure intake and output
__ Personal care and grooming
__ Shop
__ Washing lacerations
__ Other (specify)

If transfer to a non-institutional setting is practical, the team's judgement is requested about patient's needs in two categories: (1) therapeutic services and (2) support services.

Please check those services which would be needed.

THERAPEUTIC SERVICES

__ Physical Therapy
__ Speech Therapy
__ Psycho/Social Counseling
__ Occupational Therapy
__ Other (specify)

SUPPORT SERVICES

__ Food Services, i.e. Congregate Dining, Meals on Wheels
__ Transportation Services
__ Telephone Reassurance and Check Services
__ Special Program Services, i.e. Alcoholic and Drug Counseling (please specify)

Source: Malafronte, D., et al. 1977. *Appropriateness of Long-Term Care Placement.* East Orange, NJ: Urban Health Institute, Inc., appendix.
* Evaluation team consisted of physician, nurse, and social worker.

Exhibit 4-4 Medicaid Subsidizes Nursing Homecare for Individuals Ineligible for Community-based Coverage

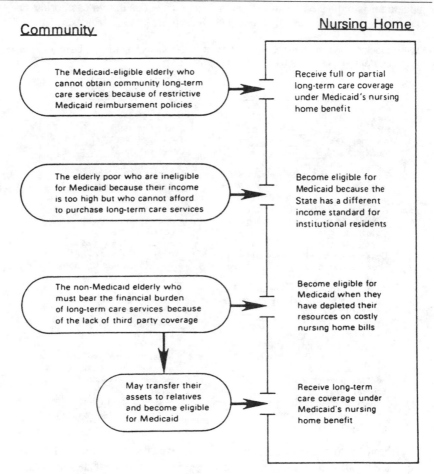

* After entering a nursing home, many elderly can never return to the community because they have depleted their financial resources and severed their community ties.

Source: General Accounting Office. Nov. 26, 1979. *Entering a Nursing Home. Costly Implications for Medicaid and the Elderly.* Washington, DC: Government Printing Office. PAD 80-12, p. 31.

mination of the patient's needs. According to Havens, Medicaid's assessment procedures were inadequate in preventing avoidable institutionalization because:

- Most of the reviews occur after admission when it is difficult to discharge the resident to the community.

- The two preadmission reviews focus primarily on medical conditions and do not include information on other factors that are critical in determining whether an institutional or community setting is the most suitable placement.

In addition to the institutional bias of some funding and/or reimbursement agencies, critics argue that the medical education system also stresses institutional care. Physicians are taught that the hospital is the choice when patients need care. However, with increasing high technology services being delivered at home and the intensive efforts of hospital management to reduce length of stay, coupled with saturation marketing campaigns by homecare organizations, that bias may change.

Resource Allocation for Homecare

Following investigations of the need for homecare services, an allocation process usually ensues. Since the allocation also involves a priority scheme, the importance of accurate data and determinations is obvious. A Canadian report (Shapiro 1980) used available data to show that 70 percent of those served by the homecare program were elderly. Acting on that information, the resources were allocated to that group first. Choices were limited by the data presented and did not use wider population-based needs assessment approaches. "Decentralized health service delivery responsive to the needs of local populations implies allocating program funds to regions on the basis of predetermined criteria that can facilitate effective planning and budgeting." This concept aptly conveys the sense of needs assessment methods and techniques.

Wolock et al. (1985) studied the post-hospital needs of patients in several New Jersey facilities. Studies of this nature contribute to resource allocation procedures because they reveal needed, concrete services. This particular investigation concentrated on the importance of discharge planning. About 70 patients were interviewed 6 to 11 months after leaving the hospital. Around 64 percent had ADL limitations; 43 percent had problems getting around outside the house; and 42 percent had problems doing things in the house, such as meal preparation and washing dishes. Sixty-five percent went home and 20 percent went to live with a relative. After 6 to 11 months, 85 percent were still on medication; 90 percent had special diets; and 29 percent still needed injections and bandages changed. Services required at that time included nursing (39 percent), medical (20 percent), homemaker (17 percent), and meals (17 percent). Almost 50 percent received from 1 to 4 services.

In a first step toward quantification, Revenson and Bell (1985) looked at homecare consumers, providers, and services in New York City. In terms of resource allocation, this study documented the fact that the number of nonprofit home health care agencies had declined; as of January 1984, there were 34 certified home health agencies in New York City. This took place in the face of Health System Agency of N.Y. estimates that 21,591 to 42,999 people will need homecare in 1990, up 96 percent; and New York State Health Planning Commission estimates that 532,352 people statewide will need homecare in 1990, up 108 percent. Again, resource allocation experts often respond to estimates of that nature in making determinations.

Responding to legislation in New York State proposing a home health care need methodology, Pettey (1985) argued for the Home Health Services and Staffing Association against the technique. This legislation projected the need for home health agencies based on the 1984 caseload of currently certified agencies. Acknowledging the growth in demand for the services of home health agencies, Pettey recommended methodological changes in need determination. She asked that a medical and health practice indicator be included; that agency growth be capped at the 1985 level; and urged a decrease in standard agency sizes to those included in early drafts of the regulations. The New York State Health Department will publish projections specifying the need for certified home health agencies and for long-term home health care programs (*Health Planner* 1984).

Staffing is also a vital part of resource allocation and Ballard (1985) discusses assessment of staffing needs in homecare. Almost 400 records were reviewed retrospectively from nine Connecticut homecare agencies employing from 3.2 FTEs to 28.2 FTEs. A Health Status Scale (HSS) was used for the record review. Following are the formulas that emerged for nursing and agency services:

$$\text{nursing service} = \frac{\text{total of nursing visits}}{\text{length of stay}}$$

$$\text{agency service} = \frac{\text{all agency visits by PT/OT/ST/SW/HHA}}{\text{length of stay}}$$

Agency visits explained 26 percent of services to cancer patients and 11 percent for cardiac patients, compared to 8 percent for both for nursing visits.

To reinforce the importance of need assessment and resource allocation, Exhibit 4-5 illustrates the scope of only the Medicare program home visits from 1969 to 1984, more than 40 million visits in that year. Furthermore, Exhibit 4-6 indicates that more than one out of every five persons

Exhibit 4-5 Trends in Home Health Care Visits under Medicare, Selected Years, 1969-1984

Year	Number (in millions)	Percent Change
1969	8.5	-
1971	4.8	-20.5%
1974	8.2	29.3
1978	17.3	10.8
1982	30.8	17.6
1983	36.8	19.4
1984	40.3	9.5

Annual Percent Increase

1975 - 1983	16.9%
1983 - 1984	7.7

Sources: Department of Health and Human Services. Health Care Financing Administration. *Medicare: use of home health services, 1980*. HCFA Pub. No. 03158, Sept. 1983, p. 6.

_____. *Health Care Spending. Bulletin 85,* December 19, 1985.

_____. Division of Program Studies. Office of Research. Unpublished data, March 5, 1986.

more, Exhibit 4-6 indicates that more than one out of every five persons receives 100 or more visits per year. If the group receiving 50-99 visits per year is added in, more than 50 percent of the beneficiaries get more than 50 visits per year.

Surely, the weight of the numbers alone indicates the tremendous attention that should be paid to calculations of reliable need assessment determinations.

Reasoned Needs Determination

An advertisement in a health care journal asked *"Who* Needs Home Health Care?" and the ad responded, *"Your* Patients Do." Then the ad proceeded to sell the services of a health care management consultant firm without attention to whether or not a need exists, as that is taken for granted by all

Exhibit 4-6 Medicare Persons Served by Number of Home Visits and Visits per Beneficiary, 1984

Number Visits	Persons Served			Visits		
	Number (thousands)	Percent		Number (thousands)	Percent	Per Beneficiary
1-9	575	38.0		2,716	6.7	4.7
10-19	345	22.8		4,811	11.9	13.9
20-29	187	12.3		4,505	11.2	24.1
30-39	113	7.4		3,840	9.5	34.0
40-49	74	4.9		3,253	8.1	44.0
50-99	149	9.8		10,214	25.3	68.6
100 and over	73	4.8		10,998	27.3	150.7
Total	1,516	100.0*		40,337	100.0*	26.6

* Do not add exactly because of rounding.

Source: Department of Health and Human Services. Division of Program Studies. Office of Research. Unpublished data, March 5, 1986.

concerned. However, need assessment is not purely a business for profit approach.

Variables, and methods, and techniques of using those variables exist. A number of formulas can be used; retrospective analysis is useful, as are anecdotal and patient assessment techniques. Nevertheless, these are only tools and dependence can lead to the "tyranny of the tool" (Eisenberg and Amerman 1985). Need assessment and resource allocation tasks require sound judgment by reasoned professionals, consumers, and community leaders.

References

Baker, M. 1980. *A selective review of client assessment tools in long-term care of older people.* Waltham, MA: Brandeis University, Heller School (Oct.).

Ballard, S. 1985. Assessing staffing needs in homecare. *Caring* 4 (3) :58

Beattie, R.T., and H.S. Jordan 1975. *Preliminary analysis of a survey of Massachusetts hospital patients who were ready for discharge and awaiting placement in other facilities on March 20, 1975.* Springfield, VA: National Technical Information Service.

Berry, N.J. 1980. Projecting demand for home health care in one health service area. *Home Health Review* 3:23-27.

Brickner, P.W. 1973. Finding the unreached patient. *Journal of the American Medical Association* 225:1645 (24 Sept.).

Buchanan, B.F. 1985. A classification system for home health care patients by functional status measures. Presentation at annual meeting of American Public Health Association. Washington, DC (Nov.).

Department of Health, Education and Welfare. 1977. *Home health care. Report on the regional public hearings. Sept. 20-Oct. 1, 1976.* Washington, DC: Government Printing Office. Pub. No. 76-135.

Department of Health, Education and Welfare. Federal Council on Aging. 1978. *Public policy and the frail elderly.* Washington, DC: Government Printing Office. Pub. No. ORDS 79-20959 (Dec.).

Department of Health and Human Services. 1981a. National Center for Health Statistics. *Current estimates from the National Health Interview Survey: U.S. 1980.* Washington, DC: Government Printing Office. Pub. No. (PHS) 82-1567, Series 10, No. 139 (Dec.).

Department of Health and Human Services. 1981b. Federal Council on Aging. *The need for long term care. Information and issues.* Washington, DC: Government Printing Office. Pub. No. ORDS 81-20704.

Eisenberg, D.M., and E. Amerman. 1985. Structural assessment for long term care. *Pride Institute Journal* 4 (4):3-13 (Fall).

Fortinsky, R.H., C.V. Granger, and G.B. Seltzer. 1981. The use of functional assessment in understanding homecare needs. *Medical Care* 19:489-497.

General Accounting Office. 1977. *Home health--the need for a national policy to better provide for the elderly.* Washington, DC: Government Printing Office. Pub. No. HRD 78-19, 124 (30 Dec.).

General Accounting Office. 1979. *Entering a nursing home. Costly implications for Medicaid and the elderly.* Washington, DC: Government Printing Office. Pub. No. PAD 80-12 (26 Nov.).

Glass, R., and M. Weiner. 1976. Seeking a social disposition for the medical patient: CAAST, a simple and objective clinical index. *Medical Care* 14:637-641.

Griff, S.L. 1984. Determining the need for home health services. *Caring* 3 (7) :15-19.

Ham, R. 1980. Alternatives to institutionalization. *American Family Physician* 22 (1) :95-100.

Hamill, C.M., and M.A. Ryan. 1985. Continuing care assessment in the acute setting. *PRIDE Institute Journal* 4 (4) :21-25 (Fall).

Hardy, J.A. 1984. A patient classification system for home health patients. *Caring* 3 (8) :26-27.

Harris, M.D., C. Santoferraro, and S. Silva. 1985. A patient classification system in home health care. *Nursing Economics* 3:276-282.

Health Planner. New York State Health Department. 1984. Home care methodology under way. 7 (4) :2.

Hospitals. 1984. Five million Americans require home health care: Government study. 58 (5) :38, 41.

House Select Committee on Aging. 1985. *Building a long-term care policy: homecare data and implications.* Washington, DC: Government Printing Office. Comm. Pub. No. 98-484.

House Subcommittee on Health and the Environment. 1980. *Community-based long-term care: Obstacles and oppor-*

tunities. Washington, DC: Government Printing Office. Serial No. 96-80.

Inguanzo, J.M., and M. Harju. 1985. Affluent consumers most discriminating: Survey. *Hospitals* 59 (19) :84,86.

Inui, T.S., K.M. Stevenson, D. Plorde, et al. 1980. Needs assessment in hospital-based homecare services. *Research in Nursing and Health* 3 (3) :101-106.

Inui, T.S., K.M. Stevenson, D. Plorde, et al. 1981. Identifying hospital patients who need early discharge planning for special dispositions: a comparison of alternative techniques. *Medical Care* 19:922-929.

Lemon, G.M., and L. Welches. 1967. Assessment of welfare clients to determine need for home health aides. *Public Health Reports* 82:729-734.

Liu, K., and K.G. Manton. 1985. Disability and long-term care. Presentation at Methodologies of Forecasting Life and Active Life Expectancy Workshop, Bethesda, Maryland (25 June).

Liu, K., K.G. Manton, and B.M. Liu. Winter 1985. Homecare expenses for disabled elderly. *Health Care Financing Review* 7 (2) :51-58.

Lloyd, E., C. Bowling, and B. Kozlowski. 1985. The Virginia long-term care information system. *Pride Institute Journal of Long Term Health Care* 4 (4) :14-20.

Lundberg, C.J. 1984. Appendix: Formula - based models for projecting home care need. *Topics in Health Care Financing* 10 (3) :88-89.

Malafronte, D., H.H. Moses, R.M. Bronson, et al. 1977. *Appropriateness of long-term care placement.* East Orange, NJ: Urban Health Institute.

Massachusetts Department of Public Health. 1975. Clients of home health agencies. *New England Journal of Medicine* 293:1261.

Morris, J.N., S. Sherwood, and V. Mor. 1984. An assessment tool for use in identifying functionally vulnerable persons in the community. *The Gerontologist* 24 (4) :373-379.

O'Shaughnessy, C., R. Price, and J. Griffith.

1985. *Financing and delivery of long-term care services for the elderly.* Washington, DC: Congressional Research Service, Library of Congress. Pub. No. 85-1033 EPW (17 Oct.).

Pear, R. 1986. *Many nursing homes are found to fail minimum U.S. standards.* New York Times (21 May).

Pettey, S.M. 1985. Letter to New York Assemblyman J. Tallon. Washington, DC: Home Health Services and Staffing Association.

Revenson, T., and D.B. Bell. 1985. *Homecare consumers, providers and services: A first step toward quantification.* New York: United Hospital Fund.

Sager, A. 1979. *Learning the homecare needs of the elderly: Patient, family and professional views of an alternative to institutionalization.* Waltham, MA: Brandeis University, Heller School.

Shapiro, E. 1980. Resource allocations for homecare. An experiment. *American Journal of Public Health* 70:77-78.

Sharma, R.K. 1980. Forecasting need and demand for home health care: a selective review. *Public Health Reports* 95:572-579.

Tidewater Regional Health Planning Council, Inc. 1974. *Home health care services survey and study.* Norfolk, VA (June).

Trager, B. 1972. *Home health services in the U.S. A report to the Senate Special Committee on Aging.* Washington, DC: Government Printing Office (April).

Warhola, C.F.R. 1980. *Planning for home health services. A resource handbook.* Washington, DC: Government Printing Office. Pub. No. HRA 80-14017 (Aug.).

Weissert, W.G. 1985. Estimating the long-term care population: Prevalence rates and selected characteristics. *Health Care Financing Review* 6 (4) :83-91.

Wolock, I., E. Schlesinger, M. Dinerman, et al. 1985. *The post-hospital needs of patients: A follow-up study.* Presentation at annual meeting of the American Public Health Association, Washington, DC.

Chapter 5

Long-Term Care, Homecare, and the Elderly

Usually, the word "homecare" is immediately associated with the old or elderly. In fact, the elderly do constitute an overwhelming portion of the population requiring long-term care and homecare. It is estimated that 40 percent of the federal budget for such care is spent on the 11 percent of the public over the age of 65 (Adams 1980). Even though homecare and long-term care is not the exclusive domain of the elderly, the group does have special issues that warrant special consideration.

Toward a Better Understanding of the Issues

Dr. Robert N. Butler (1981a, xv) outlined five imperatives leading to a better understanding of the health and social status of the elderly in America. "Imperative," implying a need for action, applies to the following:

Attitudes/Culture - Americans tend to deny their own vulnerability and realization of their own aging. Connections between present and future self need to be implanted in attitudes and culture.

Cost - Society must be aware that care for older people costs more because of the volume of services as well as the use of high technology.

Scientific research - Much needs to be learned about the natural process of aging.

Epidemiology - Interactions between the environment and genetics have a direct relation to the incidence of disease and old age; investigation is needed.

Demographics - There are simply more and more people living into old and very old age, thereby changing patterns of work, retirement, and leisure.

Combining the five imperatives into a gestalt, Dr. Butler calls them the base for a new medicine. He defines gerontology as "the discovery and application of new knowledge regarding the biologic, psychologic, and social aspects of aging" (Butler 1981a,xv).

Facts and Figures

An extensive body of literature exists on the elderly and their specific needs.

In an intensive 400+ page volume, Shanas (1982) reported on a national survey of the aged. She defined who the aged are, along with their health status and their attitudes toward health. In addition, there were details about health and welfare services for the family, family structure, living arrangements, family social contacts, isolation in old age, work, retirement, and financial resources of the elderly.

Waldo and Lazenby (1984) comprehensively review the demographic characteristics, health care use, and expenditures by the aged in the U.S. from 1977 to 1984. Areas covered include life expectancy, death rates, employment status, type of work, income, self-assessed health status, hospital discharges by diagnosis, personal health care expenditures, Medicare utilization, use of home health services, health care coverage, private insurance, and the Veterans Administration's elderly beneficiaries. These authors conclude that the aged use more health services in general and, specifically, more hospital and nursing homecare than the rest of the population: "Without changes in the reimbursement practices or coverage, the ability of government programs to finance this increased demand will be diminished greatly."

Doty et al. (1985) presented an overview of long-term care highlighting the growth in the aged population, with divisions from 65-74, 75-84, and those over 85 years of age. Projections indicate that from 1990-2010, the 85+ group will increase three to four times faster than the general population. In addition there was an analysis of helpers and helper days, a projection of the volume and source of assistance, a recording of nursing home expenditures and Medicare expenditures for skilled nursing facilities, home health care and long-term care.

As part of a series on aging in the eighties, Kovar (1986a) reviewed data from the National Health Interview Survey. This material included demographics regarding race, marital status, family size, education, and residential arrangements. Respondents gave opinions about their own health and activity limitations and use of health care. Another in the series (Kovar 1986b) looked at contacts with family, friends, and neighbors by the aged. Data addressed living arrangements, visits by children, social contacts, and health impacts. "The evidence from these preliminary data is that many of the people who had a 65th birthday and were living alone did see, or at least talk with, family frequently. They were not alienated and without social contacts" (Kovar 1986b).

Rice (1985) covered the health care needs of the elderly with attention to mortality, morbidity, life expectancy, health status, use and expenditures for medical care, activity limitations, and projections for those limitations into 2040. She concluded, "Assuming that current utilization patterns will continue, the number of hospital days, nursing home residents, physician visits, and corresponding health expenditures will need to increase to meet the needs of the elderly" (Rice, 63).

A report from the Senate Special Committee on Aging (1985) described health status and health services utilization in an aging America. Topics included how older people view their health, disability, chronic illness, mental health, death rates, causes of death, community health services, nursing homes, use of health services, and health care expenditures.

In a special issue, the Milbank Memorial Fund Quarterly's *Health and Society* (Suzman and Riley 1985) concentrated on the "oldest old," those 85 and older. Nine articles explored the demographics, the political and social importance, the search for adequate statistical data, new concepts regarding aging and disease, who is to pay for the care, and the potential changes in social and public policy.

In graphic form, the American Association of Retired Persons (1985a) details a profile of older Americans. Data is given about population trends, marital status, living arrangements, racial and ethnic composition, geographic distribution by state, income, poverty, housing, employment, education, health and health care, and functional assistance needs.

To put the narrative into illustrative form, Exhibits 5-1 to 5-5 present

Exhibit 5-1 U.S. Population (in millions) All Ages and 65 Years and Over Selected Years 1900-2000

Year	All Ages	65+ Population							
		Total	%	65 - 74	%	75 - 84	%	85+	%
				Total %		Total %		Total %	
1900	76.3	3.1	4.0%	2.2	2.9%	772,000	1.0%	123,000	0.2%
1920	105.7	4.9	4.7	3.5	3.3	1.3	1.2	210,000	0.2
1940	131.7	9.0	6.8	6.4	4.8	2.3	1.7	365,000	0.3
1960	179.3	16.6	9.2	11.0	6.1	4.6	2.6	929,000	0.5
1980	226.5	25.5	11.3	15.6	6.9	7.7	3.4	2.2	1.0
1990	249.7	31.8	12.7	18.1	7.2	10.3	4.1	3.5	1.4
2000	268.0	35.0	13.1	17.7	6.6	12.2	4.6	5.1	1.9

Source: Bureau of the Census. 1983. *America in transition: an aging society*. Washington, DC: Government Printing Office. Series, P-23, No. 128.

Exhibit 5-2 Living Arrangements of Persons 65 and Over, by Sex, 1984.

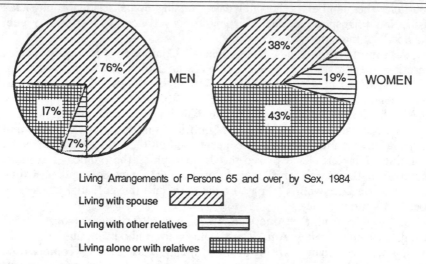

MEN

WOMEN

Living Arrangements of Persons 65 and over, by Sex, 1984

Living with spouse

Living with other relatives

Living alone or with relatives

Source: American Association of Retired Persons. 1985. *A profile of older Americans.* Washington, D.C.

Exhibit 5-3 Number of Persons Who Need Homecare per 1,000 Adults 45 Years and Over, by Type of Measure and Age, U.S., 1979 - 1980.

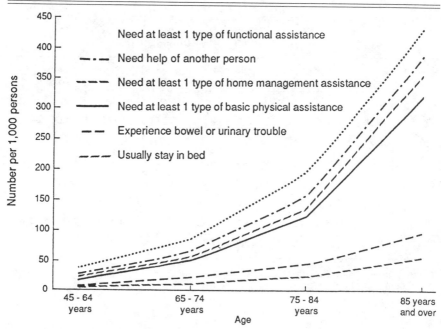

Source: Feller, B.A. 1986. *Americans needing homecare.* Washington, D.C. Government Printing Office. Pub. No. (PHS) 86-1581.

Exhibit 5-4 People Needing Assistance with ADL or IADL Activities by Percentage of Age Group.

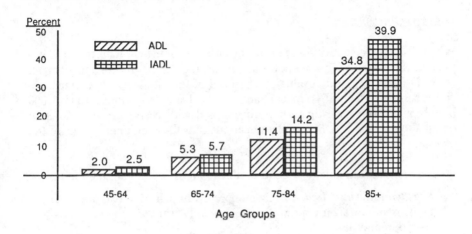

Source: Department of Health and Human Services. National Center for Health Statistics. 1983. *Americans needing help to function at home.* Washington, DC: Government Printing Office. Pub. No. (PHS) 83-1250. No. 92 (14 Sept.)

Exhibit 5-5 Americans 65 and Older in Need of Long-term Care By Nursing Home or Community Care, 1980 - 2040.

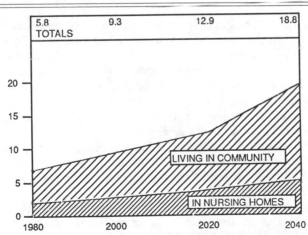

Source: Senate Select Committee on Aging. 1985. *Developments in aging:* 1984 Volume 1. Washington, DC: Government Printing Office. Report No. 99-5, p. 189 (18 Feb.)

data on the population age distribution, living arrangements, disability limitations, and nursing home and long-term care needs.

Impairment Status

When disability or activity limitations are used in statistical material, it is important that there be a common base regarding the degree of impairment. A GAO (1981,12) study evaluated the level of functioning in five areas: social, economic, mental, physical, and ADL. Data from more than 1,000 people in a prior investigation were coupled with responses to a 22-item detailed questionnaire. Seven classifications of well-being emerged from the analysis.

Unimpaired--Excellent or good in all five areas of human functioning.

Slightly/Mildly impaired--Mildly/moderately impaired in two areas or mildly/moderately impaired in one area and severely/completely impaired in another.

Moderately impaired--Mildly/moderately impaired in three areas and/or mildly/moderately impaired in two and severely/completely impaired in one.

Generally impaired--Mildly/moderately impaired in four areas.

Greatly impaired - Mildly/moderately impaired in three areas and severely/completely impaired in another.

Extremely impaired - Mildly/moderately impaired in all five areas.

There is a direct relationship between the level of impairment, the services required, and the ability to live outside of an institution. Exhibit 5-6 indicates the services required at each impairment level, with the less impaired most frequently using transportation, social/recreational, and periodic monitoring. At all impairment levels, family and friends provide more services than agencies, particularly at the greater impairment levels.

To understand the homecare needs of the elderly, Fortinsky, Granger, and Seltzer (1981) used a functional assessment technique. A modified Barthel Index measured dressing, grooming, mobility, toileting, and eating abilities. Researchers concluded that the mathematical index could be used as a screening device for potential homecare clients, as well as for allocating staff time.

A multivariate analysis was used by Greenberg and Ginn (1979) to judge impairment and subsequent home or institution placement of elderly patients. Feeding decision factors from the literature into the statistical analysis, they found the following variables linked to choices: ability to take

Exhibit 5-6 Homecare Services Required at Various Impairment Levels

Service	Unimpaired	Slightly	Mildly	Moderately	Generally	Extremely
Transportation	X	X	X	X	X	X
Monitoring	X	X	X	X	X	X
Social/recreational	X	X	X	X	X	X
Homemaker			X	X	X	X
Housing			X	X	X	X
Administrative/legal				X	X	X
Meal preparation				X	X	X
Food, groceries				X	X	X
Personal care						X
Continuous supervision						X
Nursing Care						X

Source: General Accounting Office. 1977. *Home health-the need for a national policy to better provide for the elderly.* Pub. No. HRD 78-19, p. 15 (30 Dec.).

medication; the index of ADL; client preferences; the index of medical condition; and family preferences. Applying the predictor model to a sample of people at home and in an institution, they found that 92 percent of the group was properly placed.

Semantics

Words used to describe the elderly create images that reflect how society feels about old people. Euphemistic terms such as Senior Citizens, Golden Agers, and Seniors do not disguise the fact that society may want to keep them "out of sight and out of mind." Blum and Minkler (1980) label the mechanism that achieves that effect for society a "bureaucracy of care." A historian on aging calls the condition an increasing sense of "Gerontophobia" (Fischer 1978).

An early use of the term "geriatric medicine" appeared in a textbook entitled *Geriatrics*, by Ignatz Nascher (1914). While the tone of the book was said to be slightly negative, Nascher did urge physicians to take an interest in the elderly. "Geriatric triage" was created by Dr. Isadore Rossman (1980) to indicate that the service level selected was appropriate to the individual cases. Two contemporary titles conjure up dismal images: Dr. Butler's (1975) Pulitzer prize-winning book, *Why Survive? Being Old in America*, and the chilling expose by Moss and Halamandaris (1977), *Too Old. Too Sick. Too Bad*. Both volumes illustrate attitudinal and cultural stances that classify the elderly as deviant and exploited in society simply because they are old. Dr. Butler was also given credit for coining the word "ageism" to indicate discrimination.

Health Care or Social Care?

Distinctions between health care and social/personal care have long plagued efforts to meet the needs of the elderly. Callahan (1981) noted that problems of "aging" need to be differentiated from "long-term care," referring to nonmedical problems such as work, income, loss of spouse and friends contrasted with physical and/or mental services. Americans use medical approaches to resolve an array of social needs in long term care, according to the Kanes (1980). In a progress report on key long-term care issues, the Federal Council on Aging (Department of Health and Human Services 1979,37) stated, "Long-term care is, to a large extent, a problem of living . . . Any consideration of long-term care should start with the perception that there are many people who cannot be cured in a physical sense but who require care."

For a variety of reasons, not the least of which is economic, there has been a reluctance to merge health and social services into a unified whole.

In homecare, Fortinsky, Granger, and Seltzer (1981) argue for "an emphasis on care rather than cure when addressing the needs of potential recipients of long-term home-based services."

Social/Health Maintenance Organizations. In the medical arena, the health maintenance organization (HMO) can coordinate services for the long-term care patient, including homecare. However, the social/personal services are not an integral part of an HMO's operation. Under a federal grant, Brandeis University's Heller School (Diamond and Berman 1981; Leutz, Greenberg, and Abrahams 1985) developed an entity called a Social/Health Maintenance Organization (S/HMO). "S/HMOs are agencies that provide a comprehensive range of long-term care services using management and reimbursement principles developed by HMOs to deal with the fragmentation of services in the community and to avoid unnecessary hospitalization and nursing home care" (U.S. Congress. Office of Technology Assessment 1985,229). In addition, the S/HMO enrolls both disabled and able-bodied elders in membership with prepaid premiums. Furthermore, the S/HMO is "at risk" for service costs and can profit or lose within the allocated budget (Greenberg, Levtz, Ervin, et al. 1985).

Four demonstration S/HMOs have been set up: Elderplan, Inc. at Metropolitan Jewish Geriatric Center in Brooklyn, N.Y.; Medicare Plus II at Kaiser Permanente Medical Care Program in Portland, Oregon; Medicare Partners by the Ebenezer Society in Minneapolis, Minnesota; and SCAN Health Plan, Inc. by the Senior Care Action Network in Long Beach, California (Harrington and Newcomer 1985). At Kaiser's Medicare Plus II plan, the elderly can receive long-term benefits up to $1,000 per month in home or community services above Medicare long-term care benefits for a monthly premium of $40, while Kaiser also gets a capitation rate per enrollee from the Medicare program (ICF, Inc. 1985,33). Arrangements differ at each of the plans, but the general intent is to provide health and social/personal care services under a unified case management system. Elderplan has a monthly premium of $29 with annual benefits of $6,500 in any setting. Medicare Partners also charges $29 a month with up to $6,250 in services yearly in any setting covered. SCAN has a $40 monthly premium and covers benefits up to $7,500 in any setting (Greenberg, Levtz, Ervin, et al. 1985).

In a comprehensive article, Harrington and Newcomer (1985) explained the problems with the traditional long-term care delivery system: access, costs, quality, and continuity of care. Advantages of S/HMOs for consumers, providers, and third-party payers were cited. Consumers would gain access to continuity of care; care systems would be integrated; one agency would meet all needs; institutionalization could be reduced; only one monthly payment would be required; and expanded coverage could most likely be rendered at no additional cost. Providers would have a stable clientele and income, and the freedom to offer a comprehensive range of services. Public payers would be assured of controlling costs and of establishing a system capable of meeting long-term care needs.

Interestingly, despite the apparent advantages for the elderly, many individuals "are unwilling to pay what they perceive to be the 'extra' costs for enrolling in an S/HMO . . . they incorrectly assume that Medicare and Medicare supplemental insurance will cover all their long term care needs" (Newald 1986). In fact, Brooklyn's Elderplan found that the S/HMO had to be sold. Sales people were hired and "senior ambassadors" are paid $5 an hour to promote Elderplan at community meetings (Newald 1986). In addition, there is some disagreement over the cost-saving potential of S/HMOs. Some researchers believe that the S/HMO will reduce the cost of long-term care by substituting home health and nonmedical care services for hospital and nursing homecare. Contrarywise, "the Federal Office of Management and Budget (OMB) disagrees and expects that S/HMOs will raise the cost of long-term care and create a precedent for providing nonmedical services that are not currently covered by Medicare and Medicaid" (Rich 1984a).

Hospice Care. In 1983, hospice care became a covered Medicare benefit. There are nevertheless limitations and issues yet to be resolved. Operating under the best conditions, a hospice program would blend medical and social/personal care services into an integrated activity to individuals diagnosed as terminally ill. Furthermore, services would include the family, and bereavement care would occur after the death of the person covered by Medicare. Care may be rendered at home, at a hospital, or at a hospice facility.

Generally, the problem of aging and long-term care enters into the scope of the "medicalization of aging" (Blum and Minkler 1980). With care of the elderly completely in the medical sphere, the separation of health and social/personal services creates an atmosphere in which independence and self-reliance yield to paternalization for older Americans.

Quality of Life for the Elderly

In a nationally syndicated article in Sunday newspapers, a major story featured the headline, "You Don't Have to Put Your Parents in a Nursing Home" (Robinson 1977). The author talked about ending "one of the ugliest scandals in American life; the consignment to nursing homes of old people who don't want and don't need to be in them." At the conclusion of the article, Dr. Faye G. Abdellah, then Director of the Federal Office of Long Term Care, stated, "No matter how good it is, a nursing home cannot substitute for a home environment."

Quality of care also concerned Dr. Martin Cherkasky (1955), when he wrote: ". . . it is obvious that the hospital is not the natural habitat of human beings . . . and the glamour . . . does not necessarily extend to those who are cared for in it." Even while Dr. Cherkasky cautioned that homecare was not a panacea for all the chronically ill, he did emphasize the potential for homecare in the management of long-term care to control costs while allowing the patient to remain in a personalized, warm and free atmosphere.

Personal Preference for Home. Lifestyle or quality of life is not that easy to measure. The mass media frequently carries stories about people who wish to be allowed to "die with dignity" rather than continue living with the aid of sophisticated machinery. Legal arguments often discuss quality of life for the individual as lawyers argue pro and con about "pulling the plug." Considering the role of the elderly in America, quality of life arguments take on added importance relative to health care needs. A medical educator who was also a hospital administrator commented, "Of primary importance is maintenance of personal lifestyle and social independence. Health goals are secondary and supportive" (Williams 1981,297).

That concept is not difficult to comprehend in view of the direct relationship between behavioral aspects of illness and overt disease itself. Spiegel and Backhaut (1980) cite more than 800 references in their comprehensive review of the interactions between curing and caring. Burnside authored a number of articles on the emotional aspects of caring for the elderly at home. In response to the question, "Why work with the aged?" she comments that the need is great and the gratitude profuse. "Elderly people themselves--wise, humorous, and tough--are the best reasons for choosing to specialize in their care" (Burnside 1980).

Congressman Pepper (House Subcommittee on Health and Long Term Care 1980,2) often quotes his mother: "Son, don't ever let them put me in one of those nursing homes." His mother experienced horror at the thought of being uprooted from her home with the concomitant disruption of her family life.

Noting that many older people are unaware of the availability of homecare, the American Association of Retired Persons (AARP) published *A Handbook about Care in the Home* (1984). In addition to definitions and a checklist for evaluating a home health agency, the booklet contains information about the benefits, the arrangements, community organizations, resources, and simple and inexpensive ways to make a house safe and comfortable. In cooperation with the Federal Trade Commission, the AARP (1985b) also prepared a booklet to help older people choose the homecare option. Material covered is similar, with extra attention given to other choices such as housesharing, congregate housing, and continuing care communities.

As quality of life for the elderly is a direct result of societal influences, the elderly in America have a long way to go. A quote from the classic novel, *Les Miserables* (Hugo 1979,1862,283) reiterates the dismal attitude of society toward the elderly: "The misery of a child is interesting to a mother;

the misery of a young man is interesting to a young woman; the misery of an old man is interesting to nobody."

Public Policies on the Elderly and Long-term Care

A GAO report (1981,26) concluded that "There is no federal program specifically mandated to provide long-term in-home services for the elderly." Each program and every funding source relates to its sole mission: a particular diagnosis; a specific income limitation; a special housing activity. Each program has limitations, restrictions, and a short focal lens.

Currently, public policy on long-term care has three dominant features (Department of Health and Human Services. Federal Council on Aging 1981,75):

1. Medicaid dominates the program and stresses medical and institutional care rather than community-based and support services.

2. None of the federal programs provide for an assessment of the overall needs of persons requiring long-term care, with separate criteria and eligibility required for each distinct program.

3. Community-based services under the Older Americans Act and under Title XX of the Social Security Act have not yet reached the volume level or the specific focus to make a significant impact on long-term care.

A bias toward premature admission of elderly patients to hospitals and nursing homes has been noted in a GAO study (1979,16). That study identified six reasons for the institutional bias (General Accounting Office 1979,64): lack of information about community-based services; difficulty in coordinating outside services; ineligible criteria; no alternatives available; family unable to provide services; and professional biases.

To expand Medicaid benefits, the Low Income Elderly and Disabled Medicaid Amendments of 1986 (S 2492; HR 4882) was introduced by Senator John Heinz and Representative Henry Waxman (McIlrath 1986). Only one-third of the elderly poor receive Medicaid; this legislation would make an additional two million impoverished elderly eligible for benefits. States could choose to either provide the full range of Medicaid benefits not covered by Medicare or to simply pay Medicare premiums, deductibles, and copayments.

Considering the support for community-based long-term care services, it should also be noted that critics contend that homecare and other such services will not substitute for institutional care. In fact, the issue is whether the additional services are "add-ons" to existing services (O'Shaughnessy and Reiss 1983,14). Some speculate that homecare for the elderly merely means replacing a more expensive service with a less costly but more frequent service.

Even if the institutional bias could be changed and the elderly were included in the Medicaid program as well, there would still be major public policy issues to decide relative to alternatives to governmental activities. Alternatives for those elderly not eligible for governmental programs, as well as for buy-ins using governmental monies in the areas of long-term care insurance, life care and continuing care centers and home equity conversions, are not occupying planners.

Long-term Care Insurance. About 50,000 individuals are covered by long-term care insurance policies written by at least 12 companies (Senate Special Committee on Aging 1985,1983). These insurance policies are substantially more comprehensive than standard Medi-Gap policies offering indemnity benefits from three to four years in a licensed nursing care facility. Three features are common to most of these policies: indemnity benefits ranging from $10 to $50 per day; a deductible or reduced benefit for some initial period of time; orientation to a stay in an SNF or care in a facility with a full-time nurse. Note that the policies do not pay the total costs, do not cover more frequent short stays, and frequently exclude homecare. In effect, the policy protects against catastrophic costs. These factors reduce the cost of the policies, but may also reduce their desirability to many persons and their effectiveness in reducing overall costs.

Meiners (1985) compared the policy features of 16 companies offering long-term care insurance for the following coverage: skilled care; intermediate care; custodial care; homecare; indemnity benefit; length of coverage; pre-existing conditions; prior hospitalization required; waiting period; physician referral required; renewability; premium changes. Homecare was covered by Firemen's Fund American, Equitable Life and Casualty, Blue Cross of Southern California - UltraCare, United Auto Workers. Limited homecare coverage was provided by Kemper Group, Greater Republic Life, National Foundation Life, and Merchants and Manufacturers.

A special focus on long-term care insurance appeared in *Caring* (March 1985). Articles dealt with the emerging market in long-term care insurance (Meiners 1985); the squeeze on state budgets (Curtis and Bartlett 1985); private initiatives (Lifson 1985); the Medi-Scare insurance scandal (Halamandaris, M. 1985); and steps by NAHC to get long-term care coverage (Halamandaris, V. 1985).

In response to reports of abuses in the sale of long-term care insurance policies to the elderly, Congressman Pepper undertook an investigation. Marilu Halamandaris (1985) related the Medi-Scare story about that effort. Posing as customers, investigators found only eight out of 50 insurance agents to be honest in dealings. A common sales technique was to "scare the hell out of them" while selling as many policies as possible, even though the small print states that "only one policy will pay." Agents get a 50 percent commission on new policies and only a 5 percent commission on renewals. Eight ways to avoid the Medi-Gap trap were given: understand that Medicare supplemental policies pay little more than Medicare's coinsurance and deductibles--the first $400 of the hospital bill and the first $75 of the doctor's bill; be wary of policies that "pay all your medical expenses not covered by Medicare"; do not buy more than one policy; first look to Blue Cross/Blue Shield since they return 90 cents on the premium dollar back to the insured; be skeptical about canceling an existing policy; don't talk to insurance salespeople alone; be sure to ask about limitations; if you do have a problem, complain to your state insurance commissioner.

NAHC (Halamandaris 1985b) initiated activities to bring about greater coverage of homecare and long-term care. Efforts involved employers, labor unions, commercial insurance companies, state associations, coalitions with other concerned professional groups, an operational task force, educational meetings, and a legislative lobbying focus. In conjunction with Prudential Insurance Company, AARP established the AARP Nursing Home and Home Health Care Plan (Borfitz 1986). This plan will be test-marketed in Florida and five other cities. Benefits include $20 to $25/day for skilled nursing and home health agency visits up to one year, or 60 to 80 percent of average cost/day; $40/day in nursing home up to 3 years, or 50 to 70 percent of average cost/day; maximum entry age of 79; an initial stay in nursing home required prior to homecare services; plan begins benefits after 20 combined facility days or home visits. Even with AARP endorsement, the customer still has to read the small print to discover the limits, the restrictions, and the prerequisites.

ICF, Inc. (1985,5) found a significant impact on Medicaid in simulation models. Under current funding with practically no long-term care insurance, Medicaid would pay for 43 percent of the total cumulative nursing home expenditures for age 67-69 cohort, individuals would pay for 55 percent, and Medicare for 2 percent. If about 20 percent of the age group purchased insurance reimbursing them $40/day for up to four years and costing them $480 annually, Medicaid expenditures would decline by 8 percent. If 50 percent of the group purchased insurance, Medicaid expenditures would decline by about 23 percent.

A survey of 1,000 AARP members (American Association of Retired Persons 1985c) revealed that almost half wished to learn more about long-term care and home health care insurance. Interestingly, and not surprisingly, 80 percent preferred homecare to nursing home care, even though only 5 percent had ever used homecare services, and less than 1 percent had ever been in a nursing home. There was a good deal of confusion expressed over Medicare and/or private insurance coverage, and most did not know the going rate for care.

Obviously, there is a good deal of concern with easing the worries of the elderly about the financial aftermath of an extended long-term illness. It is also apparent that much confusion exists about long-term care insurance. An investigation of private financing of long-term care (ICF, Inc. 1985) explained options such as single premium annuity, indemnity, combination life, reinsurance, pension, and IRA as mechanisms. This report also cited the barriers to private funding of long-term care: the elderly's annuity rigidity in fixed monthly income; assets that are not liquid, such as a home; laws and regulations, such as estate tax legislation, providing incentives to divest. Hopefully, the future will simplify these problems, and the elderly will be able to choose insurance options that really work.

Life or Continuing Care Communities. Life care communities are long-term care systems that provide a continuum of services for elderly residents, including homes or apartments for independent living, homecare services, an infirmary or, in many instances, nursing home care. Hospital care is usually not provided, but individuals are guaranteed that they can return to the life care community following hospitalization. A combination of monthly fees (ranging from $650 to $1,200) and entrance fees (ranging from $20,000 to $100,000) are usual for contracting with a life care community center (American Association of Retired Persons 1984,20; Laventhol and Horwath 1984,7; Winklevoss and Powerell 1984,12). Payments could also be a one-time fee-in-advance or an assignment of existing and future assets to the facility (ICF, Inc. 1985,37). There are about 275 to 500 life care communities in this country, serving some 100,000 elderly people, with expenditures of about $1 billion per year (U.S. Congress. Office of Technology Assessment 1985,230; Nassif 1985,357). Projections to the year 2000 estimate 316,000 residents, based on the assumption of 26 life care residents per 1,000 population, aged 75 to 84 (Arthur Young 1985,12). Most are privately owned and many are run by religious organizations. Proprietary companies such as Beverly Enterprises and National Medical Enterprises are already involved in the life care industry (Arthur Young 1985,12; Raper 1984,5).

ICF, Inc. cites Presbyterian Homes of Northern California as a nationally recognized example of a well-run life care facility (ICF, Inc. 1985,38). Services provided at the two facilities with 640 units include physician care, hospital care, skilled nursing care in their own SNF, and personal care services. There is a waiting list ranging from three to 10 years, depending upon the size of the housing unit. Nassif (1985,361) cites Kendal Crosslands, Kennett Square, Pennsylvania, as another example of a model life care community. Otterbein Home in Lebanon, Ohio, was also cited as an example of an established life care community (ICF, Inc. 1985,39). In addition, the ICF report compared fees for three relatively new life care facilities: Duncaster (Connecticut); the Moorings (Florida); and Roland Park Place (Maryland).

Enrolling in a life care community allows individuals to select the type of care they want before actually needing the services. There has been movement by large nursing homes to diversify into life care centers. In addition, proprietary organizations have also entered the field.

About one-third of the states have enacted legislation to govern life care communities: Arizona, California, Colorado, Florida, Illinois, Indiana, Maryland, Michigan, Minnesota, Missouri, and Oregon. Other states are considering regulatory action to address refund provisions, financial disclosures to residents, reserve requirements, and administrative operations.

A 14-point checklist includes questions that concerned consumers should ask about life care communities before signing a contract (American Association of Retired Persons 1984,23). Consumers are advised to consult their lawyers and to carefully evaluate the decision to become a life care community resident.

Life care communities and continuing care facilities represent a popular and effective approach to financing and providing residential, social, and health services for the elderly. Well-established life care organizations may have substantial waiting lists despite the high level of fees and charges. "Nevertheless, the substantial real estate and service risks facing developers of new facilities as well as the current high cost of capital may slow the rate of industry response" (ICF, Inc. 1985,43).

Home Equity Conversion. Another mechanism to finance long-term care essentially allows the elderly to borrow against the equity in their homes. In reality, the technique is similar to taking out a second mortgage. Thus, elderly who are home-rich but cash poor will be able to convert their home equity into dollars. About 65 percent of all elderly are poor, but 22 percent of the poor have $50,000 in home equity (Jacobs and Weissert 1984,83). More than 12 million homes are owned by people over 65, with a total of $600 billion in equity (Nassif 1985,174; Beirne 1985,58). Of particular relevance is the fact that in 1980 more than 50 percent of married people over 80 had $10,000 or more in home equity, with about 35 percent of the singles having likewise (ICF, Inc. 1985,15). Of course, people in that age group are much more likely to have need of long-term care.

Two types of home equity conversion are commonly used: reverse annuity mortgages (RAM) or sales/leaseback plans (Foote 1984). Under an RAM, the bank makes equal monthly payments to the elderly owners over a fixed period of time, using about 80 percent of the equity value as the borrowable amount. Homeowners can repay the borrowed money plus interest on a specific date, or after selling the house, or at death via an estate sale. In some cases, the elderly can agree to a lump sum to borrow and draw against that amount as needed, rather than receive equal monthly payments.

Sales/leaseback plans involve elderly homeowners selling their homes to an investor, but retaining guaranteed lifetime residency. An investor pays the elderly resident each month and in return receives rent from the elderly residents. Upon death or change of residence, the title of the house reverts to the investor. All appreciation in value from the time of the initial agreement also belongs to the investor. At the time of initial purchase, the investor takes over responsibility for maintenance and taxes.

ICF, Inc.'s report (1985,22) examined two sales/leaseback programs: one by Fouratt Corporation, Carmel, California, a profit-making firm; another run by the City of Buffalo, N.Y. Nassif (1985,175) also cited the National Center for Home Equity Conversion in Madison, Wisconsin, as an informational source.

Fouratt Corporation serves as a realtor for individuals or married couples over 70 who have little or no remaining mortgage on their homes. The firm finds buyers willing to make a sales/leaseback arrangement within fixed guidelines. In return for lifetime residency, the elderly owner sells the house below an independently appraised market value, usually about 20 percent below, or as a function of the seller's age. Rent is paid by the elderly resident on a fair market rental value.

Buffalo considers people over 60 for their program if they have little or no mortgage left on their homes. Cash payments to the seller are based on the house value, the life expectancy of the seller, and projected management costs over that lifespan. Sellers can choose either guaranteed lifetime monthly or lump-sum payments and retain lifetime occupancy. Maintenance, insurance, and property taxes are the responsibility of the City of Buffalo. Under death of a seller, Buffalo takes title and sells the property to regain its investment. With 65 homes in the program, Buffalo regards the program as an aid to senior citizens and as an effort to promote urban revitalization.

Exhibit 5-7 presents a summary of home equity conversion plans with examples of lump sums, monthly payments, total payments, amount due at end of program, title ownership, and coverage of taxes and maintenance.

Generally, the two forms of home equity conversion, RAMs and sales/leaseback arrangements, do not easily provide increased financing for long-term care. Typically, annuities are paid over long periods of time, while long-term care services often require lump sums over 6- to 12-month periods. It would probably be more useful if financial institutions allowed homeowners to use their home equity as a line of credit to draw upon as needed. "This option seems to have more potential to increase private financing of long-term care than RAMs or sales/leaseback arrangements" (ICF, Inc., 28).

Public Policy Recommendations. In 1983, the National Council on the Aging formed the National Institute on Community-Based Long-Term Care (NICLC) to work toward meeting the needs of functionally dependent older adults. After noting the existing limitations in public policy, such as

Exhibit 5-7 Summary of Home Equity Conversion Plans

	Lump Sum	Monthly Payment	Total Pay-Ments	Amount Due at End of Program	Title to Home at End of Program	Responsi-bility for Taxes and Maintenance
RAM with Deferred Interest[1]	0	$391	$ 46,800	$80,000	Elderly Resident	Elderly Resident
RAM with Interest Payments[1]	0	Vary from $661 to 0	$ 40,000	$80,000	Elderly Resident	Elderly Resident
Sales/ Lease back Plan[2]	$8,000	$952	$114,200	None	Buyer	Buyer

[1] Assumes a 10 year loan at 10 percent on $100,000 house with an 80 percent loan-to-value ratio.

[2] Assumes a 10 year loan at 10 percent on $100,000 house with an 80 percent sales price to value ratio and a 10 percent down payment.

Source: ICF. 1985. *Private financing of long-term care: current methods and resources. Phase II.* Washington, DC, p. 19 (Jan.).

lack of integration in services, institutional bias, insufficient funding for in-home and community-based services, and impoverishment of the elderly in order to achieve eligibility for services, the NICLC (1985) put forth 10 public policy recommendations:

1. Financial incentives, such as tax credits or reimbursement for care, should be provided by federal, state, and local governments to families and other informal providers.

2. Informal support systems should be funded with public and private funds to educate and train family caregivers, to operate family support groups, and to provide respite for family caregivers.

3. Functionally dependent older adults denied services due to eligibility requirements should be able to secure community-based homecare and institutional long-term care services via publicly funded programs, even when they are able to pay for some portion of the care.

4. Medicaid waivers for home- and community-based services should be facilitated by the federal government.

5. Medicaid programs should be reshaped by states to emphasize the use of optional services for community care as well as waivers for home and community care, and also a liberalization of eligibility requirements.

6. Regardless of payment source, states should implement case management to ensure appropriate utilization of all services, including nursing home and preadmission screening.

7. Long-term care insurance, life care communities, home equity conversion, and other private financing options should be more readily available to older adults. Federal and state regulatory barriers to developing such options should be identified, remedied, and replaced by incentives.

8. Research into the impact of private financing mechanisms, such as home equity conversion, social/health maintenance organizations, and other managed care systems, on the cost and accessibility of a full range of home-and community-based services to functionally dependent older adults, should be federally funded.

9. Research should be funded by the federal government to examine the impact of the Medicare PPS/DRG scheme on the quality of care for patients, including the appropriateness of post-hospital care settings, and the adequacy of the supply of home- and community-based services.

10. Intermittent care Medicare regulations should be modified by Congress and HCFA to permit the appropriate amount of home health services to persons discharged from hospitals with heavy daily care needs.

"Public policy reform, such as the recommendations listed above, therefore is needed to create a comprehensive, coordinated long term care system responsive to the needs and preferences of older adults and their families" (National Institute on Community-Based Long-Term Care 1985).

Continuing or Long-term Care

Thus far, we have gained some insight into the social/personal needs of the elderly by reviewing documented studies, quality of life concerns, and public policy issues. Using this information as a base, we can now examine actual hands-on care in a clearer perspective.

Long-term care is defined by the Office of Technology Assessment (U.S. Congress. Office of Technology Assessment 1985,481) as a variety of health and social services provided to individuals who need assistance because of physical or mental disability. Services can be provided in an institution, the home, or the community, and include informal services provided by family or friends as well as formal services provided by professionals or agencies. Another definition adds the critical time dimension (Arthur Young 1985,3): "Long term care refers to a wide range of services which address the social, custodial and medical needs of individuals who lack some capacity for self-care and whose continuing incapacity will necessitate the provision of care for a relatively long and indefinite period of time."

Most people immediately associate the words "long-term care," with nursing home care and high costs. Obviously, nursing home care is a large, costly component of long-term care, but it is certainly not the exclusive domain. Exhibit 5-8 lists a wide variety of long-term services, care providers, and settings. Note that the nursing home is only one of more than 20 providers and settings. Given the diversity of the two lists in Exhibit 5-8, it is apparent that a manageable network is coordinated and comprehensive services may be a wistful hope.

Speaking at the National Council on the Aging, Somers (1983) identified five major components of the long-term care dilemma: medical model vs. social model; public vs. private sector, federal vs. state/local government; technological imperative vs. geriatric imperative; and long-term care for elderly/disabled vs. national health insurance for everyone. In essence, Sommers' proposal "seeks to moderate the unacceptable growth of acute care costs . . . and broaden the Medicare package to include long-term care and preventive services."

A governmental conference on alternatives to long-term care financing and delivery systems (Feinstein, Gornick, and Greenberg 1983) also explored insurance, S/HMOs, life care communities, home equity, and other mechanisms to resolve difficulties in providing care. Regularly updated briefings are prepared for members of Congress by the Congressional Research Services of the Library of Congress (O'Shaughnessy and Reiss 1983; O'Shaughnessy, Price, and Griffith 1985). These documents are packed with facts and figures, explanations of relevant issues, proposals, and legislative actions.

Vogel and Palmer (1985) gave perspectives on long-term care gleaned from demonstration projects and research. Coordination and management was the concern of 25 of the mainly federally-funded activities: three dealt with Medicare and Medicaid coverage; five experimented with innovative reimbursement methods; and three explored certification. Other sections of the book covered population and system characteristics, community care, and the nursing home.

Exhibit 5-8 Long-term Care Services, Providers, and Settings

Long-Term Care Services

Hospice care	Job assistance
Physical therapy	Congregate meals
Respiratory therapy	Meals on wheels
Occupational therapy	Shopping assistance
I.V. Therapy	Chore services
Skilled nursing	Transportation
Physician, other medical	Friendly visiting
Nutrition/diet	Telephone reassurance
Personal care	Recreation
Mental health	Legal assistance
Day health	Protective service
Home health	Respite care
Residential care	Laundry
Foster care	Escort
Day care	Congregate housing
Sheltered workshop	Counseling
Information & referral	Preretirement counseling

Long-Term Care Providers and Settings

General hospital	Senior citizens center
Specialty hospital	Halfway house
Nursing home	Foster home
Skilled nursing facility	Community center
Intermediate care facility	Employment agency
Board and care home	Church/synagogue
Residential facility	Library
Hospice	Recreation center
Mental health center	Visiting nurse agency
Day care center	Support groups
Hospital extended care unit	Neighborhood health center
Day hospital	HMO
Vocational center	Public health agency
Home health agency	Workshop

Source: Arthur Young. 1985. *Long-term care: an industry composite*. New York, NY, p. 3.

From a clinical viewpoint, Rowe (1985) reviewed health care of the elderly for physicians. Illness behavior in the elderly often starts with failure to seek assistance and leads to multiple diseases that may be atypical and require long-term continued attention. Among the important diseases of the elderly, Rowe lists dementia, urinary incontinence, osteoporosis, and conditions leading to coronary artery bypass surgery. Importantly, physicians are advised to broaden their understanding of the clinical impact of the aging process and their comprehension of a suitable approach to elderly patients.

In a study of hospital DRGs and the need for long-term care services, Meiners and Coffey (1985) found variables distinguishing care levels for long-term services: assistance in ADL; presence of mental illness; existence of behavioral problems; and anticipated length of nursing home stay. Yet, the authors commented, "Perhaps more critical than discharge planning activities is the need to plan and develop an appropriate supply and mix of long-term care services . . ."

Obviously, long-term care is not solely an American problem. Hearings before the House Select Committee on Aging (1985b) concerned continuing care and sought international prototypes for America's aged. Presentations described programs in Belgium, Canada, England, and Denmark. Representatives from the International Association of Gerontology, the International Federation on Aging, and the U.S. Committee on World Aging also gave their counsel to Congress. Glaser (1985) submitted a paper on American problems and foreign solutions to long-term care. He told how other countries dealt with acute and extended care needs, homecare services, quality of staff, coordination and case management, the role of family, funding, and cost containment. As an overlay, Glaser noted that most of the other countries have existing national health insurance schemes for the total population and didn't start their efforts with the elderly as the U.S. did with Medicare.

Japan's aged population has increased at a rate twice that of other industrialized nations, creating long-term care situations similar to those in the U.S. (Lawrence 1985). Despite the existence of a national health insurance program, or maybe because of it, some hospitals in Japan have turned into holding stations for the sick and disabled elderly. Lawrence describes health care facilities for the elderly and comments on the high tech medical system, social welfare institutions, nursing homes, homecare, and the changes in family structure. There are a number of variations in facilities for the aged, including special hospitals for the elderly, facilities for independent ambulatory elderly, units where personal care is the major service, rehabilitation care, and retirement communities.

America's major health/medical coverage for the elderly's long-term care needs is the Medicare program. However, several comments by HHS Secretary Otis R. Bowen (1986) shed light on where we stand in America: "Medicare does not now pay for long term care per se. It does, however, provide for skilled nursing care and home health care as a transition between hospital care and full recovery . . . Medicare was originally intended only to address the consequences of acute care . . . Consequently, any new programs, such as coverage of long-term care, will be viewed with an eye carefully fixed on the solvency and survivability of Medicare as it now exists."

Nursing Home Care

In spite of any shift in attitudes and efforts at deinstitutionalization, nursing home care continues to be an overwhelmingly large part of the long-term care system. More than 23,000 nursing homes existed in 1985, with projections for 8,000 to 13,000 additional 120-bed facilities by the year 2000 (Arthur Young 1985,4). Of the existing institutions, the government manages more than 127,000 beds; nonprofit organizations over 336,000; and proprietary agencies operate 75 percent of all nursing homes with more than 1 million beds. By the year 2000, the demand for nursing home beds may double to close to three million. More than one million of the nursing home residents will be 85 or older, and over 800,000 will be 75 to 84 in the year 2000.

O'Shaughnessy and Reiss (1983,2) cite estimates of nursing home expenditures of $81.9 billion by 1990, with more than $50 billion of that being governmental funding, mainly through Medicaid. HHS Secretary Bowen (1986) stated that each American in a nursing home averages $20,000 to $30,000 a year for care expenses.

With such huge expenditures facing federal, state, and local jurisdictions, there are numerous attempts to contain costs, including facility-specific rates, uniform class rates, reimbursement ceilings, case-mix formulas, and average patient rates. Regardless of the methodology used to control costs, the issues related to the generic problems of quality of care, health vs. social care, and public policies continue to plague the provision of long-term care. Amid that atmosphere of uncertainty and conflicting demands, nursing homes are following the hospitals' lead into diversification. An advertisement in *Provider*, the official journal of the American Health Care Association, offered its own guide to the organization and operation of a home health agency (Tapia 1986).

Nursing home care has been subject to a good deal of attention in the mass media with stories of abuse and fraud. Vladeck (1980) recounted tales of unloving care in nursing home tragedies, while Mendolsohn (1975) described the tender loving greed of unscrupulous facility owners. Perhaps these conditions can be explained in part by Barker's (1986) words: "The longstanding neglect of these oldest and most vulnerable members of society by the health professions is one manifestation of the legacy of organizational and attitudinal barriers that have separated chronic care institutions and their residents from the mainstream of medical care." Congressman Claude Pepper proposed a sweeping bill to address the quality of care in nursing homes (Gapen 1986a). His legislation would require 40 percent of the nation's 15,000 nursing homes to upgrade their services with attention to establishing regulatory standards, with requirements for 60 hours of training for aides, and generally to upgrade intermediate care facilities to a skilled care level. Pepper's bill based its proposals upon a March 1986 study by the National Academy of Sciences on regulatory standards in nursing homes.

Professional organizations such as the American College of Health Care Administrators promote attention to nursing home administration. At conferences discussions center around problem solving, quality care, training, patient education, community relations, and special activity programs for residents (*Long Term Care Administrator* 1985). Perschbacher (1984) described an innovative project for nursing home residents. Elderly people in the institution used their life experiences to teach an oral history class to third grade students in a nearby school throughout the school year. This activity was given the title, "The Tiny Hearts and Aged Hands Program."

Most elderly people repeatedly express distaste at the thought of entering a nursing home and state a preference for homecare. Part of that distaste may be attributed to the belief that entering a nursing home will cause their condition to worsen: nursing home living has iatrogenic effects. However, recent research by Retsinas and Garrity (1985) contests this frequently expressed opinion of the nursing home experience. In fact, Retsinas (1985) shows that a majority of residents transfer to other nursing homes to improve their quality of life.

For a combination of socioeconomic, medical and cultural reasons, the nursing home still remains a viable long-term care option. Arguments still continue over institutional care vs. an alternative such as homecare (Pegels 1980; Powers and Burger 1985).

Homecare

Efforts to contain costs and to manage the rapidly increasing proportion of the aging population are leading many to consider homecare as a solution to the long-term care problem. There may also be a growing bias against institutionalization. "According to results of a survey released by National Research Corporation in 1984, consumers identify home health care more often than any other alternative health services as one needed in the community" (Arthur Young 1985,9).

A Long Term Home Health Consultation Service (Auerbach, Taylor, and Marosy 1985) set up a program to tackle the homecare challenge of providing care to the vulnerable elderly. A series of model long-term care programs emerged, including geriatric assessment and case management, health monitoring and maintenance for ambulatory elderly, respite services, a senior companion volunteer service, medical day care, and social day care. Jackson (1984) also spoke to home health care and the elderly in the 1980s, commenting that an individual may have to go to many agencies to obtain a variety of services because the coordination of long-term care is a problem

At a hearing in New York City arranged by the Manhattan Borough President (Stein 1985), reasons for homecare as the long-term care choice were reiterated. Witnesses spoke about the cost, the dignity, the inappropriate hospitalization, and longevity attributed to homecare. "Old at Home, Not in a Home" was the headline of the *New York Times* featuring the proceeds of that hearing.

Helping the elderly to cope at home with long-term health and social problems is at the core of the issue. Lukin (1986) details the activities of Caring Community Inc., in making the home environment a "place where frail elderly people can maximally and safely maintain independence and self-sufficiency." This organization does electrical work, plumbing, carpentry, appliance repair, painting, installation of grab bars and bedside phones, bill paying, and a myriad of vital home repairs and tasks.

In like fashion, King, Figge, and Harman (1986) found that continuity of nursing care helps the elderly to cope at home. They concluded that multiple chronic conditions of long-term care can be alleviated with nursing homecare. Critical variables related to an individual's need for certainty about his or her life situation, a comfortable level of perceived well-being, and a perceived level of care.

Newman (1985) noted three factors which largely determine the effectiveness of in-home long-term care services: the individual, the service/provider, and the housing environment. Her research into housing revealed that a substantial fraction of the target population "are living in housing units and environments that either impeded the efficient delivery of these (in-home) services or preclude their delivery altogether."

Since homecare is often mentioned as a substitute for institutional long-term care, it should be noted that there are those who do not agree with that proposition. A study by Schweitzer and Greenburg (1984) concluded that their results did not offer strong support for the substitution of social services for hospital care for stroke patients. A HCFA administrator was also doubtful: "Studies performed by HCFA and the General Accounting Office have found that expanded homecare does not substitute for institutional care unless individuals . . . are very carefully targeted" (Rich 1984b). According to Feder (Rich 1984b), "You're not substituting cheaper services for more expensive. You're serving more people."

HHS Secretary Bowen (1986) sums up the situation: "There is enthusiasm and a sense of caution that surrounds the issue of home health care. Everybody hopes that with enough know-how in targeting benefits to the right people, home health care can prove to be a humanitarian as well as cost-effective alternative to institutionalized care."

Family Caregiving and Long-term Care

Trocchio (1981) feels Americans are returning to a family orientation, again accepting responsibility for other family members. "People have started saying, 'I can give better care than an institution can.' " While Dunlop (1980) acknowledges the input of family and friends into long-term care for the elderly, he does raise doubts. He questions whether the expansion of family caregiving is a solution or a pipe dream. In his view, there is little hard evidence to bolster the contention that more families would engage in homecare if support were available.

In an extensive Medicaid study, Burwell (1986) focused on the relationships between long-term care policies and family caregivers. Areas covered included Medicaid eligibility, paying family members, tax incentives, financial contributions from adult children, and the example of the Idaho relative responsibility program. Supposedly, Medicaid eligibility policies encourage family members to seek institutional care for their elderly kin and discourage family caregiving. Payment of family members as long-term care providers is allowable in 13 states: California, Colorado, Connecticut, Florida, Kansas, Maine, Maryland, Michigan, Minnesota, North Dakota, Oregon, Virginia, and Wisconsin. There is considerable variability in the programs, although California still pays approximately 29,000 family caregivers about $900 million a year in its In-Home Supportive Services Program, funded by the Social Services Block Grant. Only Michigan uses Medicaid funds extensively to pay family caregivers. Federal tax incentives would be considered under the Child and Dependent Care Tax Credit provision. This would affect state tax, too, when the credit can be used for both. Adult children can contribute under federal guidelines which state that the law must be applicable to all adult children and not just to the children of Medicaid recipients. Idaho passed such legislation in 1983, but in March of 1984, the State Attorney General ruled that the law was not generally applicable and therefore not in keeping with federal requirements. Burwell (1986) concludes that meeting the long-term care needs of the elderly is a "shared obligation; neither the government nor families have the requisite resources to meet the demand for care."

Haug (1985) raises the question of who benefits from homecare for the ill elderly? She notes that most studies do not consider the impact upon family caregivers, mainly women. Home health care is a women's issue and Feldblum (1985) urges that services reflect the changing roles of women in American society. Benefits to family caregivers are almost entirely psychological and moral. Their reward is personal satisfaction and an avoidance of guilt by demonstrating love and affection. However, family caregivers are actually relieving institutions and health care systems of a portion of the load of geriatric care. Haug declares that "Someone needs to speak, in a voice loud enough to be heard in Washington, for the unsung family caregivers."

Homemaker-Home Aide: Essential Services for the Elderly

When family caregivers aren't available, people requiring long-term care and the elderly often need help with ADL. Tasks such as housecleaning, shopping, bathing, meal preparation, and dressing can frustrate the elderly. This does not need elaboration; it should also be obvious that if the services of a homemaker-home aide are not readily available, institutionalization may be the appropriate choice. Early on, Somers and Moore (1976) provided basic rationales for the essential nature of homemaker services. They posited that such services enable people to remain at home, relieve the burden on professionals, offer employment to mature individuals with little formal education, and may result in substantial savings for insurers and taxpayers. An Administration on Aging paper (Department of Health, Education and Welfare. Administration on Aging 1977) also provided strong backing for the use of homemaker-home health aides, noting the critical direct relation between the elderly's improved physical, mental and social status, and the help received.

A number of studies support the thesis that the use of homemaker/chore services saves money, improves functioning, and is better for long-term care of individuals. Lee and Stein (1980) use the Guale project in Georgia as a positive example. Wan, Weissert, and Livieratos (1980) compared homemaker and day care services, and raised questions. A GAO study (1981,126-129) summarized some of the better known studies: Georgia Alternative Health Services Project; Monroe County AC-CESS Project; New York State's Long Term Home Health Care Program; Wisconsin Community Care Organization Project; and Virginia Nursing Home Preadmission Screening Program.

Sentiment and instinct argue for support of homemaker-home health aide services for long-term care for the elderly and others. These are the most popular services supplied throughout the nation and also the fastest growing. Yet, the nagging questions remain: Do the services avoid institutionalization? Do they cost less? Are they effective? Are they another "add-on" to existing services?

Professional Education and the Elderly

"To date, the federal government has yet to focus significant support on education and training in geriatric care," according to the Senate Special Committee on Aging (1985,207). Fewer than 300 medical school faculty are currently involved in teaching some aspect of geriatrics. By the year 2000, at least 1,350 will be needed to adequately staff medical schools. By 1990, the following personnel will be required:

RNs in nursing homes/ECFs--150,000 (from 77,000 in 1980)

Geriatric community nurses--106,000 (from 53,000 in 1980)

Geriatricians--8,000

Geropsychiatrists--1,000

Similar increases will be needed in geriatric nurse faculty, geriatric dentistry faculty, geriatric social workers, social work faculty, social gerontologists, gerontological aides, and others. Presently, there is no certifiable geriatric specialty in the U.S. (Scheier 1986a).

In 1984, overall obligations for the Department of Health and Human Services training programs in geriatrics amounted to about $27 million; around 1 percent of expenditures for training and research in the health field. "At present, there is no effective coordinated federal approach to initiate, expand, and improve these (geriatric) types of education and training activities" (Senate Special Committee on Aging 1985,207).

Physician Education

In the provision of homecare to the elderly, the physician is the pivotal professional. Without written orders from a physician, the services are not provided and are not reimbursed. Therefore, it is essential that physicians be educated about the elderly and their use of homecare and other long-term care alternatives. In a state medical society journal, Weller (1978) detailed suggestions related to homecare. Urging doctors to learn more about services and implementation, Weller also urged medical societies to emphasize medical school training in the homecare area. In fact, a national conference addressed the subject of the teaching of chronic illness and aging in homecare settings (Clark and Williams 1976). At that conference, Dr. Ian R. Lawson (1976) set up the premise that homecare by the physician is needed and that the subject should be taught to them. "Even if not a single statistic could be produced to demonstrate the economic value resultant from it, the premises may stand as ultimately moral and attitudinal if not utilitarian as well."

A study on aging and medical education by the Institute of Medicine (1978) also recommended that medical students be instructed in the biology of aging. At that time it was reported that 61 medical schools had some type of course on geriatrics, mainly electives of two to four weeks with few students opting to take the courses. Shortly thereafter, the AAMC (Association of American Medical Colleges 1983) held regional institutes on geriatrics and medical education, and published proceedings. In addition to faculty guidelines to aid education, the report covered attitudes toward the elderly, basic knowledge in clinical skills, socioeconomic and psychosocial information, demography and aging theories, and the responsibilities of medical schools for change and expansion. Finally, Dr. Robert N. Butler told the attendees about the future of geriatric medicine and his belief that "all 126 medical schools have to have departments of geriatrics." In July 1985, in testimony (Butler 1985,34) before the House Select Committee on Aging, Butler Noted that "Our department (Mt. Sinai Medical Center, N.Y., Department of Geriatrics and Adult Development) is the only department of geriatrics in any U.S. medical school. It is not necessary that other schools establish geriatrics departments. But it is essential that they initiate geriatric training as part of the basic medical curriculum." He also pointed out that other countries, the United Kingdom and the Scandinavian countries, had expanded their efforts in geriatric training for a variety of professionals far beyond the scope of activities in the U.S.

Practicing physicians, dentists, and nurses were surveyed about their interests and concerns regarding gerontology by Anderson and Burdman (1981). Generally speaking, the health care providers did not particularly care to treat the elderly and did not express a desire for further education. Given the conflicting opinions, Anderson and Burdman proposed suggestions for the future training of professionals:

> More curriculum choices should be offered on aging that include sociological and psychological aspects as well as health and medical factors.

> Relations between health education and prevention should be emphasized in appropriate courses.

> Normal aging changes should be explained more fully so the professionals will not have unmet expectations in treating people with chronic ailments.

Dr. Butler (1981a,xvi) stated that physicians, nurses, and others have to be stimulated to "get off their apathies" to take the training and to learn more about care of the elderly. Medical students in Dr. Butler's program are required to make house calls and serve in long-term care facilities (Scheier 1986a). In a follow-up to the AAMC report, Weksler, Durmaskin, and Kodner (1983) asked how physicians could be prepared to attend to the health care needs of older persons in the hospital, the long-term care institution, and the community. Noting the importance of attitudes of health care providers while serving the elderly, the authors commented that "geriatric medical education may assert a balance between caring and curing in medical education."

Medical student attitudes toward the geriatric patient were studied by Spence, Feigenbaum, Fitzgerald, et al. (1968). They declared that an empathetic, caring attitude toward the old is past due and that appropriate teaching in the first year of medical school was indicated. In fact, Dr. Butler (1981b) advocated the use of a nursing home for teaching purposes. Exactly such an effort took place at UCLA Medical School (Jarvik, Ross, Klessing, et al. 1981) where departments of family practice, medicine and psychiatry developed a required first-year course stressing the aged patient. Students interviewed asymptomatic aged volunteers, and it appeared that prejudices about the elderly were reduced by these intimate interactions. Hopefully, the students will learn to render humane, competent care to the elderly as well as to all their patients. At George Washington University Medical Center, medical students participate in an outreach program for the elderly involving a multidisciplinary team called Case Assessment/Case Management Project (Koshes 1984). "Emphasis . . . is on promoting the positive aspects of elderly people's lives by keeping them in familiar home environment surrounded by friends, local clubs, and visitors." Benefits reported by the medical students included a better understanding of medical/social/emotional aspects of aging; an ability to work with the "well elderly"; learning how to work with a team approach to health care; and, although uncomfortable at first, the ability to come to terms with their own aging.

Eight learning modules for nursing assessment and management of the frail elderly were developed by Wahlstedt and Blaser (1986). Topics included a conceptual framework for multiphasic assessment and management; interviewing and prescreening; community assessment; multiphasic assessment; developing a plan; strategies with implementation; coordination of care; and evaluation re: outcomes of care. Butt (1986) prepared homecare protocols to deal with diseases/conditions to be used by a nurse practitioner within the sanction and guidance of the referring physician. Both of these activities could easily find their way into the training of professional nurses in homecare and long-term care.

In response to the expressed concerns of the professionals, a number of legislative bills were introduced in Congress dealing with grants for geriatric education for a variety of health professions (Senate Special Committee on Aging 1985,207-208). In addition, Butler (1985) noted that Medicare expended $2 billion a year for medical education, but little of that for geriatric training. He proposed that 3 percent of the $2 billion be devoted to geriatrics through the support of 2,000 fellows per year, with each of the 127 medical schools training 16 fellows per year in a two-year program. About $70 million per year would be for support of the fellows at $35,000 each yearly, with $250,000 to each medical school yearly for implementation and administration. This proposal would allow for reaching the estimated goal of 7,000 to 13,000 physicians training in geriatrics by 1990.

Education and training of the upcoming health care providers in geriatrics is vital. Rosow (1962) identified the dilemma some time ago: "The crucial people in the aging problem are not the old, but the younger age groups, for it is the rest of us who determine the status and position of the old person in the social order."

Planning and Research

In testifying before the House Select Committee on Aging, Trager (1984,63) stated that "It is no longer news that planning for the needs of older people in the area of long-term care has been seriously deficient in the United States." She came up with nine areas for action to improve community care:

1. Replacement of the present confusion in state and federal funding sources and eligibility requirements with a rational rearrangement.

2. Planned development of home health services in order to achieve equity of access and service range throughout the United States.

3. Realistic changes in home health care certification and eligibility requirements in order to achieve a better matching of the needs of the consumer of long-term care.

4. Requirements that all home health services require paraprofessional care to provide assistance with activities of daily living and environmental maintenance as needed as part of any reimbursed plan of care.

5. Redefinition of the concept of part-time intermittent care in order to allow for variations in intensity of need.

6. Aggressive approaches to preventive care in high risk groups using established methods of outreach, health education and health supervision based in health departments and health centers.

7. Greater emphasis on discharge planning with special attention to care in the community.

8. Implementation of the concept of the community network, with the development of services such as adult day care, meal services, special needs transportation, and the introduction of many electronic and security and monitoring devices now being used in homecare programs in other countries.

9. Serious attention to the range of innovative housing arrangements which are being developed abroad and which increase the feasibility of homecare planning.

Tagg (1986) reported on neighborhood resources for the elderly. Her survey results indicated that health was the most critical factor in independence for older people. Planning for long-term health care needs moves to the top of the list. "Ideally, senior citizens should remain independent and in their own homes for as long as possible."

Of course, reducing the health risk requires money, ofttimes coming from the elderly themselves. A House Select Committee on Aging (1985c) report studied the financial risk to the elderly. The report concluded that the Committee will work to see that Congress acts to:

- Limit the elderly's out-of-pocket costs to no more than the current level of 15 percent of income.

- Implement a coherent policy for long-term care that will protect America's aged from impoverishment in the face of chronic and disabling illnesses.

Planning for actions may be more difficult than it appears. Firstly, the goals of long-term care are difficult to articulate and often deal with functioning ability that is not simply a matter of a cure for this or that condition. Secondly, even if functioning ability could be articulated, shades of functioning are so diverse as to result in problematic agreements. Thirdly, even assuming agreement on the first two difficulties, there would be a great deal of uncertainty about the costs and benefits of achieving the goals.

Planners also argue for participation of all those concerned with the issue. Sager (1980) asked, "Who should control long-term planning for the elderly?" Professionals, patients, and family members were involved in his study. His research found that patients and family members are likely to design reasonable homecare plans within reasonable costs. In fact, their plans cost less because the families anticipate unpaid services rendered by family members. Sager concluded, "In the absence of strong evidence for or against control of homecare services by any of the three groups, and given the apparently defensible positions of all, it may be possible to devise schemes for homecare planning to permit balanced influence by patients, families, and various professionals."

Dunlop (1980) raised three vital research issues regarding expansion of homecare services: What benefits are produced via expansion? Who benefits? How much demand for services is satisfied? In addition, Dunlop noted a need for more research into the appropriate mix of agency-supplied and family/friends-supplied services. Research implications related to 17 policy issues were listed by the Federal Council on Aging (Department of Health, Education and Welfare 1979,60-61), including manpower and training in long-term care, mental health therapies, social aspects of health care, and the identification of pertinent research and demonstration projects.

A number of legal and ethical aspects of health care for the elderly requiring investigation have been elucidated by Kapp, Pies, and Doudera (1986). Topics covered include social, ethical, and political perspectives; reimbursement for long-term care; legal issues facing care providers; rights of long-term care residents; and decision-making by the elderly regarding their health care.

Policymakers and providers were advised to consider the magnitude and urgency of trends in planning for the future of long-term care (Arthur Young 1985,14). Areas of concern for planning and research related to demographic trends, traditional family-based care, alternatives to institutionalization, prospective reimbursement, homecare, S/HMOs, hospice care, life care communities, insurance, and the political and economic environment of long-term care.

A national debate on health care in Dallas, Texas, considered who should pay for long-term care and how (Gapen 1986b). Dr. Robert L. Kane, a professor at the University of Minnesota, and Robert Van Tuyle, chairman and chief executive officer of Beverly Enterprises were the participants. Both expressed enthusiasm for long-term care insurance, and Tuyle decried proposals to have the family assume more of the financial burden of paying for long-term care. Incidentally, at the meeting, Wilbur Cohen, former HHS Secretary, predicted a national health insurance scheme for the U.S. by 1995.

Long-term Care Overview

At the May 1986 annual meeting of AARP, the priority concerns were health care costs and coverage (Scheier 1986b). HHS Secretary Bowen told the 25,000 attendees, "Without a doubt the preeminent issue of our time" is the staggering cost of catastrophic and long-term care. Outgoing AARP President, Vita R. Ostrander, commented, "Health care is still too expensive and there are many gaps in the system . . . There is a serious lack out there, and if we don't fill the gap with community based services, then we're right back to the acute care system, which is more expensive." Another speaker, Governor Bruce Babbitt of Arizona, even proposed the creation of Part C in Medicare to fund nursing home and long-term care.

Stressing the need for Medicare reform to meet the threat to the elderly, the AARP passed resolutions about the top concerns (*American Medical News* 1986):

- Nationwide programs should be developed to broaden the range of in-home and community alternatives to nursing homes, including adult day care facilities.

- Medicare should be strengthened with catastrophic insurance to protect against institutionalization and to cover home-based custodial care.

- Incentives should be developed for family members providing in-home care.

The issues relative to long-term care and homecare for the elderly, as well as for the rest of the population, have been delineated by these questions of planning and research. Because of the rapid growth of homecare, some of these questions/problems have been sidestepped in order to take care of immediate needs. But they cannot be ignored indefinitely, and any time and effort used to review planning and research now is time and effort well spent.

References

Adams, J. 1980. Alternate forms of care benefit young and old. *Hospitals* 54(10:91-94.

American Association of Retired Persons. 1984. *A handbook about care in the home.* Washington, DC.

American Association of Retired Persons. 1985a. *A profile of older Americans.* Washington, DC.

American Association of Retired Persons. 1985b. *Your home, your choice.* Washington, DC.

American Association of Retired Persons. 1985c. Preferences of AARP members for specific long term care insurance product features. Report. Washington, DC (28 Feb.).

American Medical News. 1986. AARP policy session stresses health issues. 29(23):37.

Anderson, L., and G. D. Burdman. 1981. Gerontological interest and opinions of health care providers. *Educational Gerontology* 6:251-263.

Arthur Young. 1985. *Long term care. An industry composite.* Washington, DC.

Association of American Medical Colleges. 1983. *Proceedings of the regional institutes on geriatrics and medical education.* Washington, DC.

Auerbach, M., M. Taylor, and J. P. Marosy. 1985. Homecare challenge: care of the vulnerable elderly. *Caring* 4(4):38-42.

Barker, W. H. 1986. Influenza and nursing homes. *American Journal of Public Health* 76:491-492.

Beirne, K. 1985. Testimony before Senate Special Committee on Aging. *Home equity conversion. Issues and options for the elderly homeowner.* Washington, DC: Government Printing Office. Pub. No. 99-513 (28 Jan.).

Blum, S. R., and M. Minkler. 1980. Toward a continuum of caring alternatives: community-based care for the elderly. *Journal of Social Issues* 36(2):133-152.

Borfitz, D. 1986. AARP plan examined. *Home Health Journal* 7(2):3,10,13-14.

Bowen, O. R. 1986. Cost control key to Medicare's future. *Provider* 12(6):9-10.

Burnside, I. M. 1980. Why work with the aged? *Geriatric Nursing* 1(1):29-33.

Burwell, B. O. 1986. *Shared obligations: public policy influences on family care for the elderly.* Lexington, MA: Systemetrics/McGraw Hill, Inc. (May).

Butler, R. N. 1975. *Why survive? being old in America.* New York: Harper and Row.

Butler, R. N. 1981a. Foreword in *The geriatric imperative,* edited by A. R. Somers and D. R. Fabian. New York: Appleton-Century-Crofts.

Butler, R. N. 1981b. The teaching nursing home. *Journal of the American Medical Association* 245:1435-1437 (10 April).

Butler, R. N. 1985. Testimony to House Select Committee on Aging in *Continu-*

ing care: international prototypes for America's aged. Washington, DC: Government Printing Office. Comm. Pub. No. 99-523.

Butt, B. 1986. Use of protocols in homecare: an innovative approach to meet today's needs. Home Healthcare Nurse 4(2):37-40.

Callahan, J. J., Jr. 1981. How much, for what, and for whom? American Journal of Public Health 71:987-988.

Cherkasky, M. 1955. Home care of chronic illness. Journal of Chronic Diseases 1(3):346-349.

Clark, D. W., and T. F. Williams. 1976. The teaching of chronic illness and aging. Washington, DC: Government Printing Office. DHEW Pub. No. (NIH) 75-876.

Curtis, R. E., and L. R. Bartlett. 1985. High cost of long term care squeezes state budgets. Caring 4(3):28-31.

Department of Health, Education and Welfare. Administration on Aging. 1977. Homemaker-home health aide services. Washington, DC: Government Printing Office. Pub. No. (OHD) 77-20086.

Department of Health and Human Services. Federal Council on Aging. 1981. The need for long-term care. Information and issues. Washington, DC: Government Printing Office. Pub. No. ORDS 81-20704.

Department of Health and Human Services. Federal Council on Aging. 1979. Key issues in long-term care. Washington, DC: Government Printing Office (Dec.).

Diamond, L. M., and D. E. Berman. 1981. The social health maintenance organization: a single entry, prepaid long-term care delivery system in Reforming the long-term care system edited by J. J. Callahan and S. S. Wallace. Lexington, MA: Lexington Books, D.C. Heath and Co., pp. 185-213.

Doty, P., K. Liv and J. Wiener. 1985. An overview of long-term care. Health Care Financing Review 6(3):69-78.

Dunlop, B. D. 1980. Expanded home-based care for the impaired elderly: solution or pipe dream? American Journal of Public Health 70:414-419.

Feinstein, P. H., M. Gornick, and J. N. Greenberg. 1984. Long-term care

financing and delivery systems: exploring some alternatives. Conference proceedings. Washington, DC: Government Printing Office (24 Jan.).

Feldblum, C. R. 1985. Home health care for the elderly: programs, problems and potentials. Harvard Journal of Legislation 22(1):193-254.

Fischer, D. H. 1978. Growing old in America. New York: Oxford University Press.

Foote, B. E. 1984. Converting home equity into income for the elderly: issues and options. Washington, DC: Congressional Research Service, Library of Congress. Report No. 84-42 (5 April).

Fortinsky, R. H., C. V. Granger, and G. B. Seltzer. 1981. The use of functional assessment in understanding home care needs. Medical Care 19:489-497.

Gapen, P. 1986a. Sweeping bill addresses nursing homes. American Medical News 29(23):48.

Gapen, P. 1986b. Who's best qualified to determine what's best for the public? American Medical News 23(23):33-34.

General Accounting Office. 1979. Entering a nursing home: costly implications for Medicaid and the elderly. Washington, DC: Government Printing Office. Pub. No. PAD 80-12 (26 Nov.).

General Accounting Office. 1981. Improved knowledge base would be helpful in reaching policy decisions on providing long-term in-home services for the elderly. Washington, DC: Government Printing Office. Pub. No. HRD-82-4 (26 Oct.).

Glaser, W. A. 1985. Long-term care: American problems and foreign solutions in Continuing care: international prototypes for America's aged. Washington, DC: Government Printing Office. House Comm. Pub. No. 99-253 (15 July).

Greenberg, J. N., and A. Ginn. 1979. A multivariate analysis of the predictions of long-term car placement. Home Health Care Services Quarterly 1(1):75-99.

Greenberg, J. N., W. Levtz, S. Ervin, et al. 1985. The S/HMO and long-term care. Generations 9(4):51-55.

Halamandaris, M. 1985a. The medi-scare insurance scandal. Caring 4(3):42-46.

Halamandaris, V. J. 1985b. Caring thoughts. *Caring* 4(3):64.

Harrington, C., and R. J. Newcomer. 1985. Social/health maintenance organizations: new policy options for the aged, blind and disabled. *Public Health Policy* 6(4):204-222.

Haug, M. R. 1985. Home care for the elderly--who benefits? *American Journal of Public Health* 75:127-128.

House Select Committee on Aging. 1984. *Long-term care: need for a national policy.* Washington, DC: Government Printing Office. Comm. Pub. No. 98-44.

House Select Committee on Aging. 1985a. *Health care cost containment: are America's aged protected?* Washington, DC: Government Printing Office. Comm. Pub. No. 99-522.

House Select Committee on Aging. 1985b. *Continuing care: international prototypes for America's aged.* Washington, DC: Government Printing Office. Comm. Pub. No. 99-523.

House Select Committee on Aging. 1985c. *America's elderly at risk.* Washington, DC: Government Printing Office. Comm. Pub. No. 99-508.

House Subcommittee on Health and Long Term Care. 1980. *Long term care for the 1980s: channeling demonstrations and other initiatives.* Washington, DC: Government Printing Office. Pub. No. 96-234 (27 Feb.).

Hugo, V. 1979. *Les miserables.* Reprint. N.Y.: Fawcett.

ICF, Inc. 1985. *Private financing of long-term care: current methods and resources. Phase I and Phase II.* Washington, DC (Jan.).

Institute of Medicine. 1978. A study on aging and medical education. Washington, DC (Sept.).

Jackson, B. N. 1984. Home health care and the elderly in the 1980s. *American Journal of Occupational Therapy* 38:717-720.

Jacobs, B., and W. Weissert. 1984. Home equity financing of long-term care for the elderly in *Long-term care financing and delivery systems: exploring some alternatives. Conference proceedings,* edited by P. H. Feinstein, M. Gornick, and J. N. Greenberg. Washington, DC: Government Printing Office (Jan.).

Jarvik, L. F., C. Ross, J. Klessing, et al. 1981. First year medical students and the aging patient: a curricular model. *Journal of the American Geriatric Society* 29(3):135-138.

Kane, R. L., and R. A. Kane. 1980. Long-term care: can our society meet the needs of its elderly? in *Annual Review of Public Health* 1:227-253.

Kapp, M. B., H. E. Pies, and A. E. Doudera. 1986. *Legal and ethical aspects of health care for the elderly.* Ann Arbor, MI: Health Administration Press.

King, F. E., J. Figge, and P. Harman. 1986. The elderly coping at home: a study of continuity of nursing care. *Journal of Advanced Nursing* 11(1):41-46.

Koshes, R. 1984. Productive alternatives. *The New Physician.* 33(3):14-15.

Kovar, M. G. 1986a. Aging in the eighties, preliminary data from the supplement on aging to the National Health Interview Survey, U.S., Jan.-June 1984. Washington, DC: Government Printing Office. Pub. No. (PHS) 86-1250 (1 May).

Kovar, M. G. 1986b. Aging in the eighties, age 65 years and over and living alone, contacts with family, friends, and neighbors. Washington, DC: Government Printing Office. Pub. No. 86-1250 (9 May).

Laventhol and Horwath. 1984. *Life care industry.* Philadelphia, PA.

Lawrence, T. L. 1985. Health care facilities for the elderly in Japan. *International Journal of Health Services* 15(4):677-697.

Lawson, I. R. 1976. The teaching of chronic illness and aging in home-care settings in *Teaching of chronic illness and aging* edited by D. W. Clark and T. F. Williams. Washington, DC: Government Printing Office. DHEW Pub. No. 75-876.

Lee, J. T., and M. A. Stein. 1980. Eliminating duplication in home health care for the elderly. The Guale project. *Health and Social Work.* 5(3):29-36.

Levtz, W., J. N. Greenberg, and R. Abrahams. 1985. *Changing health care for an aging society: planning for the social/health maintenance organization.* Lexington, MA: Lexington Books.

Lifson, A. 1985. Private initiatives: long-term care insurance. *Caring* 4(3):33-34.

Long Term Care Administrator. 1985. Latest trends in nursing home administration. 19(12):7.

Lukin, J. M. 1986. Nonmedical care for homebound elderly in peril. *New York Times* (3 Jan.).

McIlrath, S. 1986. Expansion of Medicaid to elderly sought. *American Medical News.* 29(22):2.

Meiners, M. 1985. Long-term care insurance examples. Policy features of insurance companies. *Caring* 4(3):36-41.

Meiners, M. R., and R. M. Coffey. 1985. Hospital DRGs and the need for long-term care services: an empirical analysis. *Health Services Research* 20(3):359-384.

Meiners, M. R., and J. O. Gollub. 1985. Long-term care insurance: the edge of an emerging market. *Caring* 4(3):12-16.

Mendolsohn, M. 1975. *Tender loving greed.* New York: Random House.

Moss, F. E., and V. J. Halamandaris. 1977. *Too old. Too sick. Too bad.* Rockville, MD: Aspen Systems Corporation.

Nascher, I. 1914. *Geriatrics.* Philadelphia: Blakiston.

Nassif, J. Z. 1985. *The home health care solution.* New York: Harper and Row.

National Institute on Community-Based Long-Term Care. 1985. Public policy statement (revised). Washington, DC (5 Dec.).

Newald, J. Feb. 20, 1986. Social HMOs problems tied to marketing slips. *Hospitals* 60(4):104.

Newman, S. J. 1985. Housing and long-term care: the suitability of the elderly's housing to the provision of in-home services. *The Gerontologist* 25:35-40.

O'Shaughnessy, C., and K. Reiss. 1983. *Long term care: community base alternatives to institutionalization.* Washington, DC: Congressional Research Service, Library of Congress. Issue Brief No. 1B81013 (10 March).

O'Shaughnessy, C., R. Price, and J. Griffith. Oct. 17, 1985. *Financing and delivery of long-term care services for the elderly.* Washington, DC: Congressional Research Service, Library of Congress. Pub No. 85 1033 EPW.

Pegels, C. C. 1980. Institutional vs. nonin-stitutional care for the elderly. *Journal of Health Politics, Policy and Law* 5(2):205-212.

Perschbacher, R. 1984. An application of reminiscence in an activity setting. *The Gerontologist* 24(4):343-345.

Powers, J. S., and C. Burger. 1985. Home health care vs. nursing home care for the elderly. *Journal of the Tennessee Medical Association* 78(4):227-230.

Raper, A. T. 1984. *National continuing care directory.* Washington, DC: American Association of Retired Persons.

Retsinas, J. 1985. Nursing home nomads: a study of transfers. Presentation at annual meeting of the American Public Health Association, Washington, DC (Nov.).

Retsinas, J., and P. Garrity. 1985. Going home: the derailment of nursing home residents, unpublished.

Rice, D. P. 1985. Health care needs of the elderly in *Long-term care of the elderly, public policy issues* edited by C. Harrington, R. S. Newcomer, C. L. Estes et al. Beverly Hills, CA: Sage Publications, Inc.

Rich, S. 1984a. Aged care experiment is blocked. *Washington Post* (29 March).

Rich, S. 1984b. The old folks at home. Economizers talk about keeping them there. *Washington Post* (19 July).

Robinson, D. 1977. You don't have to put your parents in a nursing home. *Parade* (23 Jan.).

Rosow, I. 1962. Old age: one moral dilemma of an affluent society. *Gerontologist* 2:182-191.

Rossman, I. 1980. Home care of geriatric patients in *Perspectives on geriatric medicine.* Washington, DC: Government Printing Office. NIH Pub. No. 81-1924 (Oct.).

Rowe, J. W. 1985. Health care of the elderly. *New England Journal of Medicine* 312:827-835 (28 March).

Sager, A. 1980. *Who should control long term care planning for the elderly?* Waltham, MA: Brandeis University, Heller School.

Scheier, R. L. 1986a. Elderly urged to be more assertive with physicians. *American Medical News* 29(23):37.

Scheier, R. L. 1986b. Cost, coverage AARP's top concerns. *American Medical News* 29(23):2,36.

Schweitzer, S. O., and E. R. Greenburg. 1984. Do social services reduce the use of hospitals by the elderly in *Promoting the well being of the elderly* edited by M. F. Collen. Rockville, MD: International Health Evaluation Association.

Senate Special Committee on Aging. 1985. *Developments on aging: 1984 volume 1.* Washington, DC: Government Printing Office. Report 99-5 (18 Feb.).

Shanas, E. 1982. *National survey of the aged.* Washington, DC: Government Printing Office. Pub. No. (OHDS) 83-20425 (Dec.).

Somers, A. 1983. Medicare and long-term care. *Perspectives on Aging* 12(2):5-8,28.

Somers, A. R., and F. M. Moore. 1976. Homemaker services--essential option for the elderly. *Public Health Reports* 91:354-359.

Spence, D., E. Feigenbaum, F. Fitzgerald, et al. Medical students' attitudes towards the geriatric patient. *Journal of the American Geriatrics Society* 16:976.

Spiegel, A. D., and B. Backhaut. 1980. *Curing and Caring. A review of the factors affecting the quality and acceptability of health care.* Jamaica, NY: SP Medical and Scientific Books.

Stein, A. 1985. Old at home, not in a home. *New York Times* (9 Jan.).

Suzman, R., and M. W. Riley (guest editors). 1985. The oldest old. *MMF Quarterly Health and Society* 63(2):177-451.

Tagg, P. I. 1986. Neighborhood resources for the elderly. *Home Healthcare Nurse* 4(2):24-29.

Tapia, J. 1986. *Planning for home health. A guide to organization and operation.* Washington, DC: American Health Care Association.

Trager, B. 1984. Testimony at hearings. *Long-term care: need for a national policy.* Washington, DC: Government Printing Office. Comm. Pub. No. 98-44, pp. 60-63.

Trocchio, J. 1981. *Home Care for the elderly.* Boston: CBI Pub. Co., Inc.

U.S. Congress. Office of Technology Assessment. 1985. *Technology and aging in America.* Washington, DC: Government Printing Office. Pub. No. OTA-BA-264 (June).

Vladeck, B. C. 1980. *Unloving care: the nursing home tragedy.* New York: Basic Books.

Vogel, R. J., and H. C. Palmer. 1985. *Long-term care. Perspectives from research and demonstrations.* Rockville, MD: Aspen Systems Corporation.

Wahlstedt, P., and W. Blaser. 1986. Nurse case management for the frail elderly: a curriculum to prepare nurses for that role. *Home Healthcare Nurse* 4(2):30-35.

Waldo, D. R. and H. C. Lazenby. 1984. Demographic characteristics and health care use and expenditures by the aged in the U.S.: 1977-1984. *Health Care Financing Review* 6(1):1-29.

Wan, T. T., W. G. Weissert, and B. B. Livieratos. 1980. Geriatric day care and homemaker services: an experimental study. *Journal of Gerontology* 35(2):256-274.

Weksler, M., S. Durmaskin, and D. Kodner. 1983. New goals for education in geriatric medicine. *Annals of Internal Medicine* 99:856-857.

Weller, C. 1978. Home health care. *New York State Journal of Medicine* 78:1957-1961.

Williams, T. F. 1981. Clinical and service aspects of geriatric teaching programs in *The geriatric imperative,* edited by A. R. Somers and D. R. Fabian. New York: Appleton-Century Crofts.

Winklevoss, H. E., and A. V. Powell. 1984. *Continuing care retirement communities: an empirical, financial and legal analysis.* Homewood, IL: Richard D. Irwin, Inc. (Published for the Pension Research Council, Wharton School, University of Pennsylvania).

Chapter 6

Funding Homecare
Governmental & Other Sources

At least 80 federal programs assist people with long-term care problems either directly or indirectly, through cash assistance, in-kind transfers, or the provision of goods and services. Four of those sources provide the major funding for homecare: Medicare, Medicaid, Title XX, and the Older Americans Act. Exhibit 6-1 indicates the services covered, the eligibility, and the administering agency for each of the four. In addition, some homecare services are funded through projects of the Health Care Financing Administration (HCFA) or other agencies.

Private funding for homecare comes from commercial insurance companies, Blue Cross/Blue Shield plans, and prepaid group health plans such as a health maintenance organization (HMO). Hall (1981) adds to the list with United Way organizations, religious agencies, and a variety of disease/condition-related charities. Of course, individuals also pay out of their own pockets for homecare services.

According to a Congressional Research Service report, "No one program, however, has been designed to support a full range of long-term care services on a systematic basis" (O'Shaughnessy, Price, and Griffith 1985 ix). This statement also holds true for homecare. Medicare and Medicaid tend toward medical aspects, while Title XX and the Older Americans Act tend to support the social/personal services.

Cost containment policies on a governmental as well as on a private level stimulated interest in homecare with the prospect of resultant money savings. Medicare's PPS/DRG reimbursement scheme allegedly discharges from the hospital elderly people in need of community services such as homecare. However, the Gramm-Rudman-Hollings Balanced Budget legislation mandates cutbacks for homecare and sets up a Catch-22 situation. An NAHC representative asked the House Ways and Means Committee to exempt home health agencies from the one percent HCFA-ordered cutback under the Balanced Budget Law (*Home Health Journal* 1986a). Tied to the legislative mandates, the federal budget proposals for 1987 seek to curtail what is seen as excessive utilization of homecare services. In the 1987 budget, HCFA "has specifically earmarked $7 million to fund a management initiative which systematically focuses on home health utilization and the medical necessity of services" (*Home Health Journal* 1986b).

In an NAHC report, the situation was pointedly summarized: "Saving millions of dollars by moving patients out of hospitals more quickly, HHS now seems to be trying to trim the candle at both ends, rather than accepting the modest increases in the level of home health expenditures which is

Exhibit 6-1 Major Federal Programs Funding Homecare Services: Services Covered, Eligibility, and Administering Agency

Program	Services covered	Eligibility	Administering agency	
			Federal	State
Medicaid/ Title XIX of the Social Security Act	Skilled nursing facility[a] Intermediate care facility[b] Home health[c] Adult day care[b]	Aged, blind, disabled persons receiving cash assistance under SSI; others receiving cash assistance under AFDC. At State option, persons whose income exceeds standards for cash assistance under SSI/AFDC, i.e., the "medically needy."	Health Care Financing Administration/HHS	State Medicaid Agency
	2176 "waiver" services, e.g., case management, homemaker, personal care, adult day care, habilitation, respite, and other services at State option.[d]	Aged, blind, disabled, or mentally ill Medicaid eligibles (including children) living in the community who would require nursing home level care. At State option, persons living in the community with higher income than normally allowed under a State Medicaid plan.		In some cases the 2176 "waiver" program would be administered by another agency, e.g. State agency on aging.
Medicare/ Title XVIII of the Social Security Act	100 days of skilled nursing facility care Home health Hospice	Generally Social Security status. Persons 65 years and over; persons under 65 years entitled to Federal disability benefits; and certain persons with endstage renal disease.	Health Care Financing Administration/HHS	N/A

Social Services Block Grant/Title XX of the Social Security Act	Various social services as defined by the State, including homemaker, home health aide, personal care, home-delivered meals	No Federal requirements. States may require means tests.	Office of Human Development Services/HHS	State social services/human resources agency. In some cases other State agencies may administer a portion of Title XX funds for certain groups, e.g., State agency on aging.
Older Americans Act/Title III	Variety of social services as determined by State and area agencies on aging, with priority on in-home services. Also case management, day care, protective services. Separate appropriation for home-delivered meals.	Persons 60 years and over. No means tests, but services are to be targeted on those with social or economic need.	Administration on Aging/Office of Human Development Services/HHS	State agency on aging

a required for individuals over 21
b at option of state
c required for individuals entitled to skilled nursing homecare
d may be offered under a waiver of Medicaid State Plan requirements, if requested by the state and approved by HHS. May include waiver of Medicaid eligibility requirements and stipulation that services be offered on a state wide basis.

Source: O'Shaughnessy, C., R. Price, and J. Griffith. 1985. Financing and delivery of long-term care services for the elderly. Washington, DC: Congressional Research Service, Library of Congress. Pub. no. 85-1033 EPW, pp. XI–XII (17 Oct.).

the direct consequence of its own action" (*Star-Ledger* 1986). Furthermore, administration plans for catastrophic health insurance also appear to be reducing homecare benefits. While Congressman Pepper applauded the administration's concern and efforts to achieve catastrophic health insurance, he also had a complaint. "What disturbs me is that the administration is also cutting back on the most vital element of any catastrophic plan--the homecare benefit"(*Star-Ledger* 1986).

Reimbursement Basics

In discussing policy issues related to financial reimbursement for homecare, Cowart (1985) pointed out the reliance upon the medical diagnosis for payment. She suggests that "redirecting reimbursement from medical diagnosis to nursing diagnosis would allow homecare to change from services for illnesses to services for maintenance and prevention." This raises the everpresent unresolved debate over funding for medical vs. funding for personal/social services.

In a similar approach, Curtiss (1986a) identified three key concepts in home health care reimbursement: the distinction between short- and long-term care; differences between homecare services and products; and distinctions between eligibility, coverage, and payment among reimbursement categories. Short-term acute illness is more likely to be reimbursed as well as the services and products connected with and oriented toward treatment for that specific ailment. Eligibility is generally achieved through payment of premiums or by a means test for governmental benefits. Coverage is defined in the insurance policy or the regulations. Payment issues have to do with billing, claims forms, and the data for those forms. These three concepts are usually involved in any funding mechanism.

Curtiss (1986b) advised homecare providers on a practical approach toward reimbursement to make their ventures successful:

- Don't accept all patients.
- Don't provide all therapies.
- Establish joint venture relationships to share risk and incentives.
- Decentralize billing and patient recordkeeping.
- Submit no more back-up information than required.
- Track coverage and payment decisions.
- Add your name to mailing lists to receive announcements from major carriers and governmental programs.
- Insist on specific reasons for noncoverage determinations.

These pointers tend to emphasize the management aspects of reimbursement and are based on the author's experience in the funding of homecare.

Funding Sources for Homecare

Using data from the 1982 long-term care survey on noninstitutionalized elderly Americans with ADL (activities of daily living) and IDAL (instrumental activities of daily living) limitations, Liu, Manton, and Liu (1985) investigated homecare expenditures. ADL include tasks such as bathing, dressing, and toileting, while IADL tasks are of a lesser order, such as shopping and light housework. People with IADL limitations usually require less assistance with physical tasks, while those with higher ADL scores tend to require greater resources and of a more physical nature. Data about more than 5,500 people were analyzed to determine the source of funding for homecare services. Results indicated that almost 70 percent relied exclusively on nonpaid sources. Even at the highest limitation, ADL 5-6, almost 65 percent relied upon unpaid helpers. However, about 33 percent did combine paid and unpaid homecare helpers. Using only complete information about paid help, 55 percent paid for the care out of their own pockets. Medicare followed at 11 percent and Medicaid at 8 percent. For nursing care, Medicare was the most common funding source at about 39 percent, with self-pay at 16 percent, and Medicaid funding at 15 percent.

Average monthly payments, by limitation, for homecare ranged from $88 to $439, with the average for all persons at $164 per month out-of-pocket. Obviously, the average for all payers is skewed by the fact that half of those surveyed pay less than $40 per month out-of-pocket, while 10 percent report paying more than $400 per month. Exhibit 6-2 gives the source of payment for homecare services by levels of ADL limitations and IADL only. What stands out clearly is the overwhelming percentage of the elderly who pay for services out of their own pockets. Also obvious is the increase in the use of other funding sources as the level of disability increases, while still having almost 35 percent paying out-of-pocket for the care.

Public Health Values and Reimbursement

After being honored as NAHC Member of the Year, Hall (1985) spoke about homecare and the values of public health. He took the concepts of a visit, a skilled nurse, an agency, and an intermediary, and related those terms to today's homecare situation. A visit turned into a "doctored house call with a chart of procedures." *Skilled nursing* now relates to procedures;

Exhibit 6-2 Percent of Individuals with Paid Care,[1] by Payment Source and Limitation Level, United States, 1982

Limitation level	Self	Medicare	Medicaid	Insurance	Helping organization
			Payment Source[2]		
			Percent of persons		
All levels	47.8%	15.4%	8.5%	3.4%	6.7%
IADL only	54.4	6.2	7.1	1.3	7.3
ADL, 1-2	56.0	9.0	6.4	1.4	6.4
ADL, 3-4	42.0	19.2	8.6	4.2	10.1
ADL, 5-6	35.7	28.7	12.3	7.0	4.0

[1] The distribution of payment sources are based only on those cases in which a clear pattern for a person's payment sources can be determined (i.e., the "unknowns" are not included). Hence the frequencies of the specific payment sources could be higher than those presented. For example, an estimated 608,000 were self-paying, yet only 550,000 had complete payment source patterns.

[2] These are not mutually exclusive categories, because an individual may have more than one source of payment.

Note: IADL is for instrumental activities of daily living. ADL is for activities of daily living.

Source: Liu, K., K.G. Manton, and B.M. Liu. 1985. Home care expenses for the disabled elderly. *Health Care Financing Review* 7 (2):53. (winter)

Hall asked, "Who could be more skilled than the nurse who visits terminal patients and *never* performs a procedure?" "The word *agency* included an advocacy role and a commitment to change laws, regulations, and practices that are not right." HCFA and the fiscal intermediaries were accused of bypassing the intent of the public health language in the Medicare legislation and replacing the concepts with "the macho language of those interested in the bottom line, market penetration, and the biggest bang for our buck." Reacting to government organizations and their lack of comprehension of public health values vis-a-vis reimbursement, Hall was emphatic: "We must stop legislation by regulation because it is illegal, immoral, and costly." He was referring mainly to the Medicare program. Since that is the largest funding source for homecare services, it's appropriate to begin there.

Medicare

A home health agency can be reimbursed by Medicare for the following types of services:

- Skilled nursing care by a registered nurse, a licensed practical, or vocational nurse for giving injections, changing bandages, or supervising others caring for the patient.

- Physical therapy to teach the patient special exercises to regain strength and coordination.

- Speech therapy to help people with speaking, hearing, and language problems.

- Occupational therapy to provide activities and exercises to help the patient to resume self-care and normal daily life.

- Medical social services to aid the patient and family to understand problems and to assist with community agencies.

- Home health aides to help with exercise, personal care, meal preparation, and personal cleanliness.

HCFA also illustrates what Medicare will not pay for in its intermediary manual, including the following:

- Services that would not be covered in a hospital, such as 24-hour private duty nursing or television rentals;

- Meals-on-Wheels or some other program that delivers meals to the home;

- Housekeeping chores unrelated to patient care;

- Transportation.

Medicare also covers a range of homecare benefits for terminally ill beneficiaries. These hospice services were authorized in 1982 for individuals with a life expectancy of six months or less. Hospice care can include nursing care, therapy services, medical social services, home health aide services, physician services, counseling, and short-term inpatient care.

Medicare Overview

Medicare was enacted into law on July 30, 1965, as Title XVIII in Health Insurance for the Aged as part of the Social Security Act and became effective on July 1, 1966. This program covers most individuals entitled to Social Security benefits, persons under 65 entitled to federal disability benefits, and certain individuals with end-stage renal disease. With uniform eligibility and benefits throughout the U.S., the federal health insurance is available without regard to income.

Medicare focuses primarily on acute care, particularly hospital and surgical care and accompanying periods of recovery. Part A covers inpatient hospital care, services in a skilled nursing facility, homecare following a hospital stay and hospice care. There are deductibles and coinsurance for hospitalization and SNF care, certain limitations for hospice care; and Part A covers the full cost for homecare. Part B pays for physician services, homecare, outpatient hospital care, and other medical and health services such as laboratory tests, radiology, and dialysis supplies. After an annual deductible, Part B generally pays for 80 percent of approved charges.

Most people are enrolled in Part A automatically while they must choose to enroll in Part B, since there is an additional cost. About 95 percent of those eligible for Part A also elect to participate in Part B. In addition, large numbers of the elderly also purchase insurance from private companies to pay for the lacks in the Medicare coverage--the so called Medi-Gap policies.

Generally, Medicare is not regarded as a program intended to provide support for long-term care. However, Medicare does pay for some community-based long-term care services, mainly home health care services. To qualify for homecare services, beneficiaries must meet the following conditions:

- Be confined to their residences (homebound)

- Need part-time or intermittent skilled nursing care and/or physical and speech therapy

- Be under the care of a physician and have the services prescribed by a physician.

After meeting those criteria, Medicare beneficiaries may receive homecare under either Part A or Part B. Physicians are required to periodically review their written plans for the patient's homecare services.

Covered homecare services, as defined in Title XVIII, include the following:

- Part-time or intermittent skilled nursing care provided by, or under the supervision of, a registered professional nurse

- Physical, occupational, or speech therapy

- Medical social services provided under the direction of a physician

- Medical supplies and equipment (other than drugs and medicines)

- Medical services provided by an intern or resident enrolled in a teaching program in a hospital affiliated or under contract with a home health agency

- Part-time or intermittent services provided by a home health aide, as permitted by regulations.

Services must be provided by a home health agency certified to participate under Medicare following the plan of treatment developed and reviewed by the attending physician. Certification means meeting the federal conditions of participation which define the terms, set standards for personnel and agencies, detail clinical record keeping, and call for evaluation. As of the passage of the Omnibus Budget Reconciliation Act of 1980, there is no statutory limit on the number of home health visits covered by Medicare. Patients are not subject to any cost sharing via deductibles or coinsurance for covered home health services.

Definitions

A number of words used in the Medicare legislation and regulations have caused problems in the implementation of the program, starting with the definition of a home health agency and proceeding to "skilled nursing," "intermittent," "homebound," "intermediary," "part-time," and "reasonable, usual and customary charges." These terms have been used to control the homecare program covered under Medicare, particularly with regard to reimbursement.

Home Health Agency. Under Medicare, a home health agency is defined as a public or private organization primarily engaged in providing skilled nursing and other therapeutic services. Homecare professionals would opt for a definition that speaks to the delivery of comprehensive coordinated services to promote and maintain health. Trager (1980) comments that "What is contained in Title XVIII . . . is not a definition of Home Health Services. It is a description of those services which are selectively covered by the insurance system . . . This description has, however, become, for purposes of program development and service delivery, a publicly supported definition of Home Health Services . . ." In effect, the home health agencies made their programs fit into the federal definition. Emphasis shifted to curative and rehabilitative care with uncoordinated nursing and home health aide services. Services were offered to conform with those reimbursed by Medicare.

Skilled Nursing. In the federal government's homecare manual prepared for fiscal intermediaries, examples are given of the need for infrequent, yet intermittent, skilled nursing services:

- The patient with an indwelling silicone catheter who generally needs a catheter change only at 90-day intervals.

- The person who experiences a fecal impaction due to the normal aging process (i.e., loss of bowel tone, restrictive mobility, and a breakdown in good health habits) and must be manually disimpacted. Although these impactions are likely to recur, it is not possible to pinpoint a specific timeframe.

- The blind diabetic who self-injects insulin may have a medically predictable recurring need for a skilled nursing visit at least every 90 days. These visits, for example, would be to observe and determine the needs for changes in the level and type of care which have been prescribed, thus supplementing the physician's contacts with the patient.

Homecare experts would contend that governmental concepts of skilled nursing stress medically-oriented procedures and not the "caring" aspects. In fact, Hall (1985) commented that there is nothing as skilled as a nursing visit where no medical procedures are performed. Professional nursing includes such services as early identification of health problems, assessment of service needs, health monitoring, counseling, and education. Individuals, particularly those covered by Medicare, may need a nurse merely for reinforcement of care routines, monitoring of medications and diets, or for attention to incipient problems. However, these people could not receive those valid and necessary nursing services according to Medicare definitions of skilled nursing and would have to pay for that care out of their own pockets.

Under skilled nursing supervision, the services of home health aides and others would also be limited to functions similar to those performed in the hospital. Custodial care, such as shopping, cleaning, and cooking, is not reimbursed by Medicare.

Intermittent Care. Medicare manuals define intermittent care as a medically predictable, occasional need for nursing care, usually not less frequent than once every 60 days (Curtiss 1986a). Yovanovich (1985), in testifying before the House Select Committee on Aging, stated that Congress did not define intermittent care, but HCFA guidelines did.

"Under those guidelines, intermittent care would include daily care for a two to three week period and thereafter under 'exceptional circumstances.'" In her testimony before the Senate Subcommittee on Health, Mills (1984) quoted Section 204.1 of HCFA's Health Insurance Manual-11: ". . . Medicare will pay for part-time (as defined in Section 206.6) medically reasonable and necessary skilled nursing care 7 days a week for a *short* period of time (2-3 weeks). . . There may also be a few cases involving unusual circumstances where the patient's prognosis indicates the medical need for daily skilled services will extend beyond 3 weeks . . . A person expected to need more or less full-time skilled nursing care over an extended period of time, i.e. a patient who requires institutionalization, would not usually qualify for home health benefits."

Section 206.6 sets guidelines for length and frequency of different types of visits. Part-time care has been interpreted to mean that health professionals visit the home for less than one hour, with a few exceptions. For home health aides, up to four hours are included.

Although Medicare is supposed to be a uniform national program, fiscal intermediaries interpret the definition of intermittent differently across the country. A beneficiary in California could receive substantially greater homecare benefits than one living in Wisconsin. Some intermediaries consider daily to mean seven days a week, while others set daily at five or even three days a week. Some view the 2-3 week initial period as a guideline and consider extensions on a case-by-case basis. Other fiscal intermediaries are issuing denials for medically necessary daily skilled care beyond the 2-3 week period even if a physician has determined that a patient can be adequately cared for at home, does not need to be hospitalized, and no skilled nursing beds are available.

"Despite Congressional intent to expand homecare as an alternative to institutional care, as evidenced by the 1980 Reconciliation Act, fiscal intermediaries have in recent months issued interpretations of intermittent care which vary widely from state to state and have the effect of depriving Medicare beneficiaries in many states of needed medical services" (Mills 1984).

A report from the Senate Special Committee on Aging (1985,199) also addressed the intermittent care issue. Problems were traced back to the 1982 HCFA transmittal to fiscal intermediaries about the 2-3 week period. Three situations were noted: ineligibility after 2-3 weeks with claims denied retroactively; daily care ordered by physicians denied; and depending upon interpretations, the "administration of the home health benefit had become inconsistent and somewhat arbitrary. Beneficiaries with illnesses were receiving care for an extended period of time in some regions of the country, but not in others."

Several bills were introduced into Congress to define intermittent care. One bill would specifically allow daily nursing and home health aide visits for up to 90 days upon a physician's monthly certification, and after that under exceptional circumstances. Legislation of this nature did not pass, although Congress did consider the matter and debated its implications.

At a Senate Select Committee on Aging hearing in Newark, N.J., speakers told the Senators that intermittent care had been redefined, so that many who previously received care are now deemed too sick for home benefits (*American Medical News* 1986). A month later Marosy spoke for the New Jersey Health Care Coalition: "The main restriction on Medicare home health care is the intermittent care restriction" (*Star-Ledger* 1986a).

On the other side, the Inspector General's (IG) semiannual report to Congress stated that intermittent home health care visits cost Medicare more than full-time care in skilled nursing facilities (*Provider* 1986a). Using 23,000 cases from 1983 data, the IG found that homecare monthly payments exceeded nursing home care by $17 million. In 2,371 cases, payments were made for beneficiaries receiving 60 visits in one month, an average of two home visits per day. As a result of these findings, the IG recommended increased oversight by HCFA to reduce overutilization of homecare.

Homebound. HCFA manuals say that homebound usually means that the person is unable to leave the home without considerable taxing effort. A person may be considered homebound if absences from the home are infrequent, of relatively short duration, and do not indicate that the patient has the capacity to obtain health care provided outside rather than in the home. A patient may be confined to the home, but not necessarily bedridden (Curtiss 1986a).

A witness testifying before the House Select Committee on Aging told Congressman Pepper that two people assist her to a dialysis center for treatment three times a week. That is the only time she leaves the home. She is a blind, diabetic, wheelchair-bound amputee with renal failure. Joann Cooper told the panel she was denied home health coverage on the grounds that she was not "homebound" (*Star-Ledger* 1986). In another example, the New Jersey Health Care Coalition cited the case of an elderly woman recovering from a stroke but able to remain at home under her 69-year-old husband's care. She was declared ineligible for homecare benefits because she visited an adult day care center twice a week and was therefore not "homebound" (*Star-Ledger* 1986).

A HCFA survey (*Hospital Week* 1985) reported that as much as 30 percent of home health care services should not have been covered, despite only a 3 percent denial rate in 1984. In addition to care determined to be custodial as a reason, HCFA also cited inadequate support to show homebound status for noncoverage rationales. Curtiss (1986b) anticipates stricter scrutiny of homebound coverage criteria by HCFA in the future.

Fiscal Intermediary. A fiscal intermediary processes the home health agency bills for the federal government. Blue Cross plans are the most frequent intermediaries, with other private insurance companies also participating. Intermediaries assist in the billing process, consult with home health agencies, conduct audits, and do evaluations to insure adherence to regulations. Home health agencies are concerned that retroactive denials of bills by intermediaries may result in actual dollar losses since the individual may not be able to pay out of his or her own pocket for the services already rendered. Under this system, the home health agency has to decide whether or not to provide a questionable service based on the probability of reimbursement or possible denial six months later.

Reduction to no more than 10 intermediaries from the existing 47 was mandated by the Deficit Reduction Act of 1984 to take place before July 1, 1987. Congress passed that legislation to assure greater uniformity in interpretation of Medicare home health policy throughout the country. HCFA announced the designated regional intermediaries in the *Federal Register* on April 10, 1985. Criteria for selection included electronic data processing capability and past performance as measured by HCFA relative to utilization determinations, application of reimbursement principles, provider relations, and a number of other factors. Speaking for the American Federation of Home Health Agencies and the National Association for Home Care, Yovanovich (1985) protested that 4 of the 10 selected intermediaries apparently did not have the ability to process bills electronically. In addition, he noted that several of the selected intermediaries service only a relative handful of agencies. Questions were also raised about subcontracting, the actual ratings of intermediaries selected and those not selected, and omitting the provider-based agencies while including the freestanding home health agencies. Provider-based agencies will continue to be served by the intermediary of the parent provider, be it hospital, nursing home, hospice, etc.

HCFA approximated that 2,400 freestanding agencies would be reassigned to a different regional intermediary. Curtiss (1986b) says it is likely that HCFA will follow suit with the provider-based agencies after the transition of the freestanding agencies takes place. Designated regional intermediaries, as noted in the April 10, 1985 *Federal Register*, follow:

- Maine Blue Cross (Associated Hospital Service of Maine) for the Northeast (Connecticut, Maine, Massachusetts, New Hampshire, Rhode Island, Vermont);

- Prudential Insurance Co. (New York, New Jersey, Virgin Islands, Puerto Rico);

- Blue Cross of Greater Philadelphia for the East (District of Columbia, Delaware, Maryland, Pennsylvania, Virginia, West Virginia);

- Blue Cross and Blue Shield of South Carolina for the Southeast (Kentucky, North Carolina, South Carolina, Tennessee);

- Aetna Life and Casualty Company for the South (Alabama, Florida, Georgia, Mississippi);

- Blue Cross and Blue Shield of Michigan for the Midwest (Indiana, Michigan, Ohio);

- Illinois Blue Cross (Health Care Service Corporation) for the Midwest (Illinois, Minnesota, Wisconsin);

- New Mexico Blue Cross and Blue Shield for the Central South (Arkansas, Louisiana, New Mexico, Oklahoma, Texas);

- Blue Cross of Iowa for the West (Colorado, Iowa, Kansas, Missouri, Montana, Nebraska, North Dakota, South Dakota, Utah, Wyoming);

- Blue Cross of California for the Pacific (Alaska, Arizona, California, Hawaii, Idaho, Nevada, Oregon, Washington).

Reasonable, Usual, and Customary Charges. Traditionally, in reimbursement schemes the health care provider is paid a fee-for-service based upon his/her reasonable, usual, and customary charges (RUC). A reasonable charge cannot exceed the actual charge for the service, the customary charge, or the prevailing charge for the service in the community. A number of plans calculate the reimbursement using a percentage of the RUC charge for the actual payment. Since Medicare regulations now figure reimbursement at a percentage of reasonable costs, most agencies do not care to even guess at the customary cost figure. Apparently, it is common policy to use the RUC charges as the initial database upon which to determine a percentage for the cash reimbursement.

Budget Stimulation

Much of the cost containment activity in Medicare has been stimulated by budgetary actions, starting with the forecast of doom for the Hospital Insurance Trust Fund (HITF) (Pettengill 1985; Pear 1985). Reacting to the possible bankruptcy of the HITF, there was a spurt of cost-cutting activity, including the introduction of the Medicare PPS/DRG program. However, the Medicare trust fund seemed to recover, and predictions indicated solvency at least until the turn of the century (Pear 1985). However, Pettengill (1985,24) concludes that there are two points of view. One side argues for a general solution to the cost difficulties in the health care delivery system rather than a concentration on Medicare. On the other, attention is called to the rapid changes already being affected by cost containment initiatives and the need to await evaluation of those changes. Besides, the argument goes, the trust fund is not in imminent danger, and it may be desirable to see the results before embarking on any additional major reforms.

O'Sullivan (1985) reviewed the federal FY 1986 Medicare budget for distribution to members of Congress. Two items related to homecare: restructuring home health cost limits and the imposition of a copayment for a home health visit.

Home Health Cost Limits. Reimbursement for home health services has been limited to the 75th percentile of the average costs per visit incurred by all home health agencies. Separate limits were established for each type of service (skilled nursing, home health aide, physical therapy, etc.). However, the limits were applied in the aggregate to each home health agency based on its mix of services. Revision of the home health cost limits is proposed in the Reagan administration's budget proposal. HCFA issued regulations on July 5, 1985, applying the limits to each type of service and changing the 75th percentile limit to 120 percent of the mean of per visit costs. In addition, HCFA set goals of 115 percent for 1986 and 112 percent for 1987. It is estimated that this cost containment measure could reduce outlays by $5 million in 1985, $70 million in 1986, and $120 million in 1990, with a total from 1986-90 of $480 million.

Exhibit 6-3 shows per visit limits with the labor and nonlabor portions indicated as per a final notice in the *Federal Register* relative to the 115 percent effective for 1986. Additionally, Exhibit 6-3 gives the approximately 10-15 percent add-on amounts for hospital-based home health agencies as they continue to receive higher reimbursement than the freestanding agencies (*Federal Register* May 30, 1986). In the earlier notice on cost limits, HCFA stated that "more than 70 percent of the HHAs in our data base would exceed these limits in at least one discipline" unless the behavior of affected HHAs changes (*Federal Register* 1985,27748). Management and cost reporting behavior changes anticipated by HCFA included closer review of salaries, staffing levels, staff productivity, time on site per visit, travel time, and administrative costs. Under the aggregated costing limits, about 20 percent of the agencies exceed the limits (Curtiss 1986b).

In addition, HCFA (*Federal Register* March 25, 1986) opted for use of their survey-based wage index in establishing the schedule of cost limits. It was estimated that 36 percent (2,148) of the home health agencies would be disadvantaged and 48 percent (2,865) would gain from the new wage index. "Nevertheless, we (HCFA) estimate that the effect of the new wage index on total annual payments to all HHAs would be negligible because in the aggregate, increased and decreased payments would offset each other."

Exhibit 6-3 Medicare 1987 per Visit Limits for Home Health Agencies and Add-on Amounts for Hospital-based Agencies

Type of Visit	Home Health Agencies			Add-On Amount ($)	Hospital-based HHAs	
	Cost Limit ($)	Labor Portion ($)	Nonlabor Portion ($)		Labor Portion ($)	Nonlabor Portion ($)
Metropolitan Statistical Area Location						
Skilled-nursing care	$52.27	$41.31	$10.96	$6.11	$4.78	$1.33
Physical therapy	50.14	39.61	10.53	5.16	4.00	1.16
Speech pathology	56.79	44.82	11.97	6.20	4.82	1.38
Occupational therapy	52.73	41.37	11.36	5.37	4.13	1.24
Medical social services	78.37	61.36	17.01	8.51	6.57	1.94
Home health aide	33.76	26.60	7.16	3.91	3.06	.85
Rural Location						
Skilled-nursing care	57.43	47.49	9.94	6.36	5.25	1.11
Physical therapy	59.52	49.34	10.18	6.39	5.28	1.11
Speech pathology	68.71	56.69	12.02	8.31	6.83	1.48
Occupational therapy	64.69	53.16	11.33	6.20	5.15	1.05
Medical social services	81.42	67.44	13.98	11.65	9.60	2.05
Home health aide	33.77	27.89	5.88	4.09	3.38	.71

Source: *Federal Register.* 1986. Schedule of limits on home health agency costs per visit for cost reporting periods beginning on or after July 1, 1986, but before July 1, 1987. Final notice. 51(104): 19734-19741 (30 May).

Homecare trade associations reacted to the cost limits, claiming that HCFA assumed that agencies operated inefficiently, that agencies would have to drop over-cap services, that trained employees would have to be dropped, and that the beneficiaries would be hurt (Thietten 1985; Pettey 1985). Concentrated efforts are aiming at promoting legislation to allow HHAs to apply their cost limits on an aggregate rather than per discipline basis, and to end the add-on for hospital-based HHAs.

Copayment for Home Visit. Currently, home health services are not subject to coinsurance charges. Budget documents note that homecare is essentially the only Medicare service not subject to cost sharing (*Home Health Journal* 1986b). An amount equal to one percent of the inpatient hospital deductible is proposed in the administration budget to be applied to all home visits after the 20th visit in a calendar year. Copayment is estimated at $4.80 in 1986. Budget analysts expect a savings of $50 million in FY 1986, going up to $150 million in FY 1990, with a total of $590 million saved from FY 1986-1990. This copayment "is intended to insure more cost conscious utilization of this service by beneficiaries" (O'Sullivan 1985a,14,19). According to HCFA's Dr. Henry Desmarias, "approximately one-third of all home health care services since the late 1970s should have been denied as medically unnecessary or not covered by the Medicare program" (*Home Health Journal* 1986c). Sharp opposition to the copayment came from the homecare trade associations as well as from the AARP. Buddi (1985) told the House Subcommittee on Health that Medicare beneficiaries would suffer from the additional financial burden added to the already existing deductibles and coinsurance in the Medicare program. Possibly, elderly patients would forego needed homecare because of the copayment rather than incur additional debt. Furthermore, the projected savings could be dissipated by the fact that the home health agencies could be reimbursed for uncollected copayments under the bad debt provisions of the Medicare regulations. Collection of the copayment would also place an administrative burden on the home health agencies. Yovanovich (1985) made similar comments before the House Select Committee on Aging.

After emphasizing the detailed amounts that the elderly have to spend out of their own pockets for health care, the AARP representative summed it up for the House Subcommittee on Health. "This proposal would penalize those who use a less costly form of care" *Home Health Journal* 1986c).

In view of the attention to cost and utilization, an examination of homecare reimbursement expenditures in the Medicare program may elucidate the issues and problems.

Reimbursement Expenditures

Medicare expenditures for home health care services have remained fairly constant over the years, ranging between 1 and 3 percent of total Medicare outlays (Exhibit 6-4). Despite the small percent, the total dollars increased dramatically from $78 million in 1969 to almost $2 billion in 1984. Home health visits followed suit, moving from 8.5 million in 1969 to more than 40 million in 1984.

Considerable variation occurs among the states in their Medicare reimbursements (Exhibit 6-5). Alaska received only $335,000, while California, Florida, New York, and Pennsylvania all received more than $125 million; California was tops with $177 million in Medicare money. Mississippi and Vermont each got almost $2,000 in visit charges per person served, while New Hampshire and Vermont were lowest with under $500 per person served.

Proprietary home health agencies incurred the highest total charges per person served ($1,635), the highest average number of visits per person served (31.9), and were two dollars less than the highest average charge per visit ($51). At the other extreme, the governmental homecare agencies totaled $812 per person, 22.6 visits, and $36 per visit (Exhibit 6-6).

Although Medicare is a national program, Benjamin's (1986) research indicates wide variations in expenditures and utilization across the states. "HHA supply, case mix severity, costs of inputs and the availability of alternatives emerge as important in understanding variations in average expenditures per user across states. Population need, HHA supply, and the presence of service alternatives and sources of referrals are the most significant correlates of state differences in home health utilization. . . Among these findings, perhaps the most striking is the consistently strong role played by supply factors in explaining both utilization and expenditures."

Applying the 3 percent of total Medicare expenditures to budget projections from 1986 through 1990 (O'Sullivan 1985a,21), the annual costs for homecare for those years is respectively $2.3, $2.6, $2.9, $3.2, and $3.5 billion for 1990.

With the restrictive interpretations of skilled nursing, intermittent care and homebound, budget actions to curtail cost limits and to install a copayment, as well as the projected budget increases in homecare expenditures tied to rising utilization, HCFA is also attempting to curb waivers of liability and to uphold denials of payments.

Waiver of Liability for Home Health Agencies

Under current regulations, if a home health agency has 2.5 percent or less of its billed covered visits disallowed in any calendar quarter, the presumption is made that the agency has knowledge of program instructions and

Exhibit 6-4 Medicare Utilization of Home Health Agency Services, Total Medicare Reimbursement, Reimbursement for Home Health Services, and Number of Home Health Visits, Selected Years 1969 -1984

	Total Medicare Reimbursement		Home Health Agency Reimbursement			Home Health Visits	
Year	Amount (in millions)	Percent change	Amount (in millions)	Percent change	As percent of total Medicare reimbursement	Number (In millions)	Percent change
1969	$ 6,284.0	---	$ 78.1	---	1.24%	8.5	---
1973	9,637.8	17.3	92.9	40.8	.96	6.4	22.4
1977	20,890.5	17.2	366.5	24.4	1.75	15.6	15.6
1980	33,389.4	18.1	770.7	19.5	1.92	22.11	10.2
1983	55,589.0	13.1	1,657.0	31.0	2.9	36.8	19.4
1984	63,100.0	13.5	1,982.0	23.0	3.1	40.3	9.5

Source: Department of Health and Human Services. Health Care Financing Administration. Variety of material. Data for more recent years are less complete.

Exhibit 6-5 Medicare Home Health Agency Services: Reimbursement by State, 1984

Geographic Area	Total Reimbursement	
	Amount (in thousands)	Visit Charges Per Person Served
Alabama	$ 33,213	$1,536
Alaska	335	1,737
Arizona	9,732	970
Arkansas	12,559	1,111
California	177,033	1,268
Colorado	16,905	1,129
Connecticut	31,234	1,059
Delaware	5,826	1,314
District of Columbia	4,171	657
Florida	148,417	1,522
Georgia	30,784	1,526
Hawaii	3,494	1,237
Idaho	6,514	1,133
Illinois	73,657	1,261
Indiana	19,288	853
Iowa	7,844	567
Kansas	14,034	987
Kentucky	13,269	826
Louisiana	35,685	1,614
Maine	6,120	766
Maryland	27,496	822
Massachusetts	49,945	960
Michigan	58,947	1,231
Minnesota	9,920	697
Mississippi	45,388	1,972
Missouri	54,730	1,287
Montana	3,026	870
Nebraska	7,103	823
Nevada	3,800	1,199
New Hampshire	4,811	452
New Jersey	62,222	1,042
New Mexico	6,281	995
New York	126,649	1,300
North Carolina	29,317	858
North Dakota	1,943	846
Ohio	43,299	813
Oklahoma	14,319	952
Oregon	19,293	1,178
Pennsylvania	143,587	1,265
Rhode Island	9,541	947
South Carolina	21,561	1,071
South Dakota	1,232	510
Tennessee	62,806	1,965
Texas	96,367	1,507
Utah	5,707	1,339
Vermont	3,138	411
Virginia	23,930	1,020
Washington	25,077	1,047
West Virginia	10,788	993
Wisconsin	23,447	847
Wyoming	2,633	1,424
	$1,648,406	$1,215

Source: Department of Health and Human Services. Health Care Financing Administration. Division of Program Studies. Office of Research. Unpublished data, March 5, 1986.

Exhibit 6-6 Medicare Home Health Agency Services: Visits and Charges by Type of Visit and Type of Agency, 1984

Visits and Charges by Type of Visit, 1984	All[1] Agencies	Visiting Nurse Association	Combined Government and Voluntary	Government	Hospital-based	Proprietary	Private Nonprofit	Other[1]
Average Number of Visits per Person Served								
Total[2]	26.6	25.8	20.5	22.6	21.9	31.9	30.0	27.8
Nursing Care	13.8	13.5	11.0	11.8	12.2	15.7	15.2	14.4
Home Health Aide	22.1	21.8	19.6	24.0	18.1	22.7	23.9	20.1
Physical Therapy	10.7	9.9	10.7	9.4	9.3	12.1	12.2	11.7
Other[3]	6.6	6.7	7.3	8.4	5.9	6.3	6.8	8.3
Percent of HHA Clientele Receiving Specified Type of Visit								
Nursing Care	93.3%	94.0%	95.9%	95.3%	93.8%	91.4%	92.2%	85.5%
Home Health Aide	41.6	39.3	32.2	35.9	35.4	52.2	44.4	43.8
Physical Therapy	30.4	31.1	25.9	21.5	30.2	34.4	31.4	41.3
Other[3]	20.0	21.3	11.6	8.7	20.0	24.5	22.1	24.7

Exhibit 6-6 continued

Visits and Charges by Type of Visit, 1984	All¹ Agencies	Visiting Nurse Association	Combined Government and Voluntary	Government	Hospital-based	Proprietary	Private Nonprofit	Other¹
Average Charge Per Visit								
Total²	$46	$40	$42	$36	$53	$51	$48	$55
Nursing Care	50	45	47	41	57	56	52	59
Home Health Aide	39	32	32	28	45	46	42	51
Physical Therapy	52	46	48	41	60	55	53	60
Other³	54	50	49	44	63	58	55	60
Total Charges Incurred per Person Served								
Total²	$1,216	$1,037	$857	$812	$1,163	$1,635	$1,440	$1,544
Nursing Care	691	612	517	487	703	876	787	852
Home Health Aide	855	689	629	676	819	1,046	1,009	1,018
Physical Therapy	555	463	517	384	563	672	653	695
Other³	360	335	352	368	374	365	372	502

1. Includes rehabilitation and skilled nursing facility agencies not shown separately.
2. Detail does not add to total since persons may receive more than one type of service.
3. Includes speech or occupational therapy, medical social services, and other health disciplines.
Source: Department of Health and Human Services. Health Care Financing Administration. Division of Program Studies. Office of Research. Unpublished data. March 5, 1986.

exercises due care in rendering covered care. HCFA then allows those HHAs to be reimbursed for acting in good faith to provide services found not to be covered at a later date. "This presumption is important because predicting coverage decisions is very difficult for home health, as shown by the fact that 32.4 percent of home health claim denials are subsequently reversed" (Pettey 1985). In fact, in supporting the preservation of the waiver of liability for HHAs, the American Public Health Association (Daubert 1985) resolution noted that the regulations, guidelines, directives, and memos do not usually clearly and consistently convey coverage policy.

HCFA attempted to eliminate the presumption of waiver of liability in proposed rules in the *Federal Register* on February 12, 1985 and again on February 21, 1986. Under HCFA's new proposals, liability would be handled on a claim-by-claim basis "without the general assumption that the provider did not know or could not be expected to know that the services were not covered" (Curtiss 1986b). Not covered usually means that services were not reasonable and necessary or constituted custodial care.

There was reaction from the homecare trade associations, who argued that HHAs would have to be much more selective in accepting patients; paperwork would be increased enormously; claims processing would be slowed down; costs to intermediaries and agencies would increase; subjective determinations by intermediaries would continue; and in the end, the Medicare beneficiary would suffer (Daubert 1985; Lenz 1985; Pettey 1985; Yovanovich 1985). Congressman Edward Roybal attacked HCFA's actions as "an affront to Congress's stated objection to dropping the waiver and jeopardizes the elderly patient's ability to get the nursing home and home health care they need" (*Provider* 1986b).

HCFA efforts to eliminate the waiver of liability for home health agencies have been derailed. Both the House and the Senate approved retention of the 2.5 percent waiver of liability provision in the budget reconciliation meetings (*Home Health Journal* 1986d). Congressional revisions call for HCFA to maintain the waiver "until 12 months after the date on which the 10 regional intermediaries have commenced operations to service home health agencies."

Denials

In responding to questions from the House Select Committee on Aging (1985,10-11,26), HHS responded that there has been only a slight increase in denial of home health agency claims expressed as a percentage of claims processed; from 1984 to 1985, the percentage went from 1.6 to 2.0. On appeal, HHS reported 21.1 percent reversals in 1985. This contrasts with the 32.4 percent claimed by the homecare trade associations.

A rule in a Medicare evaluation of carriers may be causing denials with greater frequency (*Medical Economics* 1986). "For every $1 a carrier receives to process claims, it's expected to deny at least $5 in claims." "Intermediaries who fail to meet this standard are in danger of losing their contract with the government" (*American Medical News* 1986). Yovanovich (1985) stated that the FY 1985 HCFA contractual mandate also ordered intermediaries to subject at least 37.5 percent of all claims to medical review. In addition, he expected the $5 return and the medical reviews to increase in the future. Connecticut and New Jersey use legal teams to appeal denials of home health care benefits by Medicare intermediaries. New Jersey's Human Services Commissioner, Geoffrey Perselay, told a Senate Select Committee on Aging that his state will fight back against an intensive HCFA effort to deny care "to some of the sickest individuals with the highest care needs" (*American Medical News* 1986).

In response to critics, HCFA is preparing a series of model denial notices for use by Peer Review Organizations (PROs). These sample denials will explain in accurate and easily understandable terms the rationale for noncoverage of a home health agency's service currently or in the future (*Home Health Journal* 1986e).

Medicare's Future

According to former HHS Secretary Margaret M. Heckler (1985), "Medicare is a social contract this government has made with the elderly and disabled. It is not a welfare program. . . We have a duty to ensure that these benefits are secure for each eligible American when he or she turns 65 or becomes disabled."

In the June 1986 issue of *Provider*, the theme was "Medicare. A Dream Lost?" Articles dealt with the lessons of Medicare's history, the DRG challenge, the effects of policies upon reimbursement, the quality of care, cost containment, and solutions to problems after the dream.

Is Medicare a dream lost? If not lost, there is still no denying that the original dream requires considerable alteration. To that point, a Harvard Medicare Project reported on the future of Medicare (Blumenthal, Schlesinger, Drumheller, et al. 1986). More than 40 recommendations emerged to be implemented within the next 10 to 15 years dealing with physicians, administrative simplification, hospital payments, prepaid health care, and beneficiaries. In reference to homecare, the report proposed that "Medicare provide more generous coverage of long-term care in outpatient settings, especially of home health care and mental health services." Researchers noted that 10 to 30 percent of the elderly in nursing homes are there because they could not find adequate outpatient care.

Critics have accused the federal government of trying to dismantle Medicare's home health care benefit (*Home Health Journal* 1986), seen in the waiver removal efforts; the restrictive intermittent and homebound interpretations; technical denials of payment; bonding and escrow requirements;

reduction of fiscal intermediaries; disallowing appropriate administrative costs; poorly designed forms; and coverage for benefits. As a result of the tight homecare policy, Senator Frank Lautenberg says that money will not be saved and that, "The policy shows a lack of compassion" (*American Medical News* 1986). Vladeck (1986) also stated that, by regulation, HCFA was slashing reimbursement for homecare. This happened despite the original Congressional intent to provide care, the existence of statutory Medicare entitlements, and the fact that the 15 percent of Medicare beneficiaries (who account for more than 25 percent of the total long-term care expenses) are eligible for both Medicare and Medicaid.

Senator Bill Bradley held hearings in New Jersey to evaluate Medicare homecare programs (*Star-Ledger* May 22, 1986). Senator Bradley detailed his new bill, the Medicare Home Care Improvement Act, designed to prevent HCFA from restricting eligibility for homecare services. Bradley said that HCFA, "through a variety of administrative mechanisms, has made it very difficult--and frequently impossible--for elderly patients to receive the homecare services that they need and are entitled to under Medicare."

In a time of cost containment and austerity, liberalization of benefits under Medicare is problematic. Undoubtedly, there will be many suggestions for reforming Medicare emanating from a variety of concerned sources, including Congress. At the official signing into law of the Medicare program, President Lyndon Johnson put it succinctly: "No longer will older Americans be denied the healing miracle of modern medicine. No longer will illness crush and destroy the savings that have so carefully been put away over a period of time so that they might enjoy dignity in their later years" (Hartwell 1986).

Medicaid

Medicaid, Title XIX of the Social Security Act, is a joint federal/state program providing medical assistance for certain low-income people. Coverage must be provided to all recipients of Aid to Families with Dependent Children (AFDC), most beneficiaries of Supplemental Security Income (SSI), and people in programs for the blind, the disabled, and the aged. Each state administers its own program subject to federal guidelines, but each state has wide latitude in determining eligibility, scope of benefits, administration, and reimbursement. Program costs are shared between the federal government and the states based on per capita income in each state. Sharing ranges from a minimum of 50 percent in high per capita income states to 78 percent in low per capita states.

States must provide Medicaid benefits to cover hospital and skilled nursing facility care, home health care physician services, laboratory, X-ray, and family planning services. They must also cover early and periodic screening, diagnosis, and treatment of children under 21, and rural clinic services. At the state's option, additional services such as outpatient prescription drugs, dental care, eyeglasses, prosthetic devices, and care for patients over 65 in tuberculosis and mental institutions can be added.

Federal Medicaid law does not define "home health services." However, Medicaid regulations require the states to include a minimum range of home health services in their state medical assistance plans. Services include intermittent or part-time nursing care, home health aide services, and medical supplies and equipment. Optionally, states can offer audiology, occupational, physical, and speech therapy. Regulations specify that services will be provided upon written recommendation of a physician and that the plans have to be reviewed every 60 days.

Medicaid programs generally follow Medicare's example in requiring that home health agencies meet the federal conditions of participation. Legislation itself does not define "home health agency."

In the cost containment surge, many states utilize restrictions similar to Medicare's. More than 75 percent of the states limit part-time nursing services, home health aide care, medical supplies and equipment, and physical, occupational, and speech therapy (Feldblum 1985). Some states require that prior authorization be granted to home health care providers to assure reimbursement. Most commonly, limits are placed on the number of visits or hours of service to be rendered by nurses and home health aides. Additionally, reimbursement rates set by the states may be lower than Medicare's for similar services, causing providers to limit or not accept Medicaid patients.

Homecare services reimbursed under Medicaid have not thrived for a few major reasons:

- State policies are restrictive and services are limited.

- Reimbursement dollars for homecare services are extremely low in some states.

- Increases in Title XX monies have directly affected the expansion of Medicaid homecare services.

Medicaid Homecare Expenditures

Homecare expenditures constitute a small part of the Medicaid budget compared with the more than 40 percent that goes for nursing home care, more than $10 billion in 1984. From 1974 to 1983, homecare expenditures went from $13 million to $600 million, under 2 percent of total Medicaid outlays. In only 11 states did home health benefits exceed more than 1 percent of the total Medicaid expenditures. New York State alone accounted for nearly 80 percent of total Medicaid home health costs (O'Shaughnessy 1985,15). Using the 2 percent estimate for homecare services, Medicaid homecare expenditures can go from $840 million in 1985, to more than $1 billion in 1988 (O'Sullivan 1985b,5). Exhibit 6-7 shows the variations among the states in Medicaid vendor payments for 1984. Expenditures ranged from Oklahoma's $8,159 to New York's $522,958,000.

A study by Liu, Manton, and Liu (1985) showed that Medicaid was the source of payment for a small percentage of all paid helpers and nursing helpers: 8.1 and 14.8 percent respectively.

Section 2176 Waivers

In 1981, Congress enacted legislation that allowed HHS to reimburse states for a broadened range of community-based services by waiving certain Medicaid requirements. Specifically, Section 2176 of the Omnibus Budget Reconciliation Act of 1981 authorizes the HHS Secretary to approve 2176 waivers. Under the waivers, states can provide a variety of community-based and home services for individuals who would require the level of care provided in a skilled nursing facility or intermediate care facility without such services. HCFA can waive two specific Medicaid requirements: one, that Medicaid services be available throughout a state; and two, that covered services be equal in amount, duration, and scope for certain Medicaid recipients. States then have flexibility to provide 2176 services in only a portion of the state and selected services to particular eligible Medicaid groups. In addition, more liberal Medicaid income eligibility rules can be extended to waiver participants.

Services can also extend beyond medical and medically-related care to include social/personal services. Importantly, case management can also be provided. Case management is commonly understood to be a system having a designated person or organization responsible for locating, coordinating, and monitoring a group of services for a specific individual. Homemaker-home health aide and chore services, adult day health care, rehabilitation services, and respite care are also included under the waiver. Other services may be offered if the states can show that the additional care would be cost effective and necessary to prevent institutionalization.

Due to the possibility of skyrocketing costs, the legislation also requires that states demonstrate that the costs of services for individuals receiving home and community-based services not exceed the cost to Medicaid of care in institutions.

A report from the Queen's Medical Center (1985) in Honolulu, Hawaii, reported on the use of a 2176 Medicaid waiver to establish a foster family to care for individuals in need of intermediate care. Under the waiver, the Hawaii State Medicaid Program supplements the income of eligible clients for personal care and homemaker services provided by the foster family,

Exhibit 6-7 Medicaid Medical Vendor Payments for Home Health Services by Locality, FY 1984

Locality	Amount
Alabama	$ 8,468,659
Alaska	41,097
Arizona (no Medicaid program)	
Arkansas	2,667,400
California	4,565,544
Colorado	11,609,462
Connecticut	6,331,219
Delaware	1,016,722
District of Columbia	4,075,980
Florida	21,177,263
Georgia	19,197,740
Hawaii	366,760
Idaho	389,981
Illinois	19,431,482
Indiana	2,138,613
Iowa	1,878,426
Kansas	892,009
Kentucky	15,809,657
Louisiana	2,263,067
Maine	5,236,331
Maryland	6,641,515
Massachusetts	21,534,239
Michigan	5,938,535
Minnesota	5,292,285
Mississippi	1,923,664
Missouri	1,756,102
Montana	289,123
Nebraska	1,320,582
Nevada	2,006,412
New Hampshire	529,052
New Jersey	17,197,303
New Mexico	1,069,571
New York	522,958,000
North Carolina	5,567,848
North Dakota	1,918,625
Ohio	2,184,317
Oklahoma	8,159
Oregon	406,242
Pennsylvania	3,251,481
Rhode Island	683,930
South Carolina	1,860,565
South Dakota	4,330,054
Tennessee	5,026,197
Texas	1,612,026
Utah	384,545
Vermont	1,602,075
Virginia	5,532,340
Washington	4,584,915
West Virginia	451,503
Wisconsin	9,383,619
Wyoming	42,450
Puerto Rico	0
Virgin Islands	12,469
	$764,847,155

Source: Department of Health and Human Services. Health Care Financing Administration. Medicaid data Fiscal Year 1984.

and the case management services provided by the Queen's Medical Center. In six years of operation, the program served 133 clients. Investigators concluded that "foster family care appears to be a less costly, quality alternative to nursing home placement for some ICF patients."

An evaluation of Connecticut's Medicaid 2176 waiver program (Ycatts, Steinhardt, and Capitman 1985) in Fairfield County looked at the cost and effectiveness of the activity. Components of the program included preadmission screening, assessment, care plan development, and case management. While the findings were tentative because of extraneous factors, the researchers did conclude that the 2176 program helped to reduce nursing home use; did serve some clients who would otherwise have to be institutionalized, and cost Medicaid about 50 percent less per waiver client than nursing home client.

States may be cautious in requesting 2176 waivers because adequate assurances have to be presented supporting the decreased state expenditures. Homecare cost savings have been open to debate, and the question involves many complex issues. Additionally, states may be reluctant to provide services that could increase their costs of sharing in the federal Medicaid program. These issues surfaced in 1984 as states encountered lengthy delays in gaining waiver approval and HCFA asked some states to meet arbitrary cost reductions not required by the law (Senate Special Committee on Aging 1985,201). On the other hand, HCFA contends that there was a gradual tightening up of management and accountability relative to 2176 criteria and no substantial change in regulations.

Waivers are a small Medicaid program with under $200 million allocated for FY 1985. Most of the 2176 Medicaid waivers are for fewer than 500 persons located in limited geographic areas. As of June 30, 1985, HCFA had approved 107 waivers in 46 states (O'Shaughnessy, Price and Griffith 1985,23). However, only nine regular waivers were approved in 1984, as opposed to the first two years when states enthusiastically responded (Senate Special Committee on Aging 1985,200). Responding to questions from the House Select Committee on Aging (1985,7-9) later in that year, HHS stated that the final regulations published in the *Federal Register* on March 13, 1985 will not decrease state participation in the 2176 waiver program. In fact, HHS said that there was a 25 percent increase in waiver applications. From July 1, 1984 through June 26, 1985, 30 waivers were approved, 10 withdrawn and 16 disapproved; 30 were for new programs and 20 were for extension of existing waivers.

In talking about the 1987 federal budget, HHS Secretary Bowen (*Home Health Journal* 1986b) commented on the Medicaid 2176 waiver program. He said they were "highly successful programs that allow older and disabled persons on Medicaid to receive less costly home and community-based care instead of going into a nursing home." Nevertheless, there are critical questions that have to be resolved regarding the waiver activities.

Does the program identify and serve those people who would otherwise have to enter an institution? Does the program improve the quality of life and care for the individual on home and/or community care? Does the individual use fewer services and avoid hospitalization? Are the home and community care services substitutes or merely add-ons? Does home and community care cost less than nursing home care? These questions are similar to those considered by Weissert, Wan, Liveratos, et al. (1980) in the well-discussed comparison study of homemaker and day care services to the chronically ill (*Home Health Care Services Quarterly* 1980.

Federal legislation has liberalized the 2176 Medicaid waiver program and states may have more opportunity to engage in innovative approaches. What remains to be seen is if the Medicaid program will extend the homecare benefit to significant numbers of people.

Social Services Block Grant--Title XX

Title XX providing for federal/state social service programs to the aged, disabled, and children was implemented in 1975, after Congressional passage the prior year. In 1981, the Omnibus Budget Reconciliation Act (PL 97-35) significantly changed Title XX, reformulating it into a Social Services Block Grant (SSBG), reducing the budget, and making the program entirely federally funded (Blancato 1986). States were given much more freedom in determining the population to be served and the kinds of services to be provided. PL 97-35 eliminated requirements that states expend a portion of funds for welfare recipients; that services be limited to families with incomes below 115 percent of the state median income; and that fees be charged to persons with specified income levels. Previous state planning requirements were lessened, but the law still requires states to develop and make public a report on how funds are to be used, prior to the state plan period, including the types of activities to be funded and the characteristics of the individuals to be served. States are allowed considerable discretion in providing services as long as the services are structured to meet the following goals: achieving or maintaining economic self-support and self-sufficiency; preventing or remedying neglect, abuse, or exploitation; preventing or reducing inappropriate institutional care by providing for community-based care, home-based care, or other forms of less intensive care; and securing referral or admission for institutional care when other forms of care are not appropriate, or providing certain services to individuals in institutions (excluding room and board).

Generally, Title XX reimburses only for social services. However, when medical care is "integral and subordinate" to the provision of a social service, coverage will be provided. Title XX services can be supplied directly by the state or local agency; through contracting with a public or private provider; or through independent providers not affiliated with an agency. While the federal regulations do not specify standards for homecare providers, some states use licensing or accreditation requirements as the basis for provider participation. In 1983, home-based services were provided to about 307,000 persons of all ages, 11 percent of the total Title XX recipients (O'Shaughnessy 1985,27). A GAO report (1986) found that Community Services Block Grant funds supplement short-term local needs not met by the social services agencies.

Services

An HHS analysis of the FY 1985 state pre-expenditure reports on intended use of funds revealed that all the states planned to provide homecare services including home health, homemaker, chore and home management assistance to adults and children; that 26 states were offering adult day care; that 24 states reimbursed for home-delivered meals; and 16 states supported adult foster care (Wills and McKeough 1986,19). Eleven of the states offer 70 percent or more of the 26 identified SSBG services, as of FY 1985. Other related homecare services include social support services (socialization, recreation, living skills, family management), transportation, housing services, protective and emergency care, counseling and prevention, and intervention services (assessment, family-centered early intervention, and home evaluation and supervision.

Funding and Expenditures

States receive allotments of SSBG funds on the basis of population within a federal expenditure ceiling. There are no requirements for use of Title XX funds, and state money can be spent on service needs at the state's discretion. Legislation set the expenditure ceiling at $2.7 billion in FY 1985. Exhibit 6-8 shows the state-by-state allocation for 1985, along with the total funding and the percent of the total program funds supplied by the state. Note that SSBG funds represent a range from 28 percent (Massachusetts) to 99 percent (North Carolina) of a state's total service program funds. In addition, Exhibit 6-8 shows the approximate amount of funds allocated by each state for homecare services using the percentage figures from 1980 and an overall 14.3 percent of total expenditures. However, it is important to realize that 28 of the states spent between .7 and 10 percent on homecare; 15 spent 11-20 percent; 5 spent 21-29 percent; and two states spent 32-36 percent on homecare services. Therefore, the overall 14 percent is overweighed by the 20 states that exceed 10 percent. Even so, the data are more indicative than actual because of the lack of actual reporting by the states.

Exhibit 6-8 Social Services Block Grant Estimates of Funding by State, by Percent of Total, by Homecare Allocations, and by Percentage, 1985.

States	SSBG Allotment	Total Funding	Percent of Total	Homecare Percentage Allocation*	Applied to 1985 SSBG Estimate
Alabama	46,148,632	52,923,455	87%	7.9%	3.6 million
Alaska	5,126,326				
Arizona	33,473,266			5.0	1.7
Arkansas	26,813,724	37,061,071	72%	6.0	1.6
California	289,368,191			35.9	104.1
Colorado	35,638,495			14.9	5.3
Connecticut	36,902,520			4.2	1.5
Delaware	7,045,771	9,723,545	72%	5.2	.364
District of Columbia	7,385,166			11.0	.814
Florida	121,908,230	163,060,794	75%	4.3	5.2
Georgia	65,998,513			5.7	3.8
Hawaii	11,633,715			12.0	1.4
Idaho	11,294,301			6.6	.746
Illinois	133,986,696	296,437,984	45%	10.6	14.2
Indiana	64,032,251	89,882,000	71%	7.3	4.8
Iowa	33,999,943	61,347,277	55%	25.7	8.7
Kansas	28,183,085	42,413,127	66%	12.2	3.4
Kentucky	42,918,345	63,160,877	68%	6.7	2.9
Louisiana	51,052,582	64,234,288	79%	7.6	3.9
Maine	13,260,563	27,436,436	48%	9.4	1.3
Maryland	49,917,301	83,688,900	60%	7.6	3.8
Massachusetts	67,660,472	244,730,391	28%	19.3	13.1
Michigan	106,611,182			27.6	29.4
Minnesota	48,372,380			9.4	4.5
Mississippi	29,856,749			5.8	1.7
Missouri	57,946,203			7.5	4.3
Montana	9,374,856			5.3	.498
Nebraska	18,562,448	22,471,230	83%	16.8	3.1
Nevada	10,311,171			9.0	.927
New Hampshire	11,130,446			16.2	1.8
New Jersey	87,053,900			11.3	9.8
New Mexico	15,905,653	31,360,700	51%	17.3	2.8
New York	206,679,862			5.7	11.8
North Carolina	70,446,010	71,301,904	99%	10.9	7.7
North Dakota	7,841,640			32.4	2.5
Ohio	126,297,207			8.9	11.2
Oklahoma	37,183,414			.7	.260
Oregon	31,003,735			9.2	2.9
Pennsylvania	138,867,238	147,552,000	94%	3.8	5.3
Rhode Island	11,212,374			21.6	2.4
South Carolina	37,487,717	52,930,963	71%	9.2	3.5

*Based on 1980 percentage spent on homecare

Exhibit 6-8, continued

States	SSBG Allotment	Total Funding	Percent of Total	Homecare Percentage Allocation*	Applied to 1985 SSBG Estimate
Tennessee	54,435,021	88,344,000	62%	5.6	3.0
Texas	178,836,190	505,227,055	35%	25.6	45.8
Utah	18,187,922			3.3	.600
Vermont	6,039,223			3.7	.810
Virginia	61,266,329	91,917,879	67%	13.5	8.3
Washington	49,683,221			16.5	8.2
West Virginia	22,799,274			23.7	5.4
Wisconsin	55,769,270	58,257,625	96%	10.0	5.6
Wyoming	5,875,376	10,250,130	57%	16.1	.950
			U.S.	14.3	372.5

*Based on 1980 percentage spent on homecare
Source: Department of Health and Human Services. 1986. *Social services block grant pre-expenditure reports. Fiscal year 1985*. Washington, DC: Government Printing Office. Pub. No. 918-997, pp 23 - 24

Impact

Although the SSBG represents the major social service program funded by the federal government, its impact on the population needing long-term care is relatively limited. Because Title XX provides a variety of social services unavailable from Medicare and Medicaid, there are competing demands from a diverse population. Some feel that many of the social services for the sick poor could be integrated into the homecare benefits supplied by Medicaid. Of course, the limited amount of money available to the states severely restricts efforts to provide the scope and amount of homecare services needed in the community. Compared with nursing home expenditures, the Title XX dollars are a miniscule piece of the pie.

Older Americans Act

In 1965, the Administration on Aging (AOA) was established by Congress to administer the mandates in the Older Americans Act (OAA) to improve the lives of older persons in the areas of income, emotional and physical well-being, housing, employment, social services, civic, cultural, and recreational opportunities. Title III of the Act, Grants for State and Community Programs on Aging, aims to strengthen and/or develop a coordinated and comprehensive program to help elderly Americans maintain an independent lifestyle. Under Title III, grants are made to state agencies on aging, which in turn award funds to 664 area agencies on aging (AAAs) to plan, coordinate, and advocate for a comprehensive service system for older persons.

Certain supportive services under Title III have been given priority by Congress, including in-home services such as homemaker and home health aide, visiting and telephone reassurance, and chore maintenance. Each state agency is required to spend a portion of its supportive services allotment on these services. Community-based services that may be provided under Title III include case management, assessment, adult day care, and respite care. Title III also supports congregate and home-delivered meals and nutrition services. A report from the National Association of Meal Programs (1985) indicates that the 500+ members serve an average of 650 meals a day, 264 days per year in congregate and home-delivered programs.

Services

Services under the Title III program are provided to older persons regardless of income, although concentrated on those with the greatest social or economic need. Older persons are to be given the opportunity to contribute to the cost of services, but failure to do so cannot be a basis for denial of service. Unlike Medicare and Medicaid, the AOA is not hampered by restrictions or income tests, and can serve people whose benefits in those programs have been exhausted.

State agencies on aging are required to operate a statewide ombudsman program. To help carry out the mandates, state agencies created about 400 subarea ombudsman programs as of 1984. Required ombudsman activities include the investigation and resolution of complaints relating to the health, safety, welfare, and rights of institutionalized persons; the monitoring of federal, state, and local laws, regulations, and policies with respect to long-term care facilities; the providing of information to public agencies regarding problems of older persons in long-term care facilities; and the establishment of procedures for access to facilities' and patients' records, including protection of the confidentiality of such records. Obviously, the ombudsman programs concentrate on institutions and boarding homes, but the transition to homecare activities is easy to make.

Some state AOAs have acted as catalysts to reorganize community-based health and social services systems to serve the population in need more effectively. Coordination with other programs such as Title XX is usual. In some states, the state AOA has administered the Medicaid 2176 waiver program. Comprehensive case management and assessment systems through AAAs have been developed in some states, allowing support of services otherwise unavailable to the elderly.

More than nine million unduplicated persons were served in 1984, about equally divided between those with the greatest social need and those with the greatest economic need. Numbers of people served by specific activities include the following: health, 977,000; visiting/telephone reassurance, 969,696; homemaker, 653,594; escort service, 358,095; chore/maintenance, 255,691; home health aide, 178,002; residential repair/renovation, 86,579 (House Select Committee on Aging 1985,24-25).

Additionally, Title IV of the AOA provides for research and demonstration projects. These activities are directed to models or alternatives for living and service delivery arrangements for older Americans who, without such services, would otherwise be institutionalized.

Funding and Expenditures

Unlike the Title XX program where states are given a block grant for unspecified services, Congress makes separate appropriations for Title III funds for specific services. However, the law does give the state and area agencies flexibility to define the supportive services and to transfer funds among the three services: supportive services, congregate nutrition services, and home-delivered nutrition services. Funds are allocated according to the number of older persons in the state as compared to all states.

FY 1985 appropriations for Title III totaled $785 million, with $336 million for congregate nutrition services, and $265 million for supportive services. About $68 million of the federal appropriation is devoted to home-delivered nutrition services. Budget authorizations for 1986 and 1987 allocate $377 and $395 million for congregate nutrition; $342 and $362 million for supportive services; and $72 and $76 million for home-delivered nutrition services. Federal administration budget proposals have suggested reductions in OAA funds, particularly in Title III monies, of about 5 percent. Congress rejected the budget cuts and proceeded to restore adequate funding (Senate Special Committee on Aging 1985,266-267).

Homecare services clearly represent an expenditure priority for the Title III program. According to the National Data Base on Aging, about 25 percent of funds controlled by AAAs, both OAA and non-OAA monies, was directed at in-home services in 1984. While a substantial portion of the funds was spent on home-delivered meals, almost an equal portion was spent on homecare services devoted to housekeeping, personal care and chore services (O'Shaughnessy 1985,29).

Increasingly, states have shifted federal funds from the congregate nutrition program to home-delivered and supportive services components. By 1987, legislation will allow for the transfer of up to 30 percent among the funding categories (Senate Special Committee on Aging 1985,260). In FY 1984, states transferred more than $41 million from the $321 million allocated to congregate nutrition. Part of the shift is due to the increase in the number of "old old" and the resultant greater demand for homecare services.

About $12.1 million was spent for ombudsman activities in FY 1983 ($8.9 million in federal funds and $3.2 from state and local funds).

Impact

Due to the low level of financial resources, as compared with other programs, the OAA does not have the ability to make a significant impact on the homecare service system. Formal coordination and changes in the benefit and reimbursement structures of Medicare, Medicaid, and the Social Services Block Grant programs are needed to have the OAA fit into an improved mechanism to provide homecare services. Despite the lack of resources, many state and area aging agencies have made strides to bolster homecare through their coordination activities. They have brought together health and social service agencies and developed a social service infrastructure for the elderly at the local level. Flexibility to fill in the gaps has a good deal to do with the impact of the OAA and its state and local counterparts in moving beyond the narrow confines of monetary restrictions.

Critics of the OAA contend that the activities foster a separate network of services that isolate and segregate older persons from the mainstream of America and from other age groups (Estes 1980,19). Others argue that the federal, state, and local OAA agencies lack the statutory mandate to perform the coordination and advocacy roles necessary to provide services in an effective and efficient manner.

"In the long run, the development of a national policy on aging under the OAA remains uncertain. . . It is clear that Congress will need to go beyond the incremental changes in reforming the Act, to enhance and further the goals it set for itself and the Nation back in 1986" (Senate Special Committee on Aging 1985,270).

Government-funded Projects

Over the last decade, the federal government has funded a wide range of demonstration and research projects designed to test the provision and coordination of homecare-related services, as well as achieve savings in the provision of care. Initially, many were sponsored by HHS through HCFA and the AOA. For some projects, Medicare and Medicaid eligibility and service waivers were obtained to allow benefits to persons who would not ordinarily receive them under the existing program. Most projects aimed to provide or access a range of health and health-related social services for specified client groups, such as homemaker, home health, chore, home-delivered meals, adult day health, and transportation. Common features of the activities included multidisciplinary teams, case management, assessment, and follow-up. A prominent effort funded by HHS for the first time during 1980 was the National Long-Term Care Channeling Demonstration Program. Ten states initiated multi-year programs to manage and coordinate (channel) community-based services for the benefit of clients. Attention focused on preventing institutionalization and hospitalization, utilization of community health and social services, services provided by family caregivers, costs of case management, and the relation of costs incurred to overall well-being. Data indicate that a large majority of those living in the community need help with preparing meals, shopping, and other household activities (House 1980,40).

State-level initiatives have involved the control of institutional access through screening/assessment procedures to identify the "at risk" population and provide community and home-based alternatives. To avoid duplication and fragmentation, some states reorganize access to community services with case management or "gateway" services. Cost control mechanisms in some states limit the amount of funds available to alternatives to a percentage of institutional care. Community and/or homecare cannot be provided unless the cost is below that percentage of institutional care. In addition, some states allow a form of dependent tax credit when dependents are cared for in the home by family members.

Private Funding of Homecare

For homecare services alone, about 14 percent of the elderly paid, out of their own pockets, from $360 to $1,680 per year, based on 1982 data from the National Long-Term Care Survey. Nursing home care can cost from $12,000 to $50,000 per year (Senate Special Committee on Aging 1985,197). Furthermore, the House Select Committee on Aging (1985) reported the range of costs for specific visit and hourly charges to private pay patients by type of service and the percentage of agencies in each charge grouping (Exhibit 6-9). With those costs in mind, the private funding of homecare can be examined.

Homecare services are funded by commercial insurance companies, Blue Cross plans, United Way agencies, voluntary nonprofit health/disease oriented organizations, and a variety of religious sponsorship agencies. In many instances, the services offered could hardly be called comprehensive, coordinated, or efficient.

Exhibit 6-9 Visit and Hourly Charges by Provider to Private Pay Patients

	Per Visit		Per Hour	
Registered nurse	$26-$40	(32%)	$10-$25	(16%)
	$41-$55	(42%)	$26-$45	(49%)
	$56 or more	(12%)	$46 or more	(27%)
Physical therapist	$21-$35	(18%)	$25 or less	(16%)
	$36-$50	(38%)	$26-45	(36%)
	$51 or more	(16%)	$46 or more	(29%)
Occupational therapist	$21-$35	(9%)	$25 or less	(5%)
	$36-$50	(32%)	$26-$50	(29%)
	$51 or more	(12%)	$51 or more	(10%)
Speech therapist	$21-$35	(11%)	$25 or less	(7%)
	$36-$50	(44%)	$26-$50	(43%)
	$51 or more	(15%)	$51 or more	(13%)
Medical social worker	$21-$35	(5%)	$25 or less	(3%)
	$36-$50	(32%)	$26-$50	(29%)
	$51 or more	(23%)	$51 or more	(15%)
Homemaker-home health aide	$20 or less	(22%)	$10 or less	(16%)
	$21-$35	(37%)	$11-$20	(25%)
	$36-$50	(23%)	$21-$35	(26%)
			$35 or more	(19%)

Note: This information is based on a survey conducted by the U.S. Select Committee on Aging in cooperation with the National Association for Home Care. Data reflect the responses of 292 agencies (Medicare-certified only) and do not total 100% because of nonresponse rate to some survey questions.

Source: House Select Committee on Aging. 1985. *Building a long term policy: home care data and implications.* Washington, DC: Government Printing Office. Comm. Pub. No. 98-484.

Insurance Companies

In *A Physician Guide to Home Health Care* (1981), the AMA noted that the Health Insurance Association of America recommended that its member companies "make homecare insurance benefits available under their medical expense policies." While insurance companies may have followed the advice, few individuals are aware of whether or not their health insurance covers homecare services. Policies that provide for private duty nursing in the home will also usually cover skilled nursing care services. The public may be well-advised to read the small print in their health insurance policies.

With the advent of the PPS/DRG scheme and the national emphasis upon containing health care costs, more private insurance companies are considering coverage of homecare. Their emphasis is on saving money by offering homecare as an alternative to high cost hospitalization. In addition, there is legislative interest in mandating homecare coverage for all policies written within specific states. Recently, Colorado passed a law requiring all policies sold after July 1, 1985 to offer home health and hospice coverage. That state joins about a dozen others which already mandate such coverage (Rothman 1985). Coverage usually carries an additional charge. In the article it was noted that "insurance companies are very unfamiliar with home health. They know what hospitalization is, but they don't know what homecare is." Some insurance companies benefit from a model for state legislation regarding homecare drafted by the AMA (1981,31). That model speaks to definitions, number of visits, deductibles and coinsurance, and application to short-term policies.

Blue Cross Plans

Early on, an article in *Hospitals* proclaimed that homecare can be reimbursed (Koncel 1979). He mentioned Blue Cross programs and the money saved in dollars and bed days. However, the Blue Cross Association (1974,1978) had already prepared and revised a manual detailing a model home health care benefit and guidelines for its members. By 1981, 60 of the 69 Blue Cross plans offered homecare services to their 60 million subscribers, although the services were adaptable and flexible in their variety. Regardless of the model, "The Blue Cross/Blue Shield Association believes that home health care can be an effective and cost-efficient means of providing health care services to patients" (Koncel 1979).

A home health care survey report from the Blue Cross/Blue Shield Association (1985; *Hospitals* 1985) reported on the provision of home health care benefits, the providers, patient characteristics, utilization management, cost effectiveness, and statistical data on each plan. Of the 61 out of 90 plans in the organization responding to the questionnaire, 55 had home health care benefits covered under their basic contracts. Hospice care is included in the core benefits of 21 plans. Twenty-six of the plans have cost-sharing provisions for their home health care benefits. In addition, nearly all the plans limit benefits, with the most common being an imposition on the number of home visits.

While coverage, payment and management vary considerably, most plans offer skilled nursing visits, physical, occupational, and speech therapy, medical social services, home health aide visits, and supplies. Physician visits and durable medical equipment are usually covered under other benefits. Eligibility is similar to Medicare in most cases: patient must be under the care of a physician; be essentially homebound; and custodial care is excluded.

Forty-seven of the plans have participating agreements with various sponsored home health agencies. In order of total number of contracts, the agency aegis is public, hospital, private nonprofit, proprietary, VNA, and skilled nursing facility. Fifteen plans have pilot or demonstration programs in the areas of hospice care, early maternity discharge, chronically ill children, expansion of high technology services, and postsurgical ambulatory care.

Prepaid Group Health Plans

Prepaid group health plans, no matter what they are labeled, usually provide comprehensive health care to enrolled members for a fixed annual fee. Plans include HMOs (Health Maintenance Organizations), PPOs (Preferred Provider Organizations) and PHPs (Prepaid Health Plans), to cite only a few. Comprehensive benefits usually include homecare without additional cost or with a nominal charge. Frequently, the homecare may be offered in lieu of hospitalization or for earlier discharge.

Thus, prepaid group health plans compete with existing home health agencies for clients. With the emergence of the PPS/DRG scheme and patients leaving hospitals in need of homecare, the prepaid plans have stepped up their activity in recruiting membership among those covered by Medicare. In fact, the Florida Association of Home Health Agencies (Borfitz 1986) said that "HMOs have nearly put freestanding home health agencies out of business in South Florida."

Reimbursement Variations

Based upon data from 30 home health agencies in western Pennsylvania, Shuman, Wolfe, Whetsell, et al. (1976) considered three variations: retroactive payment with a ceiling limitation; prospective payment without a ceiling; and prospective payment with a ceiling and a 50/50 sharing of surpluses and deficits. Retroactivity proved to be most restrictive of the reimbursement methods, while prospective was the most costly. Prospective with a ceiling and cost sharing contained the best attributes of the other two methods.

With the federal government evidently pleased with the success of prospective payment as a cost control mechanism in inpatient hospital care, it is evident that an application to home health care will be sought. Several alternatives have emerged for consideration, such as RUGs (Resource Utilization Groups), AVGs (Ambulatory Visit Groups), RIMs (Relative Intensity Measures), and SI (Severity of Illness) Index. RUGs (Fries and Cooney 1985) essentially integrate activities of daily living into a prospective reimbursement scheme. There are classifications based on the utilization of resources for attending to the needs of long-term care patients.

AVGs (Kavaler 1986) were developed by the same group of Yale University researchers that generated the diagnosis-related groups being used for inpatient hospital reimbursement. Using similar techniques, ambulatory care has been classified into about 700 categories, with reimbursement based on per visit charges.

RIMs (Shaffer 1984) focus upon the reimbursement of nursing services in hospitals. However, many of the elements in the classification scheme could just as easily be transferred to the nursing care required in homecare situations.

The Severity of Illness Index has been the target of a number of investigations, in regard to reimbursement methods. The contention is that patients require differing resources based upon the severity of illness, even within the same diagnostic classification. Horn and Horn (1986) discuss the validity and reliability of the index. Again, the application to homecare is obvious because so many patients having the same condition can require a wide variety of services.

Homecare, as with other types of ambulatory care, provides special reimbursement issues. Should care be paid for per visit? Should care be paid for per episode of care? How can acute care and long-term care services and resources be combined in reimbursement? Will there be abuse and fraud because care is rendered in the home, out of direct observation and administrative control? Reimbursement variations will have to consider these and other questions as the problems of payment methods are resolved.

Fraud and Abuse

Homecare has moved from being a charitable enterprise into being a large, lucrative business with a good number of proprietary agencies participating. Carpenter (1986) summed up the situation: "Essentially, the purpose of a for-profit home health agency is to make money for its owners by performing a service that people *want* ; for a nonprofit agency, it is to meet socially desirable *needs*." Earlier experience with nursing home investigations provided knowledge of unethical and illegal practices. Administrative excess and fraud could include the following (Stewart 1979,155):

- Billing twice for the same service.

- Billing more than one funding source for the same service.

- Billing for services never provided.

- Billing for a higher level of care than actually provided.

- Offering kickbacks, bribes, or rebates for client referrals to a specific home health agency for services.

- Offering kickbacks, bribes or rebates for client referrals to other agencies for additional services or supplies.

- Hiring too many executive staff.

- Paying excessive salaries to administrative staff.

- Providing lucrative employee expense accounts.

- Leasing or buying luxury automobiles to make home visits.

Randall (1985) discussed charting a course through the gray areas of criminal charges of fraud and abuse in the homecare industry. She identified four situations to be viewed with concern:

1. A joint venture where the HHA incurs little or no financial risk and where no services are required of the HHA.

2. An agreement linking rate of return to volume of patients referred.

3. An agreement where the HHA gets employee time, equipment, etc. free or at way below market costs; or a reversal where the HHA is charged way above market costs.

4. An arrangement where the HHA performs "extra services" for physicians who refer patients.

All of these abuses and fraudulent activities have been revealed in investigations of homecare agencies (General Accounting Office 1979, 1981; Weinraub 1977; Hall, Tufts, and Ricker-Smith 1977; Linz 1985; Fine 1984). Congress passed the Medicare-Medicaid Anti-Fraud and Abuse amendments in 1977 (P.L. 95-142) allowing for fine or imprisonment or both, with abuse being a felony. Sections of the amendments dealing with criminal sanctions, monetary penalties under the 1981 Omnibus Budget Reconcilia-

tion Act (Teplitsky 1985), exclusion procedures, and disclosure requirements were covered in *Caring* (June 1985). Most of the homecare trade associations also have codes of ethics that specifically prohibit fraudulent activities; the Medicare Conditions of Participation also allow for the termination of certification of agencies engaging in such practices. Nevertheless,
there are always some who must try to beat the system.

In its investigation of eight Florida and three Louisiana home health
agencies, the GAO (1979,19) cited the following questionable reimbursements:

- Undocumented and/or unrelated costs to patient care that were for
  substantial amounts.

- Excessive costs for office space where the owner of the property had
  a common business interest with the home health agency.

- Costs were claimed for what appeared to be the seeking of patient
  referrals from other facilities/providers.

- Fringe benefits were claimed without the required prior approval of
  the fiscal intermediary.

Undocumented/unrelated costs included a 14-country European tour
for an agency's officers and their spouses, unexplained restaurant charges, a
fishing trip, flowers for a variety of people, and membership in a local
country club. The question of referrals aroused suspicions about the difference between program promotion and patient solicitation, as Medicare
was billed for gifts to physicians and to hospital social workers, and for
memo pads, pens, desk organizers, and letter openers. Interestingly, the
home health agencies did not see anything wrong with giving gifts to
physicians and social workers and charging them to Medicare.

Halamandaris (1985) reviewed the case history of a massive fraud involving a $7.5 million homecare empire in California. There were seven in-
terlocking corporations, with the owner drawing salaries and expenses from
three of the companies, with salaries also being paid to three sisters, one
nephew, and one daughter. In addition to leased Cadillacs and a $35,000
luxury mobile home, the company car was a luxury Mercedes 450SL. An
auditor for the fiscal intermediary was hired by the owner, and political contributions were made on behalf of the homecare agency. After the collapse
of the empire in the late 1970s, the owner was convicted of fraud and sent
to jail. However, Halamandaris comments that there have been only seven
such convictions of homecare providers in the history of Medicare/
Medicaid.

Title XX fraud was reported by Hall, Tufts, and Ricker-Smith (1977)
wherein one homemaker/chore agency realized a 982 percent profit--
$178,092 on an investment of $18,140. Reimbursement was made for

$77,405 in expenses and $11,843 for liquor and tobacco. Another agency's initial investment of $27,282 yielded a 347 percent return, $94,598, in one year, with $22,803 being paid for automobile, parking, and gasoline credit card expenses.

Independent contractors can also be perpetrators of fraud and abuse because they are not subject to regulation. Cabin (1985) points out the problems of liability coverage for the agency hiring independent contractors; the issue of reimburseable tasks that may not be subject to Medicare/Medicaid standards; and the lack of requirements for workers to meet. Some states do have qualifications and regulations for independent contractors, but essentially the hiring agency has a great deal of leeway.

Embarrassingly, the former head of the American Federation of Home Health Agencies was convicted of embezzling from his former home health agency employer and passing those fraudulent expenses on to federal fiscal intermediaries for reimbursement (*Home Health Line* 1983). This was a dramatic reminder to homecare providers that the burden of perception of fraud and abuse falls most heavily upon the proprietary homecare agencies. Whether or not this is true is unimportant, for the profit motive is being questioned throughout the health care delivery system and is not restricted to homecare agencies. Legislative and regulatory decision-making proceeds from that point and the homecare industry must take steps to remove fraudulent and abusive practices.

In his role as Inspector General of HHS, Kusserow (1985) explained the attention to fraud and abuse. He noted that home health care is a minute part of the overall budgeted activities of HHS: only two-thirds of one percent. However, he did say, "One of the things that we're focusing very heavily on in the Office of the Inspector General is to do more studies in the area of home health."

HCFA initiated the Program Administration to Reduce Overpayments and Losses (PATROL) in September 1984, which yielded REINs (reduced expenditure initiatives) and PIW (program initiative work group). Because all of these activities cause delay in reimbursement to homecare agencies, Congress has been urged to look into the reimbursement issue (*Home Health Journal* 1986g). Some home health agencies are now waiting 120 days or more for payment. Yet, Dr. William Roper, new HCFA chief, told contractors that 95 percent of claims will be paid within 27 days (McIlrath 1986). However, HCFA may still continue to maintain a bottom limit for waiting before reimbursement.

Funding and Homecare: Impact

It is true that reimbursement for homecare services is still a minor portion of the federal expenditure. It is also true that a majority of consumers still pay for homecare from their own pockets. Yet, events on the federal level often filter down into all aspects of homecare reimbursement. Note that PPS/DRGs are being picked up by insurance carriers and other funding sources. What appears to emerge from the reimbursement battle is a basic concern over paying for services that may turn into runaway expenditures simply because nobody can really estimate future homecare costs. Furthermore, the debate over whether or not to reimburse for social/personal services without a direct medical/health link is also disconcerting. These critical situations are not readily resolvable. Unfortunately, and ironically, the people in need of care are the ones being hurt in the interim.

References

American Medical Association. 1981. *Physician guide to home health care.* Chicago, IL (July).

American Medical News. 1986. N.J. eyes legal team to appeal denials of coverage for home health benefits. 29(19) :24.

Benjamin, A.E. 1986. Determinants of state variation in home health utilization and expenditures under Medicare. *Medical Care* 24:535-547.

Blancato, R. 1986. The Older Americans Act as a vehicle. *Pride Institute Journal* Special Issue:29-32.

Blue Cross Association. 1978. *Home-health care. Model benefit program and related guidelines.* Chicago, IL (June).

Blue Cross/Blue Shield Association. 1985. *Home health care survey report.* Chicago, IL (April).

Blumenthal, D., M. Schlesinger, P.B. Drumheller, et al. 1986. The future of Medicare. *New England Journal of Medicine* 314:722-728 (13 March).

Borfitz, D. 1986. Florida home care blasts top HMO. *Home Health Journal* 7(6) :1,5.

Buddi, J. 1985. Testimony before House Subcommittee on Health on the Medicare 1986 budget. Washington, DC: American Federation of Home Health Agencies, Inc. (16 April).

Cabin, W. 1985. The problem with independent contractors. *Caring* 4(6) :32-34,63.

Caring. 1985. Key federal statutes on fraud and abuse issues. 4(6) :56-62.

Carpenter, S.S. 1986. Profit versus nonprofit: Comparisons and considerations. *Home Healthcare Nurse* 4(1):18-23.

Cowart, M.E. 1985. Policy issues: financial reimbursement for home care. *Family and Community Health* 8(2):1-10.

Curtiss, F.R. 1986a. Financing home healthcare products and services. *American Journal of Hospital Pharmacy* 43:121-131.

Curtiss, F.R. 1986b. Recent developments in federal reimbursement for home health care. *American Journal of Hospital Pharmacy* 43:132-139.

Daubert, E.A. 1985. Personal communication. Connecticut Association for Home Care, Inc. Wallingford, CT (9 Dec.).

Estes, C.L. 1980. *The aging enterprise.* San Francisco: Jassey-Bass Publishers.

Federal Register. 1985. Medicaid program: home and community-based services. Final rule. 50(49) :10013-10028 913 March).

Federal Register. 1985. Medicare program: assignment and reassignment of home health agencies to designated regional intermediaries. 50(69) :14162-14165 (10 April).

Federal Register. 1985. Medicare program: hospice payment cap. 50(221) :47278-47279 (15 Nov.).

Federal Register. 1986. Medicare program: use of HCFA wage index for setting schedule of limits on home health agency costs per visit reporting periods

beginning on or after July 1, 1986.
51(57) :10267-10274 (25 March).

Federal Register. 1986. Schedule of limits on home health agency costs per visit for cost reporting periods beginning on or after July 1, 1986, but before July 1, 1987. 51(104) :19734-19741 (30 May).

Fine, D.R. 1984. The home as workplace: prejudice and inequity in home health care. Position paper prepared for Visiting Nurse Association, San Francisco, CA (Jan.).

Fries, B.E., and L.M.Cooney, Jr. 1985. Resource utilization groups: a patient classification system for long term care. *Medical Care* 23:110-122.

General Accounting Office. 1979. *Home health care services. tighter fiscal controls needed.* Washington, DC: Government Printing Office. Pub. No. HRD 79-17 (15 May).

General Accounting Office. 1981. *Response to U.S. Senate Subcommittee on abuses in the home health care industry.* Washington, DC: Government Printing Office. Pub. No. HRD 81-84 (24 April).

General Accounting Office. 1986. *Community services: block grant helps address local social service needs.* Washington, DC: Government Printing Office. Pub. No. HRD 86-91 (7 May).

Halamandaris, V.J. 1985. Homecare fraud. A case history. *Caring* 4(6) :16-20.

Hall, H.D. 1981. Homemaker-home health aide services in *Handbook of the social services,* edited by N. Gilbert and H.S. Pecht. Englewood Cliffs, NJ: Prentice-Hall, Inc., pp. 35-49.

Hall, H.D., J.A. Tufts, and K. Ricker-Smith. 1977. Formulation of a national policy for in-home health and supportive services. Presentation at annual meeting of American Public Health Association. Washington, DC.

Hartwell, S. 1986. From the editor's desk. *Provider* 12(6) :2.

Heckler, M.G. 1985. Medicare turns 20 as America grays. *Hospitals* 59(3) :59-60,62.

Home Health Care Services Quarterly. 1980. Comments on the Weissert report. 1(3) :97-121.

Home Health Journal. 1986a. Congress

asked to exempt one-percent cost cutbacks. 7(4) :5.

Home Health Journal. 1986b. '87 federal budget proposes cutback on homecare service. 7(3) :8.

Home Health Journal. 1986c. Co-payment call brings charges. 7(4) :1,3.

Home Health Journal. 1986d. Deadline update. 7(4) :2.

Home Health Journal. 1986e. PRO model denial notices. 7(4) :1.

Home Health Journal. 1986f. National association says Reagan out to dismantle Medicare home benefit. 7(4) :5,8.

Home Health Journal. 1986g. Congress looks at payment delay problems. 7(6) :3,4.

Home Health Line. 1983. Reck guilty plea rocks industry; home health leader confesses fraud. Port Republic, MD (17 Oct.).

Horn, S.D., and R.H. Horn. 1986. Reliability and validity of the severity of illness index. *Medical Care* 24:159-178.

Hospital Week. 1985. Many ineligible home health agency services covered by Medicare: Davis. 21(13) (20 March).

Hospitals. 1985. Most Blue Cross/Blue Shield plans cover home care: study. 59(18) :62,64.

House Select Committee on Aging. 1985a. *Health care cost containment: are America's aged protected?* Washington, DC: Government Printing Office Comm. Pub. No. 99-522.

House Select Committee on Aging. 1985b. *Building a long term policy: home care data and implications.* Washington, DC: Government Printing Office. Pub. No. 98-484.

House Subcommittee on Health and Long-Term Care. 1980. *Long-term care for the 1980s: Channeling demonstrations and other initiatives,* Washington, DC: Comm. Pub. No. 96-234 (27 Feb.).

Kavaler, F. 1986. Personal communication (Sept.).

Koncel, J.A. 1979. Home health care can be reimbursed. *Hospitals* 53(20) :44-45.

Kusserow, R.P. 1985. Protecting the public. *Caring* 4(6) :4-8,53.

Lenz, E.A. 1985. Letter to Henry Desmaris, MD. Washington, DC: Home Health

Services and Staffing Association (14 March).

Linz, J. 1985. Homecare audits. *Caring* 4(6) :54-55.

Liu, K., K.G. Manton, and B.M. Liu. 1985. Homecare expenses for the disabled elderly. *Health Care Financing Review* 7(2) :51-58.

McIlrath, S. 1986. New HCFA chief promises to speed payment of MD's Medicare claims. *American Medical News* 29(23) :1, 49.

Medical Economics. 1986. Some patients just can't win under Medicare (14 April).

Mills, M. 1984. Testimony on intermittent care before Senate Subcommittee on Health. ABC Home Health Services, Brunswick, GA (22 June).

National Association of Meal Programs. 1985. *Partners in nutrition for seniors.* Washington, DC.

O'Shaughnessy, C., R. Price and J. Griffith. 1985. *Financing and delivery of long-term care services for the elderly.* Washington, DC: Congressional Research Service, Library of Congress, 85-1033 EPW.

O'Sullivan, J. 1985a. *Medicare: FY 86 budget.* Washington, DC: Congressional Research Service, Library of Congress. Pub. No. IB85047 (8 Nov.).

O'Sullivan, J. 1985b. *Medicaid: FY86 budget.* Washington, DC: Congressional Research Service, Library of Congress. Pub. No. IB85057 (14 Nov.).

Pear, R. 1985. Medicare trust fund is seen as healthy until '98. *New York Times* (29 March).

Pettengill, J. 1985. *Medicare: the financing problem in the hospital insurance program.* Washington, DC: Congressional Research Service, Library of Congress. Pub. No. IB85013 (1 Aug.).

Pettey, S. 1985. Letter to Congressman James R. Jones. Washington, DC: Home Health Services and Staffing Association (12 Dec.).

Provider. 1986a. IG recommends home health controls. 12(4) :55.

Provider. 1986b. HCFA eliminates Medicare waiver of liability. 12(4) :53.

Queen's Medical Center. 1985. Community care program. Sixth annual report. Honolulu, HI (Oct.).

Randall, D.A. 1985. Charting a course through the grey areas of criminal charges of fraud and abuse. *Caring* 4(6) :28-30.

Rothman, H. 1985. Insurance companies must offer homecare/hospice policies. *Home Health Journal* 6(3) :17,19.

Senate Special Committee on Aging. 1985. *Developments in aging: 1984 volume 1.* Washington, DC: Government Printing Office. Report 99-5 (18 Feb.).

Shaffer, F.A. 1984. Relative intensity measures and the state of the art of reimbursement for nursing services in *DRGs: changes and challenges.* New York: National League for Nursing. Pub. No. 20-1959, pp. 57-64 (20 June).

Shuman, L.J., H. Wolfe, G.W. Whetsell, et al. 1976. Reimbursement alternatives for home health care. *Inquiry* 13(3) :277-287.

Star-Ledger (Newark, NJ). 1986. Pepper maintains health insurance should include home care coverage (20 March).

Star-Ledger (Newark, NJ). 1986. Bradley acts on health care (22 May).

Star-Ledger (Newark, NJ). June 11, 1986. Health Coalition rallies Medicare support.

Stewart, J.E. 1979. *Home health care.* St. Louis: C.V. Mosby Co.

Teplitsky, S.V. 1985. Civil money penalties. *Caring* 4(6) :22-27.

Thietten, G.L. 1985. Testimony before Senate Finance Committee on Medicare deficit reduction proposals. Washington, DC: American Federation of Home Health Agencies, Inc. (12 Sept.).

Trager, B. 1980. Home health care and national health policy. *Home Health Care Services Quarterly* 1(2) :1-103.

Vladeck, B. 1986. Federal inaction on long term care to hurt PPS. *Hospitals* 60(6) :120.

Weinraub, B. 1977. Charges of widespread fraud in California Medicare program made at Congressional hearing on health. *New York Times* (9 March).

Weissert, W.G., T.T.H. Wan, B.B. Liveratos, et al. 1980. Cost effectiveness of homemaker services for the chronically ill. *Inquiry* 17(3) :230-243 (fall).

Wills, I., and M. McKeough. 1986. *Social Services Block Grant pre-expenditures reports. Fiscal year 1985*. Washington, DC: Government Printing Office. Pub. No. 918-997.

Yeatts, D.E., B.J. Steinhardt, and J. Capitman. 1985. Evaluation of Connecticut's Medicaid home- and community-based care waiver program. Presentation at annual meeting of American Public Health Association, Washington, DC (Nov.).

Yovanovich, S. 1985. Testimony before House Select Committee on Aging. Visiting Nurse Association, Butler, PA (5 July).

Chapter 7

Does Homecare Curtail the Costs?

The underlying question in this discussion is whether or not homecare is less costly than hospitalization or nursing homes or other alternatives utilizing facilities, particularly in a "climate of cost containment" (Knollmueller 1984). Judging from the large volume of material in the mass media as well as in professional journals, apparently most agree that homecare costs less. On the face of it, this seems to be common sense. If an individual does not have to spend time in an expensive hospital or nursing home, the costs should be less. However, problems related to the application of cost effectiveness and cost benefit analyses in comparison studies compound the findings. In addition, there are those who say that homecare is not a substitute for institutionalization, but rather an "add-on" to existing services. Hay and Mandes (1984) go even further and raise the issue of substantial economic inefficiency in an analysis of home health care cost functions. "If these empirical results are to be believed, cost-based reimbursement may not be appropriate in the home health care market."

General Approval

Support for homecare as a cost containment measure has been expressed for a long time. A family physician from Beaver Dam, Wisconsin (Bush 1977), added his comments to "cost-saving pearls" in a journal devoted to patient care: "We've hardly scratched the surface as far as exploiting health care at home as a cost-saving device . . . What's required is for physicians to support this activity more widely than they do at present." A physician writing in a California medical journal (Schrifter 1980) seconded the point, as he stated that costs are less and patients feel better. A multidisciplinary team (Silver, Majorie, Romain, et al. 1984)--physician, nurse, dietitian, pharmacist--noted that, "Homecare is the ultimate extension of the cost reduction principle: that it generally costs less to treat patients in a nursing home than in a hospital and still less to treat them at home." At nationwide regional hearings on homecare (Department of Health, Education and Welfare 1976, 51), consumers, service providers, health and social service providers, advocates, and third-party insurers agreed that homecare was more cost effective than institutional care. In a magazine directed to the over-50 age group, Ognibene (1980) declared that homecare is better and cheaper. A headline in the Wall Street Journal (Schorr 1981) proclaimed, "Home Care Services for the Elderly and Disabled are Advocated as

Cheaper than Nursing Homes." At a later date, the Journal of Commerce (Lawson 1984) noted that "Home Health-Care Idea Catching On" with employers offering the benefit. In Newsweek, Seligmann (1980) heralded the fact that "Home Care Pays Off." Even an official federal government publication for health and welfare workers noted that "Nursing Home Costs Halved by Home Maintenance Program" (Shepherd 1978). After a review of 20 studies, Hammond (1979) concluded that "the preponderance of evidence from the studies summarized suggests that from the standpoint of third-party underwriters, homecare is indeed less expensive than extended hospitalization." In a question and answer fact sheet on a piece of federal legislation on home health care distributed by Senator Orrin Hatch's (1981) office, there was a strongly worded response to a query about cost: "To date, however, every published study suggests that home health care costs less than nursing home care." A review of 70 studies (Health Policy Alternatives, Inc. 1983, 28), reported the possibility of savings in 40 reports, but the overall impact was inconclusive.

Generally, many segments of the American public have expressed themselves on the side of homecare as a less costly method of meeting the health and social needs of the population. While numerous studies can and will be cited comparing homecare costs with hospital inpatient care, nursing home care, adult day care and other alternatives, there are vital underlying problems and issues. These issues deal with the type of data collected, interpretations of cost-effectiveness and cost benefits, and the assumptions girding the initiation of the homecare activities.

Basic Premises

Doty (1984) identifies four key assumptions that must be valid before determinations can be made about cost savings via alternatives to institutional care:

1. *Appropriate Targeting* -- High-risk individuals can be identified who would use nursing homes "but for" the availability of alternatives; services can be targeted to that specific population.

2. *Substitutability* -- Home- and community-based services can substitute for institutional care in a "significant" percentage of cases for "significant" periods of time.

3. *Regulation of Institutional Care Services* -- Institutional beds and services can be influenced or regulated to keep within legitimate medical need expectations and allow for an appropriate type and amount of alternative care to develop.

4. *Lower Per Capita Cost* -- Providing home- and community-based care to persons who would otherwise require institutional placement is less costly per individual served.

Obviously, being able to identify the "but for" group, achieving real substitute alternatives, controlling the institutional bed supply, and curtailing cost per individual is not an easy task. Nevertheless, Doty (1984, 41) commented that "it appears reasonable to conclude that well-designed and carefully implemented alternative programs are capable of preventing or postponing some nursing home use that would otherwise occur."

Three cost-saving objectives of homecare are listed in the study by Health Policy Alternatives, Inc. (1983, 3):

1. Speed discharges from hospitals and nursing homes.

2. Prevent admissions to institutions, especially nursing homes.

3. Serve individuals requiring care at home even though they are not likely to enter an institution in the near future.

Both sets of premises contain similarities relating to the identification of a high-risk population, the add-on factor, and the prevention of institutionalization. To measure the impact of the application of these assumptions, it is appropriate to discuss cost-effectiveness and cost-benefit analysis.

Cost-Effectiveness

From the viewpoint of a medical economist, Klarman, Francis, and Rosenthal (1968) define cost-effectiveness:

In cost-effective analysis, the costs of alternative ways of achieving a specific set of results are compared. Interest focuses on the alternative that either (a) incurs the least cost for a given outcome or (b) for a given cost, renders the highest level of outcome.

A majority of the comparison studies usually measure cost-effectiveness in terms of differences in the expenditures between homecare services and hospitalization, nursing home confinement or some other type of facility. Medical and health benefits are assumed to be the same regardless of location of care. Social and personal care benefits are routinely added on to the homecare ratio. For meaningful cost-effectiveness analysis, Day (1984) argued for consideration of outcome (mortality) and the separation of services at entry and exit from the series of formal and informal providers on a continuum of care. Rogatz (1985) examined the social and economic considerations of home health care. He went beyond the question of homecare merely being cheaper to the issue of homecare being more effective. Interestingly, he also asked what if homecare was more expensive and also more effective? In fact, Saltzman (1985) says exactly that: "Based on experience the cost per patient is certainly less than that of hospitalization or institutionalization. But in the long run, the cost of health care will not be less." He further comments that regardless of the increased cost, homecare is cost-effective "since our purpose is to serve the health needs of our population."

In the Health Policy Alternatives study (1983, 8), a list of potential cost-saving and cost-increasing factors emerged in considering cost-effectiveness. Saving variables included shorter hospital and nursing home stays, fewer hospital and nursing home admissions, reduced use of other health care services, reduced use of support services, increased use of family and other nonpaid services, and savings from early rather than later treatment services. Cost increasing factors, to be deducted from the saving factors, included additional patients, additional services, substitution of less efficient services, increase in early detection costs, higher cost per unit of service including travel costs, reduced use of family and unpaid help, inadequate management and coordination of services, and incentive for unnecessary services.

Even with data on the cost plus and minus factors, cost-effectiveness measurement techniques may have significant weaknesses according to Ruby, Banta, and Burns (1985). They note that the lack of efficiency data may improve and thus bolster calculations as more research is accomplished. Yet, cost-effectiveness investigations stress quantifiable factors, such as death rates and financial costs, to the exclusion of nonquantifiable factors, such as ethics and equity. "In effect, this weakness means that cost effectiveness analysis cannot in most cases be the dominant factor in a decision." Despite these drawbacks, health economist Fuchs (1982) felt that cost-effectiveness is the most rational approach available for effective, efficient allocation of resources.

Returning to the basic premises about the objectives of homecare services, Weissert (1985) contends that the programs are not likely to pass the cost-effectiveness test. He makes this statement after a decade of research and the realization that homecare services can't meet their underlying assumptions for being. While noting the appeal and intuitiveness of arguments that it is cheaper to care for sick old people at home, Weissert comes up with seven reasons for the difficulty of making community-based long-term care cost-effective:

- Community care is a complement to existing care and not a substitute for institutional care. Those people using community care are not at risk of institutionalization.

- Even those at risk are at risk for only a short stay, not long enough to produce major savings.

- Community care has not been effective in reducing or avoiding even those short stays.

- Patients at risk of institutionalization are very difficult to find in the community.

- High screening and assessment costs continue to be a major outlay for many community care programs.

- High per units costs in community care services exist because of the few clients served.

- Community care has limited effectiveness in producing changes in health status beneficial to patients. Patient contentment was one area positively affected by community care services.

After that discouraging picture, Weissert concludes, "Community care rarely reduces nursing home or hospital use; it provides only limited outcome benefits; and to this point, it has usually raised overall use of health services as well as total expenditures." He suggests that community care supporters redirect their efforts toward those who need palliative care using a functional definition of old age rather than counting birthdays.

Obviously, cost-effectiveness in homecare does have its detractors and its supporters. What remains is to find the happy medium allowing for valid and reliable interpretations.

Cost-Benefit Analysis

Whereas cost-effectiveness may be used to determine the best way to reach a defined objective, cost-benefit analysis may be used to determine how to get the best care for the least amount of money. A monetary value is assigned to the accrued benefits, and that figure is related to the dollar costs of the program. Direct, indirect, and intangible costs are calculated in the evaluation. Direct costs include items such as medical care providers, pharmaceuticals, laboratory tests, and actual resources used in caring for the patient. Indirect costs include the loss of earnings of family caregivers and the value of volunteer efforts. Intangible costs can include pain, suffering, and inconvenience.

Homecare is a difficult area for cost-benefit application because of the intangibles involved in the improvement of the patient's quality of life and functioning. In many cases, the calculation is based on a functional assessment, where the dollar value related to incremental improvement may be quite small. There are also ethical and moral overtones in cost-benefit decisions relating to how our society treats the elderly, the disabled, the handicapped, and other stigmatized population groups.

Exhibit 7-1 lists dollar expenditures that should be included in cost-benefit analysis comparisons of home health care, acute inpatient hospital care, and SNF/HRF care. Note that household and personal maintenance costs are included where appropriate. Apparent problems arise when seeking the details of what is included in a daily rate for comparison. Laundry, cleaning, and meal preparation are only a few services directly involved in running a home that may not automatically be included in the dollar values.

Of course, dollar values for pain, suffering, inconvenience, lost wages, volunteers, family chores, and the like raise similar difficulties in cost-benefit analysis. Stewart (1979) asks if there are accurate measures of equal qualities and quantities of care? Are hourly or per visit services the same as 24-hour-per-diem services? Can quality of life be given a monetary value? Hughes (1984) points out that there is a difference between hospital charges and hospital costs that also tends to confuse the cost-benefit analysis.

These are not idle questions, and court decisions regularly place a value on some of these intangibles in lawsuit determinations. It is apparent that cost and benefit should be linked for evaluations of achieving the best

---

Exhibit 7-1 Cost Inclusions Necessary for Comparison of Home Health, Skilled Nursing Facility/Health Related Facility, and Acute Hospital Care

Home Health Care
- All services delivered through a program of home health care.
- All health and health related goods and services obtained through sources other than a home health agency, e.g., physician visits.
- Household and personal maintenance costs.

SNF/HRF
- Daily rate.
- Health and health related goods and services not included in daily rates, e.g., usually physician visits.
- If household is maintained, household costs.

Acute Hospital Care
- Daily rate.
- Health and health related goods and services not included in daily rates, e.g. usually physician services.
- Household maintenance, or daily rate if SNF or HRF.

Source: Watson, A.L., and A. Thom. 1977. *Home health care utilization, costs, and reimbursement.* New York: Health Systems Agency of New York City, p. 58 (Nov.).

value for the expenditure. What is not so clear is whether the techniques for making the judgments enhance the decision-making process.

Substitution or Add-on

Using the outcomes of cost-effectiveness and/or cost-benefit analysis, planners have to decide whether or not to expand homecare programs. Directly linked to that decision is the problem of deciding if homecare is a substitute for other more expensive care or merely an addition to existing services. Critics have also expressed the opinion that if homecare services were expanded, family members would happily relinquish their caregiving tasks to paid workers, thereby adding to expenditure.

To achieve substantial savings for the health and social care delivery system, community-based homecare must be substituted for institutional care. "If alternatives supplement rather than substitute for institutional services, the additional services will add to the cost" (Skellie, Mobley, and Coan 1982). It may be a truism that the total cost of homecare services may be limited only by the available supply. A *Wall Street Journal* article (Schorr 1981) applies political overtones to the same expectation:

> Some Reagan administration officials privately support more home support for the elderly. But like their Carter administration predecessors, cost-conscious Reaganites fear that millions of elderly currently getting by on their own or with family help might line up for the federal homecare aid. Government health care costs could soar at a time when the administration is seeking to cap the surge in Medicaid outlays.

Doty (1984) also found that people were probably receiving homecare services who would not have entered nursing homes without the additional care. She questioned how large the add-on population would be and whether the costs would outweigh savings. Pointedly, Doty felt that the political "will" of governmental program administrators to limit services to persons imminently at risk of institutionalization would be an important factor in the volume of add-on services.

Cost and Impairment Level

A number of studies indicate that homecare may be less costly than institutional care for patients with lower levels of impairment. However, as the impairment level becomes more severe, the cost savings tend to disappear. A GAO (1977, 12) report listed seven impairment levels: unimpaired, slightly, mildly, moderately, generally, greatly, and extremely. A break-even point is reached as the patient moves into the greatly impaired level. At that point, the cost of homecare approximates the cost of institutionalization. After that point, homecare costs jump to more than 50 percent higher than the facility's costs. Exhibit 7-2 illustrates the cost changeover, showing that as the impairment level exceeds the average, the cost of homecare rises. Exhibit 7-3 gives the percentage breakdown of costs, related to the impairment level, borne by family as compared to the agency. At the greatest impairment levels, the family and friends are paying for 70 and 80 percent of the total cost. In dollars, a Senate Special Committee on Aging report (1985, 3) noted that annual out-of-pocket expenses by the elderly with mild, moderate, and severe impairment was $1,022, $1,418, and $5,266 respectively.

As infirmity increases and additional services are required, the advantages of centralization and the spreading of costs among many patients reduces the cost of that type of care. However, institutional costs also rise with impairment level severity, although the per person expenditure will still remain below homecare costs.

Willemain (1980) interprets the GAO data differently. He claims that the GAO did not properly locate a break-even point due to calculation underestimates, scale economies, and inappropriate use of impairment levels.

Exhibit 7-2 Homecare Costs Vs. Nursing Home Costs as a Function of Service Requirements

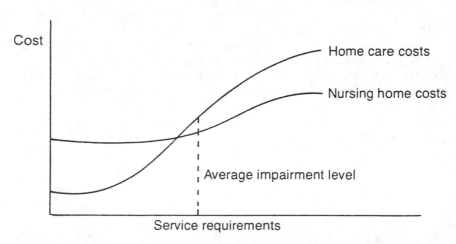

Source: Katzper, M. 1981. *Modeling of long-term care.* Rockville, MD: PROJECT SHARE. Human Services Monograph Series, No. 21 (July).

Exhibit 7-3 Assigned Average Monthly Percentage of Cost per Person by Impairment Level

Impairment level	Cost borne by family and friends	Cost borne by agency
	Percentage	Percentage
Unimpaired	59%	41%
Slightly	57	43
Mildly	63	37
Moderately	70	30
Generally	67	33
Greatly	71	29
Extremely	80	20

Source: General Accounting Office. 1977. *Home health – the need for a national policy to better provide for the elderly.* Washington, DC: Government Printing Office. Pub. no. HRD 78-19 (Dec.).

His contention is that the analysis showed that it is not necessarily an efficient strategy to target the highest risk groups if the goal of homecare is to avoid institutionalization. That interpretation seems similar to Weissert's (1985) later remarks.

In a comparative study of case mix at nursing homes and in home health agencies, Kramer, Shaughnessy, and Pettigrew (1985) found that greater impairment levels do relate to costs. "From the standpoint of cost effectiveness, it would appear that home health care might provide a substitute for acute care hospital use at the end of a hospital stay, and appears to be a more viable option in the care of patients who are not severely disabled and do not have profound functional problems."

Cost Evaluation Problems

Considering cost-effectiveness, cost-benefit analysis, impairment levels, the add-on factor, and other variables, it is easy to understand why critics question conclusions about savings. However, it should be noted that cost-saving judgments are related to the totality of social benefits as well as costs. Decisions cannot be made solely on calculated direct costs without thinking about the overall value to society. Some of the problems in cost evaluation concern a consensus on elements necessary for comparison; confusion as to where and how homecare fits exactly into the health care delivery system;

the subjectivity of analyses; the social value costs that defy calculation; and the basic insufficiency of data on costs and values.

This situation is not unique to homecare. Health care research has often been criticized in this way, regardless of the subject matter under review. Until homecare investigations can compare apples with apples instead of with oranges, the true cost savings will not be universally accepted.

Homecare Cost Comparisons

With all that has been said so far, why proceed with comparisons of the cost of homecare services vs. inpatient hospital care, nursing home care, and other facility care? Despite the critics, investigators are still reporting cost savings. Of particular concern, companies in business to make a profit for their stockholders, such as insurance companies, are reporting large savings in expenditures. In addition, high technology homecare services stimulated by the PPS/DRG reimbursement plan are also finding huge savings. Therefore, it is appropriate to examine the studies that report saving dollars through the use of homecare services as a substitute for institutional care. A cautionary note: the date of the study is important, since the actual dollar value will have changed; the ratio between the figures will still be critical.

Inpatient Hospital Care vs. Homecare

An eight-hospital coalition in the Midwest established a homecare program and Emerson (1985) reported that homecare costs averaged about 25 percent of hospital day costs. Lawson (1984) adds the dollar value by noting that the average cost of a hospital stay is between $350 to $400 per day, while homecare averages $35 to $70 per day. The National Association for Home Care (NAHC) reported (Home Health Journal 1986) an average cost of $53 for each day a homecare visit occurs as against an average $310 per day for inpatient hospital care. However, Hughes (Intravenous Therapy News 1985) did say that "it is not clear whether home health care is less expensive and more economical than hospital care." A GAO report (1982) also stated that homecare may cost more despite being beneficial. Nevertheless, most would agree that in considering only dollar amounts, inpatient hospital care is more expensive than homecare.

Insurance Companies. "Most (commercial insurance) companies see homecare as a way to cut costs," according to Donna Sanctis of the Health Insurance Association of America (HIAA) (Anderson 1986). Don Thomas, also of HIAA, said, "As long as employers have an interest in saving dollars, homecare will be encouraged" (Cabin 1985a). Speaking for Blue Cross and Blue Shield Association, Bernard Tresnowski commented, "Nine out of ten Blue Cross and Blue Shield Plans now offer home health care as an answer to high health care costs" (Cabin 1985a).

Using an Individual Case Management (ICM) program, Aetna Life and Casualty reported that 600 people benefited in 1985 at a savings of $36.8 million (Matus 1986). According to Matus, the ICM Coordinator, "The ICM program is designed to help patients faced with huge expenses of acute care to receive quality care in an alternate setting. The home is an ideal alternative." Aetna has accrued substantial savings using high technology homecare services in place of hospital care. In the case of a young man with a spinal cord injury from an automobile accident, the insurance company secured a waterbed for his home and allowed him to leave the hospital. The waterbed enables the patient to turn himself and improves muscle strength. Savings to the company: about $27,000 a month (Woodbridge 1984). Aetna also reported a $78,000 per case savings from using the ICM program for victims of catastrophic accidents (Cabin 1985a; Caring 1984a).

CIGNA (Connecticut General Life Insurance Company) estimates that it saves five days of hospital bills for each homecare situation. "It comes to an average of $1,000 per hospitalized employee," says Kathleen M. Dayley, a marketing director for the company (Business Week 1984). As an incentive to employers to control costs, CIGNA allows them to offer employees the choice of 100 percent coverage for homecare and only 80 percent payment for inpatient care costs (Lawson 1984).

Blue Cross/Blue Shield of Maryland saved $1.2 million in 1982 by reducing the average subscriber's inpatient days through its Coordinated Home Care Program. Since 1973, the program claims a net saving of $6.3 million for the homecare program (Cabin 1985a). In a joint cost-cutting effort, Blue Cross of Greater Philadelphia, Pennsylvania Blue Shield, and the Philadelphia Council of the AFL-CIO saved about $31.1 million for union members in five local counties. Activities included preadmission testing, ambulatory surgery, home health care, and benefit coordination to provide for other party liability (Cabin 1985a; Ozga 1984).

High-Technology Savings. "Anecdotal evidence suggests that high technology homecare can be provided for about one-third the cost of the same care in a hospital" (Anderson 1986).

IV Antibiotic. Homecare intravenous antibiotic therapy as a cost containment measure was the subject of a symposium for pharmacy professionals. Six articles covered cost containment, the role of the pharmacist, implementation, evaluation, and pitfalls *(Drug Intelligence and Clinical Pharmacy 1985)*. "Perhaps the most effective method of cost containment is home administration of antimicrobials" (Barriere 1985).

Using intravenous antibiotics at home as an alternative to a long hospital stay, Newman (1985) found a 73 percent saving compared to care in the hospital. Citing nine studies, Harris (1984) said, "Published reports indicate that a home parenteral antibiotic program may result in savings ranging from 68 to 78 percent over hospital costs for similar therapy." Pelletier (1985) found an average per day patient savings of $200 to $300 when antibiotics were administered at home. Bowyer (1986) noted a study which showed an average savings per patient on home antibiotic intravenous therapy of $3,658.20 for 18.2 days of care. In home treatment of osteomyelitis with IV antibiotic therapy, for 30 days, Grizzard (1985) calculates minimal savings of more than $9,000. "An extremely conservative estimate of savings for a patient who is able to return to work while receiving IV antibiotic therapy is $312 per day.

Hughes (1984) cited three studies in his review of the economics of home health care dealing with IV antibiotic therapy. One investigation of 150 patients showed costs reduced by at least $142 per day. Another saved $1,600 per patient per course of therapy. Comparative costs in another study found homecare IV antibiotic therapy costing $69.35 per day while inpatient hospital care was $243.22 per day.

With data from 23 patients, Harris, Buckle, and Coffen (1986) found substantial savings in home vs. hospital IV antimicrobial therapy. Daily cost ranges and averages for individuals follow:

Hospital Cost	Home Cost	Savings	Total Savings
$288 - $538	$52 - $365	$142 - $313	$993 - $10,419
$428	$207	$221	$5,034

Individual daily homecare costs ranged from 20 to 68 percent of individual daily hospital charges and averaged 48 percent. "Since institution of our program of home therapy in February 1984, we have saved third party payers $115,783."

Total Parenteral Nutrition. Home parenteral nutrition also seems to save money compared to inpatient hospital care. Dzierba, Mirtallo, Graver, et al. (1984) reported that annual costs were 60 percent lower and cost about $119 per day. In treating 13 patients for one year, $651,651 was estimated to be saved. Silver, Majorie, Romain, et al. (1984) cite similar evidence from a Michigan facility where inpatients receiving total parenteral nutrition incurred charges of $338 daily as compared to home therapy at $150 daily. "Most studies have shown a minimum of 40 percent and maximum of 75 percent reduction in costs treating the same hospitalized patient with nutritional support at home." Brakebill, Robb, and Ivey (1983) noted a daily charge of $205.68 per infusion day in the hospital compared to $48.19 per homecare infusion day.

Respiratory/Ventilator Dependent Care. Home respiratory care for ventilator-dependent individuals was examined by the American Association for Respiratory Therapy (AART) in a 20-state survey in 1984 (Fox 1984; Milligan 1984). Investigators found 258 people medically able to go home; 48 were under 17 years of age. Almost 2,000 people were being cared for in hospitals at a cost of about $270,830 per year. Treatment at home was about $21,000 per year. Savings for the 258 people able to go home was calculated at $64.4 million. It was noted that the huge savings were based upon data from only 20 states and could be considerably larger with information from the 30 states not surveyed. Probably due to this huge savings, the AART cost figures have appeared often (Callas 1985; Cabin 1985a; Weinstein 1985). Focusing upon ventilator dependent children, Kahn (1984) compares the cost from acute care hospital ICU, to hospital intermediate ICU, to rehabilitation hospital, to independent living center, to homecare by an RN, to homecare by a certified homecare giver. Respective monthly patient care costs for 1981-1982 were $35,000; $22,000; $14,300; $14,300; $7,200; $8,000; and $5,400. There was a 77 percent difference between acute care ICU and RN homecare.

Pediatric Homecare. It is estimated that there will be a 75 percent drop in expenses when a child is brought home. Cabin (1985b) reviewed the cost-effectiveness of pediatric homecare and cited about 15 examples of cost-saving programs. Almost all the activities dealt with home respiratory care and exhibited the large volume savings already noted. During a four-year period, for example, Illinois saved more than $4 million treating only 10 ventilator dependent children who returned home.

Early Maternity Discharge. By 1985, the early maternity discharge program became so popular that Blue Cross/Blue Shield of Vermont doubled its incentive from $50 to $100. In addition to the incentive, mothers receive three skilled nursing visits at home and nine hours of homemaker services from participating VNAs. Eligible mothers can also be reimbursed up to $50 for taking an approved prenatal course. At an estimate of $700 saved per case with 250 women participating, total savings are figured at $175,000. Insurance officials calculate that saving one-half day of the usual three-day maternity stay could result in savings of between $40 and $50 million nationally on the one million births covered by the 15 plans (Cabin 1985a).

Diagnosis-Specific Homecare. Homecare at Park Nicollet Medical Center is physician-owned and clinic-based, with activities designed to treat certain conditions that normally require a hospital stay: newborn family care; bilirubin phototherapy; low back pain; and psoriasis (Roeder 1984c). Of a total savings of $2 million, the newborn and low back programs contributed more than 40 percent each, with psoriasis 16 percent, and bilirubin 3 percent. Comparative data for each activity follows:

Program	Hospital Cost	Home Cost	Savings
Low back pain	12 days @ $452 $5,452	12 days $852	$4,573
Newborn	Mother/child $480	$161	$ 319
Psoriasis	3 weeks @ $452/day $9,450	12 days $852	$8,650
Bilirubin	2.5 mother/child days $690	2.5 days $200	$ 490

In a later article, Roeder and Skovbroten (1985) reported that the bilirubin program treated 77 patients and saved more than $30,000.

Health Maintenance Organizations. HMOs have maintained for many years that they save money with preventive medicine and prompt attention, thereby keeping their members out of the hospital. Brazil (1986) told of one HMO that paid its participating physicians an additional $300 to take care of specific illnesses at home. For example, a patient with low back pain might receive a hospital bed, traction equipment, and nurse visits from the HMO instead of seven to eight days in the hospital. For making housecalls as necessary and for supervising care, the physician receives the additional $300, and the HMO may save about $1,500.

Nursing Home Care vs. Homecare

Because of the assumption that individuals who cannot secure homecare will have to be placed in nursing homes, this area of comparison has received considerable attention. Some investigations have questioned this idea, contending that homecare is an add-on service and not a substitution for nursing home care. However, funding policies and medical practices do appear to encourage the placement of the chronically ill and disabled in nursing homes (Brazil 1986). This results in inappropriate placements for a percentage of nursing home residents. Yet, "the Medicare skilled nursing facility is likely to continue to have a crucial role in post-hospital care as the treatment modality of choice for individuals who require both highly skilled care and functional assistance" (Kramer, Shaughnessy, and Pettigrew 1985). Of the estimated 26 million patients who may need assistance, NAHC calculates that 2 million get homecare, while 1.3 million are in nursing homes (*Hospitals* 1985a).

NAHC brochures claim that homecare is less expensive because it does keep people out of nursing homes. University of North Carolina, Chapel Hill, researchers found, however, that bills for certain patients were much lower when cared for at home, but that homecare agencies "don't keep many elderly patients out of expensive institutions" (*Hospitals* 1985b). Tightening of Medicare eligibility requirements regarding "homebound" and "intermittent care" to contain costs may also send people into institutional care. According to homecare proponents, "whatever Medicare saves will be spent many times over to pay for more expensive hospital or nursing home care of patients who could have been treated at home" (Whitlow 1985).

In spite of the questionable premise that "but for" homecare, the individual would have to enter a nursing home, articles are still reporting comparative cost data.

Cost Overview. The cost of care in a nursing home can range from $12,000 to more than $25,000 per year per person. As Congressman Claude Pepper often notes, the federal government is spending billions to keep people in facilities and only a few million for homecare (House Select Committee on Aging 1985, iii). Allen (1985) cites a $1,000 per month cost for SNF care and $300-$400 per month for a rest home. NAHC (Home Health Journal 1986) notes that the average Medicare reimbursement for a day of homecare is $53, compared to $62 per day on a continuing basis for nursing home care. Even at that minimal savings ($9 per day), there could be an annual savings of more than $3,000 per patient.

Cost Comparisons

Gateway II. In Maryland, the Gateway II Project found that a client who received funds to fill gaps in community care services cost the state $222 per month. If that same client entered a nursing home, the cost to the state would be $482 per month, a savings of $260 per month. Total local, state, and federal costs to maintain a Gateway II client in the community totaled $398 monthly, compared to $959 in a nursing home, a savings of $561 per month for the same client (Cabin 1985a; Interagency Aging Committee 1984).

Chelsea-Village. A long-running homecare program, the Chelsea-Village Program of New York City's St. Vincent's Hospital and Medical Center consistently reports considerable savings over nursing home care. For example, an 84-year-old homebound woman requiring pain medication, leg soaks, and infection control along with meals-on-wheels, shopping, cleaning, and cooking is able to be maintained at home. Lipsman, Brickner, Scharer, et al. (1984, 197) report her health and living care costs as follows:

Service Source	Monthly Costs	Payment Source
Professional health care team MD, RN, MSW	$ 235	Chelsea Village Program
Personal care worker	593	New York City
Dressing supplies	29	New York City
Rent	94	Patient
Utilities	25	Patient
Telephone	30	Patient
Food	120	Patient
Total	$1,126	

In November 1982, the New York State Department of Social Services put the average 30-day Medicaid reimbursement for a skilled nursing facility in New York City at $2,686. In this case, the monthly savings would be $1,560.

This model homecare program serving frail, semi-ambulatory elderly patients of an average age of 80 maintains people in their own homes for about half the cost of nursing home care (Bricker and Scharer 1977).

Medicaid 2176 Waivers. Medicaid home- and community-based waivers saved money, according to a report to Congress from HCFA (Department of Health and Human Services 1984). "In aggregate, the approved waiver programs are projected by the states to reduce expenditures for nursing home care by $705.9 million (6.1 percent of expenditures for covered levels in year one)." Savings estimates projected are $235.5 million for FY 1983; $615.3 million for FY 1985; and $697.4 million for FY 1986. Savings over the five years, 1982-1986, are estimated to total $2.04 billion. Greatest savings are noted in community care for those who are developmentally disabled and/or mentally impaired; $9,815 vs. $5,089 per patient per year for those with less severe limitations are estimated for 1984.

Considerable variation occurs among individual state waiver programs. Florida estimates that its program, with two waivers, will save $144 million (25 percent) by 1986. Six other states calculate savings over $25 million in 1986: California, $65 million; Louisiana, $57 million; Illinois, $48 million; Colorado, $42 million; New Jersey, $28 million; and Alabama, $27 million. Savings of less than one million are projected by 14 other waiver programs. This level of saving is contingent upon the states' actually serving the projected number of waiver recipients at projected costs, and effecting the projected reductions in nursing home use through the home- and community-based waivers.

Based on an evaluation of the waiver program in Connecticut, Yeatts, Steinhardt, and Capitman (1985) found supporting evidence for the savings. "Total average monthly Medicaid expenditures for waivered service users ($745) was far less than nursing home users ($1,480). If the waiver clients are indeed the "but for" population, this indicates that Medicaid is experiencing close to a 50 percent reduction in expenditures for these persons." However, the authors do state that the conclusions are speculative, since unknown factors in existence at the time could have influenced these observations.

HCFA's 1982 data showed Medicare expenditures of about $300 million for SNF care, while Medicaid spent $4.3 billion. Average annual Medicaid costs per client were $7,854 for nursing home care; $6,395 for ICF care; $2,179 for general inpatient hospital care; and $1,251 for home health care (House Select Committee on Aging 1985, 7). Furthermore, a national homecare cost survey revealed that homecare services rarely extended beyond one month at an average cost of $352.26, compared to a monthly nursing home cost of $1,564.06 (Shannon 1985).

Nursing Home Without Walls. New York State's Nursing Home Without Walls (NHWW) program began in November 1978 as "the most viable alternative to institutional care" (Lombardi 1986). There are 84 approved programs in 48 counties, including New York City, serving more than 4,000 patients. While legislation allows NHWW program costs to go up to 75 percent of nursing home care, experience has shown that the cost per patient is about 50 percent of institutional care. Exhibit 7-4 shows monthly cost comparisons as of May 1984 for patients in New York City. At that date, total costs for NHWW patients were 63.6 percent of the allowable cap and only 47.7 percent of the cost of institutional care. For May 1984 alone, the potential savings of NHWW compared to nursing home care could amount to as much as $1,755,413. A New York State Department of Social Services report for 1983 estimated Medicaid savings at $20,418,736. Almost $300,000 was appropriated to the Home Health Care Grant Program by the New York State Legislature for FY 1984-85 to stimulate NHWW programs. Lombardi (1986) stated that, "The Nursing Home Without Walls program continues to serve as a truly viable cost effective alternative to institutional care for people who want to be cared for in their own home."

Brazil (1986) noted that New York State will pay over $2,000 per month to keep a patient in an SNF but "absolutely nothing if the family takes care of such patients in their own homes." He suggests that the state pay the family $700 to $800 per month for care; they still would accrue considerable savings.

Exhibit 7-4 Cost Comparisons for Nursing Home Without Walls (NHWW) Patients in New York City for May 1984

Level of Care	No. of NHWW Patients	Approved NHWW Patient Budgets	Monthly Cost Ceiling (CAP)	Potential RHCF Costs for These Patients	Potential NHWW Cost Savings
SNF	893	$1,184,021	$1,887,802 (62.7%)	$2,517,367 (47%)	$1,333,346
HRF	483	$ 419,802	$ 631,281 (66.5%)	$ 841,869 (49.8%)	$ 422,067
Totals	1,376 (63.6%)	$1,603,823 (47.7%)	$2,519,083	$3,359,236	$1,755,413

Averages:

· Average Cost for SNF Level NHWW Patient: $1,325/month (47% of SNF Care)
· Average Cost for HRF Level NHWW Patient: $ 869/month (49.8% of HRF Care)
· Average Cost for NHWW Patient: $1,165/month (47.7% of Institutional Care)

SNF = Skilled Nursing Facility
HRF = Health Related Facility
RHCF = Residential Health Care Facility
Source: New York City Human Resources Administration. Long-term Home Health Care Program. Monthly Statistics for May 1984.

Veterans Administration. A GAO (1981) study of VA hospitals found homecare a cost-beneficial alternative to institutional care. Per diem charges in 16 VA hospitals ranged from $91.81 to $256.82 in 1979. Six VA nursing homes cost from $51.49 to $86.13 per day. Home visit costs ranged from $25.59 to $109.21. The GAO therefore urged expansion of homecare, but with attention given to the improvement of program management.

Alternative Health Services Project. Researchers compared alternate living services, adult day rehabilitation, and home-delivered services to provide community-based long-term care. Skellie, Mobley, and Coan (1982) found that costs for those at risk of entering a nursing home were somewhat lower, but were add-ons for those not at risk. Their data suggest the possibility of community-based services substituting for nursing home care for the population likely to enter an institution.

Homemaker vs. Day Care vs. Combined Services. Weissert, Wan, and Livieratos (1980) conducted a one-year cost comparison of groups receiving homemaker care, day care, or both. Homemaker costs for patients in the study were 60 percent higher ($9,189) compared to the control group ($5,757), a $3,432 difference. Day care costs increased 71 percent despite reduced institutionalization for the study group. Costs were $6,501 and $3,809 for the control group, a difference of $2,692. Patients receiving both services in the study group cost $8,566 per year, compared to $6,228 for the controls, a 38 percent increase of $2,338. These investigators concluded that the homemaker services were not cost-effective. However, significantly lower proportions of the study group receiving homemaker services died. The conclusions of this study were challenged frequently during Congressional hearings citing savings data from California, Massachusetts, New Jersey, and Washington (O'Shaughnessey and Reiss 1981, 13).

Private Practice Comparison. A matched group of 10 homecare and 10 nursing home patients in the care of a private practice internist in Tennessee were compared. While Powers and Burger (1985) found that the total cost during the six-month observation was $10,524 for nursing home patients, compared to $7,514 for homecare, the results were not statistically significant. Costs for these groups did not differ for medication, hospitalization, laboratory tests, housing, and maintenance. However, $2,922 was added to the homecare costs as estimated living expenses. Nevertheless, despite the dollar cost misgivings, the authors did comment that "family and patient satisfaction is a key consideration in the choice between homecare and nursing home placement."

This last study again focuses on problems often noted in comparative cost investigation; for instance, only using official costs/charges rather than including all types of unpaid service contributions to care. The add-on or substitute issue also remains an important consideration.

Hospice Care vs. Homecare

Supportive care for terminally ill patients at home "has enabled many such patients to preserve personal dignity and to maintain a significantly better quality of life than would otherwise be possible" (Rogatz 1985). Buckingham and Lupu (1982) estimated the number of hospices operating in the U.S. at 500 to 700 in 1982. By 1984, the National Hospice Organization estimated nearly 1,400 organizations providing care (*Hospice News* 1985). No matter the number, the hospice movement is growing rapidly. Hospices are organized in a variety of structural forms, which poses a problem for cost comparisons. However, the usual comparison is made with care at an inpatient hospital and a less intensive facility, such as a nursing home.

A study by Case Western Medical School found that hospice care saved from 39 to 51 percent of the costs for nonhospice care patients (Weinstein 1985; *Caring* 1984a; Hospice Council of Northern Ohio 1983). Saltzman (1985) reported that hospital care for the hospice patient is $335 to $409 per day, while home hospice care ran $53 to $286 per day, including medical emergencies. Freudenheim (1986) cited additional savings in his *New York Times* article on hospice as an option. A Congressional Budget Office report estimated that Medicare saved $330 on those beneficiaries electing hospice care, and the National Hospice Organization called that figure "very conservative." Cabrini Hospice in New York states that it costs $66 per day for hospice homecare for cancer patients. AIDS patients cost more than $800 per inpatient hospital day in San Francisco, Atlanta, and New York, and health professionals find that homecare costs much less.

Insurance Coverage. Blue Cross/Blue Shield of Vermont started hospice coverage in a 1981 pilot program and expanded the coverage in 1985. Patients stay in the program an average of 36 days at a 1984 cost of $36.30 per day, compared to a hospital per diem cost of $440 (Cabin 1985a). Hospice coverage is offered by 64 of the nation's Blue Cross/Blue Shield plans as an alternative to hospital stays (*Medical Economics* 1986). A 1985 survey by the Washington Business Group on Health found that 59 percent of the Fortune 500 companies offered the hospice benefit under their coverage (Freudenheim 1986).

Hospice homecare cost savings to third-party insurers was investigated by Brooks and Smyth-Staruch (1984). Almost 1,400 nonhospice care patients were compared to 153 Cuyahoga County, Ohio, patients who received hospice homecare while dying of cancer. "Hospice cost savings to third-party insurers were substantial, representing a relative savings of approximately 40 percent as indicated by the differences between the hospice and the nonhospice study subjects." Differences and savings in the last 2 weeks, 4 weeks, 8 weeks, and 12 weeks before death between hospice homecare and nonhospice patient care were as follows:

Period	Homecare	Nonhospice Care	Savings	
Last 2 weeks	$1,067	$1,910	$ 843	44%
Last 4 weeks	1,890	3,313	1,423	43%
Last 8 weeks	3,081	5,715	2,634	46%
Last 12 weeks	4,192	7,872	3,680	47%

The authors concluded from these results, that hospice homecare was less costly than nonhospice homecare.

Hospice of North Shore. In suburban Chicago, the Hospice of the North Shore (HONS) compared home hospice care to inpatient hospice care. Haid, Fowler, Nicklin, et al. (1984) reported on a 20-month period up to the end of 1981, that HONS cared for 22.3 percent of all those dying of cancer within six communities, at a cost of $14.26 per day, with an average cost of care at $946.86 per patient, and a median cost of $449.19 per patient. An average of 11.05 hospital days per patient were avoided. At a 1983 Evanston Hospital per diem cost of $438, the savings per homecare hospice patient are $4,839.90 ($438 X 11.05 days saved). Subtracting the average homecare hospice cost of $946.86, a net savings of $3,893.04 is achieved. Projecting that savings to the 44,000 cancer-related deaths expected nationally, HONS homecare hospice-type programs serving about 23 percent of those terminal patients could achieve savings of $381,985,084.80 for the nation.

National Hospice Study. A multisite, multiyear, quasiexperimental national hospice study compared costs for hospice care at home (HC) or in a hospital (HB) to the costs of conventional care (CC) (Greer, Mor, Morris, et al. 1986). Total costs per study day were $101 for HC, $146 for HB, and $149 for CC. For Medicare patients, HC patient costs were lower than for HB patients. In the last two months of life, HC patients had lower costs than CC patients, but CC costs were lower in earlier months. In the last year of life, "nonetheless, a large ($2,221) estimated savings conservatively attributable to hospice was observed." Average costs in the last year of life were $10,798 for HC; $12,698 for HB; and $14,799 for CC (Mor and Kidder 1985). Despite HB patients having lower costs than CC patients only in the last month of life, the net savings for HB care was $585. Medicare patient costs for the last month of life were $2,270 for HC; $2,657 for HB; and $6,110 for CC (Mor and Kidder 1985). "The HC model is less costly than HB or CC because HC substitutes homecare for inpatient care, relying on family members to provide up to 12 hours a day of direct care" (Greer and Mor 1986a). In an inpatient setting, ancillary services are also reduced during the stay of a terminally ill patient.

Noting the complexity of evaluating cost factors, Greer and Mor (1986) called the cost savings impact "mixed." While the HC model reduces costs, the HB model may not. Length of stay appears to be a critical variable. As patients stay longer in hospice care, the costs mount, reducing the savings impact. In addition, if hospice care becomes an industry, "the commitment, integrity, and restraint that was observed in the demonstration may diminish" (Mor and Kidder 1985). "A crucial factor affecting future hospice costs will be the quality of management" (Birnbaum and Kidder 1984).

In discussing the use of hospice homecare by business concerns, David L. Glueck, a management consultant, commented: "Hospice is definitely a cost saver if administered properly. It needs to be accepted as a means of offering humane and supportive care. For the employer and the doctor to be encouraging it for cost reasons is a ghoulish approach. Employees become apprehensive and cynical, as they well might be" (Freudenheim 1986).

Family Assurances. For families to participate in homecare hospice and other homecare programs, there must be assurances of 24-hour access to help, a facility bed if necessary, and respite care to relieve them of the burden for a brief time.

Around-the-clock help need not mean a home visit, but could mean having telephone access to a physician, nurse, or other professional. An emergency response system can also provide a calming effect. Ruchlin and Morris (1981) described the cost-effectiveness of an electronic device allowing the owner to push a button that automatically dials a 24-hour emergency number.

If there is a need for the patient to be readmitted to the facility, the family would like to know that a bed will be provided without a wait. In some cases, this means having swing beds available, depending upon the needs of the population at risk in the community.

Caring for ill, disabled, and terminally ill people at home is a physically and mentally draining task. Family members need to know vacations, however brief, are possible from time to time. At times, the patient can be returned to an institution or others can be employed to come into the home.

Cost-saving Strategies

Based on a review of 70 cost-saving studies, Health Policy Alternatives, Inc. (1983, 32) came up with specific cost-saving strategies for homecare:

- Develop program capacity for assessment of high-risk individuals, of services to supplement unpaid care, and for coordination of care.

- Provide for patients whose hospital stay can be shortened, for nursing home patients whose level of care can be provided efficiently outside the facility, and for patients applying for nursing home admission in the near future.

- Identify levels of aid needed for patients who can be cared for at home through functional and psychological evaluations.

- Assess the resources of the patient, including the residence, family aid, other unpaid care resources, community agencies for help, financial capabilities, and other factors.

- Evaluate limitations on the cost of covered services to protect against the possibilities of aggregate cost increases by considering the cost of all alternatives.

Cost-Saving and Social Policy

It appears that many organizations and individuals are jumping on the homecare bandwagon as a cost containment measure. Cynics would say that the right thing is happening for the wrong reason. Rogatz (1985) believes it is a mistake to consider homecare primarily in cost containment terms. Interestingly, Rogatz and Crocetti (1958) made that same observation more than 25 years ago, when homecare was being widely touted as an economy measure. Still holding this view, Rogatz (1985) says, "Home health care must not be seen as a cost-saving technique, but rather as a vital component of the broad spectrum of institutional-based ambulatory and community-based services which an enlightened society must make available to its members. There is no free lunch." In a similar vein, Greer and Mor (1986) spoke about the results of their hospice study, commenting that social policy determines further applications of homecare.

References

Allen, S. L. 1985. Cost containment projects could reduce health costs. *Home Health Journal* 6(4):11-12.

Anderson, H. J. 1986. High technology services help cut lengths of stay, save money. *Modern Healthcare* 16(4):90, 92.

Barriere, S. L. 1985. Cost-containment of antimicrobial therapy. *Drug Intelligence and Clinical Pharmacy* 19:278-281.

Birnbaum, H. G., and D. Kidder. 1984. What does hospice cost? *American Journal of Public Health* 74:689-697.

Bowyer, C. K. 1986. The complex care team: meeting the needs of high technology nursing at home. *Home Healthcare Nurse* 4(1):24-29.

Brakebill, J. I., R. A. Robb, and M. F. Ivey. 1983. Pharmacy department costs and patient charges associated with a home parenteral nutrition program. *American Journal of Hospital Pharmacy* 40(2):260-263.

Brazil, P. 1986. Cost effective care is better care. *Hastings Center Report* 16(1):7-8.

Brickner, P. W., and L. K. Scharer. 1977. Hospital provides homecare for elderly at one-half nursing home cost. *Forum* 12:6-12.

Brooks, C. H., and K. Smyth-Staruck. 1984. Hospice homecare cost savings to third-party insurers. *Medical Care* 22:691-703.

Buckingham, R. W., and D. Lupu. 1982. A comparative study of hospice services in the U.S. *American Journal of Public Health* 72:453-463.

Bush, C. 1977. Cost cutting pearls from reader reviewers. *Patient Care* 4(5):48-53.

Business Week. 1984. The insurers' big push for home health care (28 May).

Cabin, B. 1985a. Cost effectiveness of pediatric homecare. *Caring* 4(10):62-70.

Cabin, W. 1985b. Some evidence of the cost-effectiveness of homecare. *Caring* 4(10):62-70.

Callas, T. 1985. Home mechanical ventilation: restoring independence. *Rx Home Care* 7(7):45-50.

Caring. 1984a. Blue Cross finds hospice saves insurers money. 3(1):8.

Caring. 1984b. Aetna reports new homecare benefit saves $78,000 per case. 3(5):65.

Day, S. R. 1984. Measuring utilization and impact of homecare services: a systems model approach for cost effectiveness. *Home Health Care Services Quarterly* 5(2):5-24.

Department of Health and Human Services, Health Care Financing Administration, Office of Research and Demonstrations, 1984. *Studies evaluating Medicaid home- and community-based care waivers.* Washington, DC: Government Printing Office (Dec.).

Department of Health, Education and Welfare. 1976. *Home health care: report on the regional public hearings 9/20-10/1/76.* Washington, DC: Government Printing Office. Pub. No. 76-135.

Doty, P. 1984. Can home and community based services provide lower cost alternatives to nursing homes? Working paper. Washington, DC: Health Care Financing Administration (Dec.).

Drug Intelligence and Clinical Pharmacy. 1985. Antibiotic cost-containment in the home health care environment. 19(4):278-296.

Dzierba, S. H., J. M. Mirtallo, D. W. Grauer, et al. 1984. Fiscal and clinical evaluation of home parenteral nutrition. *American Journal of Hospital Pharmacy* 41:285-291.

Emerson, D. 1985. Hospitals' home health coalition improves care, cuts costs. *Health Progress* 66(5):26.

Fox, J. E. 1984. Home respiratory care seen cheaper, better. *U.S. Medicine* 20(5):28 (1 March).

Freudenheim, M. 1986. Hospice care as an option. *New York Times* (4 Feb.).

Fuchs, V. R. 1982. Foreword in *Cost-benefit and cost-effective analysis in health care: principles, practice and potential,* edited by K. E. Warner and B. R. Luce. Ann Arbor, MI: Health Administration Press.

General Accounting Office. 1977. *Home health--the need for a national policy to better provide for the elderly.* Washington, D.C.: Government Printing Office. Pub. No. HRD 78-19 (30 December).

General Accounting Office. 1981. *Veterans Administration's home care program is a cost beneficial alternative to institutional care and should be expanded, but program management needs improvement.* Washington, DC: Government Printing Office. Pub. No. HRD 81-72 (27 April).

General Accounting Office. 1982. *The elderly should benefit from expanded home health care but increasing those services will not insure cost reduction.* Washington, DC: Government Printing Office. Pub. No. GAO/IPE-83-1 (7 Dec.).

Greer, D. S., and V. Mor. 1986a. An overview of national hospice study findings. *Journal of Chronic Disease* 39(1):5-7.

Greer, D. S., V. Mor, J. N. Morris, et al. 1986b. An alternative in terminal care: results of the national hospice study. *Journal of Chronic Disease* 39(1):9-26.

Grizzard, M. B. 1985. Home intravenous antibiotic therapy. *Postgraduate Medicine* 78(6):187-196.

Haid, M., M. Fowler, O. Nicklin, et al. 1984. People and dollars: the experience of one hospice. *Southern Medical Journal* 77(4):470-472.

Hammond, J. 1979. Home health care cost effectiveness: an overview of the literature. *Public Health Reports* 94:305-311.

Harris, L. F., T. F. Buckle, and F. L. Coffen, Jr. 1986. Intravenous antibiotics at home. *Southern Medical Journal* 79(2):193-196.

Harris, W. L., Jr. 1984. Home parenteral antibiotic therapy. *Topics in Hospital Pharmacy Management* 4(3):43-55.

Hatch, O. G. 1981. Community home health services act of 1981. *Congressional Record-Senate* S5600-S5610 (22 Jan.).

Hay, J. W., and G. Mandes. 1984. Home health care cost-function analysis. *Health Care Financing Review* 5(3):111-116.

Health Policy Alternatives, Inc. 1983. *Expansion of cost effective home health care.* Washington, DC (May).

Home Health Journal. 1986. New statistics from NAHC. 7(2):5.

Hospice Council of Northern Ohio. 1983. *Cost savings of hospice home care for third party insurers.* Cleveland, OH (Nov.).

Hospice News. 1985. 3:1. National Hospice Organization, Arlington, VA.

Hospitals. 1985a. Five million Americans require home health care: government study. 59(5):38, 41.

Hospitals. 1985b. News at deadline. 59(14):21.

House Select Committee on Aging. 1985. *Building a long term care policy: home care data and implications.* Washington, DC: Government Printing Office. Comm. Pub. No. 98-484.

Hughes, T. F. 1984. The economics of home health care. *Topics in Hospital Pharmacy Management* 4(3):9-15.

Interagency Aging Committee. Maryland Office on Aging. 1984. Gateway II--cost effective community care in Maryland. *Caring* 3(5):62-63.

Intravenous Therapy News. 1985. Economic implications of home care uncertain. 12(9):1, 14.

Kahn, L. 1984. Ventilator-dependent children heading home. *Hospital* 58(5):54-55.

Klarman, H. E., J. O'S. Francis, and G. D. Rosenthal. 1968. Cost effectiveness applied to the treatment of chronic renal disease. *Medical Care* 6:48-54.

Knollmueller, R. N. 1984. Funding homecare in a climate of cost containment. *Public Health Nursing* 1(1):16-22.

Kramer, A. M., P. W. Shaughnessy, and M. L. Pettigrew. 1985. Cost-effectiveness implications based on a comparison of nursing home and home health case mix. *Health Services Research* 20(4):387-405.

Lawson, J. C. 1984. Home health care idea catching on. *The Journal of Commerce* (25 June).

Lipsman, R. P. W. Brickner, L. K. Scharer, et al. 1984. The Chelsea-Village program in *Hospitals and the aged,* edited by S. J. Brody and N. A. Persily. Rockville, MD: Aspen Systems Corporation.

Lombardi, T., Jr. 1986. Nursing home without walls--an update. New York State Senate Health Committee, Albany, NY (1 Jan.).

Matus, B. 1986. Personal communication. Aetna Life and Casualty, Hartford, CT (12 Feb.).

Medical Economics. 1986. The terminally ill may spend less time in hospitals (28 April).

Milligan, S. 1984. Survey finds respiratory home care saves $250,000 per person annually. *Caring* 3(5):58-60.

Modern Healthcare. 1985. Home health agencies overstate savings. 15(26):5.

Mor, V., and D. Kidder. 1985. Cost savings in hospice: final results of the national hospice study. *Health Services Research* 20(4):407-422.

Newman, W. A. B. 1985. Intravenous antibiotics at home: alternative to a long hospital stay. *Rx Home Care* 7(7):41-43.

Ognibene, P. J. 1980. Health care at home: better and cheaper. *Fifty Plus* 20(2):90-93.

O'Shaughnessey, C., and K. Reiss. 1981. *Long term care: community-based alternatives to institutionalization.* Washington, DC: Congressional

Research Service, Library of Congress. No. 1B81013 (23 June).

Ozga, J. 1984. Health care coalitions focus on home care. *Caring* 3(5):64-65.

Pelletier, G. 1985. DRGs and home care. *National Intravenous Therapy Association* 8(1):19-21.

Powers, J. S., and C. Burger. 1985. Home health care vs. nursing home care for the elderly. *Journal of the Tennessee Medical Association* 78(4):227-230.

Roeder, B. 1984. Diagnosis-specific home care: a model for the future. *Caring* 3(12):39-42.

Roeder, B., and B. Skovbroten. 1985. Park Nicollet Medical Center. *Caring* 4(5):92-94.

Rogatz, P. 1985. Home health care: some social and economic considerations. *Home Healthcare Nurse* 3(1):38-43.

Rogatz, P., and G. Crocetti. 1958. Home care programs -their impact on the hospital's role in medical care. *American Journal of Public Health* 48:1125-1133.

Ruby, G., H. D. Banta, and A. K. Burns. 1985. Medicare coverage, Medicare costs, and medical technology. *Journal of Health Politics, Policy and Law* 10(1):141-155.

Ruchlin, H. S., and J. N. Morris. 1981. Cost benefit analysis of an emergency alarm and response system: a case study of a long-term care program. *Health Services Research* 16(1):65-80.

Saltzman, B. N. 1985. Is home health care cost effective? *The Journal of the Arkansas Medical Society* 81(8):429-431.

Schorr, B. 1981. Home care services for the elderly and disabled are advocated as cheaper than nursing home. *Wall Street Journal* (26 March).

Seligmann, J. 1980. Home care pays off. *Newsweek* (10 March).

Senate Special Committee on Aging. 1985. *The cost of caring for the chronically ill: the case for insurance.* Washington, DC: Government Printing Office. Pub. No. S. Hrg. 98-1224.

Shannon, K. 1985. Home health care study paves way for fixed homecare benefits. *Hospitals* 59(5):72.

Shepherd, R. 1978. Nursing home costs halved by home maintenance program. *HCFA Forum* 2(2):33-35.

Shrifter, N. 1980. The physician and home health care -costs are less and patients feel better. *LACMA Physician* 110:23-26 (6 Oct.).

Silver, C., D. Majorie, C. S. Romain, et al. 1984. Home setting to play greater role in medical care. *Journal of the Louisiana State Medical Society* 136(11):25-26.

Skellie, F. A., G. M. Mobley, and R. E. Coan. 1982. Cost effectiveness of community based long term care: current findings of Georgia's alternative health services project. *American Journal of Public Health* 72:353-358.

Stewart, J. E. 1979. *Home health care.* St. Louis: C. V. Mosby Company.

Weinstein, S. M. 1985. The how-tos of homecare. *National Intravenous Therapy Association* 8(3):227-230.

Weissert, W. G., T. T. H. Wan, B. B. Livieratos, et al. 1980. Cost effectiveness of homemaker services for the chronically ill. *Inquiry* 17(3):230-243.

Weissert, W. G. 1985. Seven reasons why it is so difficult to make community-based long-term care cost effective. *Health Services Research* 20(4):423-433.

Whitlow, J. 1985. Medicare cuts called threat to aged home care. *Star Ledger,* Newark, NJ (5 Dec.).

Willemain, T. R. 1980. Beyond the GAO Cleveland study: client selection for homecare services. *Home Health Care Services Quarterly* 1(3):65-83.

Woodbridge, M. 1984. Individual case management - "doing well by doing good". *Aetnasphere* (Oct.).

Yeatts, D. E., B. J. Steinhardt, and J. Capitman. 1985. Evaluation of Connecticut's Medicaid home and community-based care waiver program. Presentation at annual meeting of American Public Health Association, Washington, DC (Nov.).

Chapter 8

The Quality of Homecare

An American maxim avers, "You get what you pay for." This implies that if the cost of what you buy is too low, it's really not worth much. Homecare has been put into that position by the side effects of the cost containment motives stimulating the growth of the field, particularly the Medicare PPS/DRG reimbursement plan for hospital inpatient care. On top of that, homecare has often been put into the same category of care as nursing homes, and attitudes toward nursing homes continue to be negative. Henry (1986) reported the latest attack on nursing homes at hearings on a Senate Special Committee on Aging study, "Nursing Home Care: The Unfinished Agenda." Among the 8,900 facilities examined, 11 percent gave grossly substandard care, 7 percent chronically substandard, and 34 percent substandard. Quality, or lack of quality care was a major topic at the hearings. A Senior Citizens Law Center representative called for "effective methods of surveying and determining the quality of service provided, solid enforcement procedures to eliminate bad practices and promote good ones and adequate reimbursement properly focused on quality care and services." That remark could apply equally well to homecare.

Hospice homecare is also concerned with issues of quality as a separate entity. A GAO report (1979) focused on the increased growth of hospice homecare in the U.S. and detailed the concept. Torrens (1985) concentrated on quality care issues such as licensure, accreditation, ethics, administration, education, and planning.

Noting that the U.S. health care system has turned extremely entrepreneurial, Egdahl and Taft (1986) identify the key issue as quality of care. Although acceptable patterns of medical practice can vary considerably, "the focus should be on clinical results and on whether the incentives lead to appropriate medical and social outcomes." In this case, the authors are referring to the financial incentives that may limit the use of resources for patient care. Similarly, Dolan (1986) complained about Health Care Financing Administration (HCFA) homecare action that "clearly demonstrates the cruelty and inhumanity of current Medicare policies." He noted that "a mere six hours of in-home care hardly meets the required level of service."

Quality of Care Generics

A national conference sponsored by the American Association of Retired Persons (AARP), the American Hospital Association (AHA), the American Medical Association (AMA), and the American Nurses Association (ANA) (Simmons 1986) set quality of care for older Americans as the theme. A basic question was, "What is quality of care and what is the best way to measure it?" Additional questions considered at the conference included:

- What kind of care do the older patients themselves want?
- Is health care for the elderly being rationed?
- Who will oversee care that is given outside hospitals?
- How can future physicians be better prepared to care for the elderly?

Individuals want "competent and compassionate" help, often willing to limit high technology for simple "curing and caring" (Spiegel and Backhaut 1980). Preference for homecare is also a common response. Rationing services adds overtones of moral judgment to quality of care problems; there is also the possibility of people being denied care. Homecare or other care rendered outside of facilities may lose its traditional assuring quality of "peer supervision." Obviously, since the physician is pivotal in the delivery of quality care, medical schools should integrate educational offerings into their curriculums. All these areas have a direct relation to the quality of homecare services. Interestingly, one of the conference participants pointed out that the political clout of the elderly would work to assure more than a minimum of care but would require taking services away from other age groups.

Homecare Industry and Quality of Care

Basically, the issue is whether or not the homecare industry applies quality assurance mechanisms, either voluntary or regulatory, as in other health and social service systems. Therefore, concerns about lower cost treatment and care services should become secondary to the manner in which high quality care is attained for the protection of the public and for the cost containment mandates of those paying the bills. This is not a simple matter. Altman (1982) reviewed the problem of health costs and quality and headlined the situation as a delicate balance. In that article, Altman quoted a Rand Corporation researcher, Dr. Robert H. Brook, on quality care as it exists in the health care delivery system generally:

In the past 65 years about 500 research studies have been published assessing the level of quality care delivered, and virtually all these studies have detected basic problems in the level of quality delivered.

Pointedly, the question arises as to whether homecare can then claim to deliver high quality care at a lower cost when experts continue to discover basic problems. Nationally recognized homecare groups and individuals are moving to establish mechanisms similar to those used in the rest of the health care system to achieve high quality care. Areas of concern include patient rights, accreditation, licensure, Medicare conditions of participation, certificate of need, service standards, quality assurance programs, personnel standards, and relations with physicians.

In Congressman Roybal's Quality Assurance Reform Act of 1985 (House Select Committee on Aging 1985, 145), the proposed legislation mandated that Professional Review Organizations (PROs) conduct quality assurance reviews on home health agencies similar to their other evaluations; that PROs set up a 24-hour "hot line" to receive questions and complaints; that PROs set up a Consumer Advisory Board; that a National Council on Quality Assurance be convened; and that the PROs study the impact of DRGs on health care quality. A bill with similar provisions is being proposed by Senator John Heinz and Representative Pete Stark (*Home Health Journal* 1986a). That bill would also establish national standards for discharge planning as part of the Medicare conditions of participation, Senator Heinz noting that patients may not be getting adequate posthospital care.

Within its budgetary orientation, HCFA (*Home Health Journal* 1986b) seeks to institute an enhanced review of the appropriateness and medical necessity of home health services with a $7 million allocation. Is it aimed at quality of care? Critics will contend that cost containment comes first, followed by some concept as to the minimal, adequate, optimal, or maximal level of care to deliver to program beneficiaries.

In discussing cost-effectiveness, Brazil (1986) urges physicians to ensure that the new system produces quality care. "We should distinguish between luxury health care and quality health care. And while we obviously cannot afford the former, we must insist on the latter."

Impediments to Quality Homecare

The fact that services are delivered in the privacy of the home immediately raises a monumental barrier to assuring high quality care. On-site monitoring could require untold hours of personnel time and incur huge costs. Clients are in locations scattered over wide geographic areas. Possibly, homecare staff members may also be dispersed geographically without daily supervision or regular meetings to review their experiences. Clients are isolated at home and dependent upon homecare workers for their daily needs. That isolation and dependence builds up a reluctance to question the quality of care being received. Both clients and homecare workers could be exploited in this setting (Stewart 1979, 153). In a home setting the opportunity exists for the provision of poor services, for overutilization, and for totally inadequate surveillance of the quality of care.

Another major barrier exists in the diseases and conditions afflicting homecare clients. Illnesses may be chronic, incurable, intractable, and terminal. Multiple diagnoses evoke a complex mixture of treatment modalities with causes and effects difficult to distinguish. Even when detectable, the incremental health and social changes may be small with a majority of the outcomes in the area of functional ability--improvement in the patient's activities of daily living. Therefore, quality measurements in homecare should stress functional status and not concentrate on health status alone, as in inpatient care. Measuring functioning requires instruments more complex than a lab test, a medical observation regarding temperature or vital signs, or an X-ray. Tools to determine the quality of homecare may be more subjective than objective in nature. Data may come from verbal expressions of patients and the observations of homecare workers, both subjective.

Community mental health and rehabilitation programs use functional assessment techniques for quality evaluations. However, the instruments vary from the very simple to the very complex. Often, the person making judgments chooses from five to seven gradations in rating dressing, eating, walking, toileting, and other ADL factors. Examples of these techniques, along with the limitations, can be found in Hagedorn, Beck, Neubert, et al. (1976); Hargreaves, Atkinson, and Sorenson (1977), and Spiegel and Podair (1981).

Directly related to quality measurement using functional assessment is the dichotomy between medical/health care and personal/social care--the science of medicine and the art of medicine. These views appear to be antithetical in the U.S. health care system. Spiegel and Backhaut (1980) review more than 800 separate references in the literature on "curing and caring" and comment extensively on the paucity of measurement tools to evaluate the subjective elements of the quality of care.

Allgaier (1980) commented that, "Many physicians think homecare is inferior care and that patients are better off in the hospital." Even though insurers encourage the use of homecare as a cost-saving alternative, "the commercial insurers are apprehensive about the quality of care rendered in the home" (Sandrick 1986a). With those attitudes, poor quality homecare could become a self-fulfilling prophecy: if you believe it to be so, then it is so. Should that belief remain dominant among health care providers, it could easily be the major impediment to high quality homecare.

Recurring Themes in Quality Homecare

At national public hearings on home health care (Department of Health, Education and Welfare 1977, 56), there was agreement that better quality homecare was needed. Four themes were repeated throughout the testimony:

- Inherent difficulties in assuring the delivery of high quality care in the home.

- Variability of quality care under the differing standards of existing support programs.

- Importance of clearly defined, measureable, and enforceable standards for personnel and institutions.

- Need to protect both the patient receiving services and the public's tax dollars from abuse and exploitation.

Suggestions from those testifying included strengthening medical and utilization reviews; requiring standards as a condition of reimbursement; requiring paraprofessional homecare staff to be employees rather than independent contractors; encouraging increased intermediary supervision; establishing uniform record keeping and accounting methods; and promoting consumer education activities. Using the Medicaid program for data, numerous monitoring techniques such as utilization review, medical record audits, computer surveillance, and patient simulations address similar efforts to assure quality care (Spiegel and Podair 1975; Spiegel 1979).

In practical terms, Brodsky (1979) lists visible signs of inferior quality care, such as bedsores, foul odors, unexplained weight loss, no emergency equipment, minimal activity, excessive restraints, unnecessary transfer to an acute care facility, limited or missing physical and/or occupational therapy, and no social services.

Another oft-heard theme is that voluntary nonprofit homecare agencies supposedly render higher quality care because of their traditional altruism and their lack of economic profit motivation. A Congressional Budget Office report (1977) considered the charge and stated that there is no evidence that proprietary agencies delivered poorer quality services than voluntary agencies. Warhola (1980, 39) also noted that for-profit homecare agencies were purported to provide lower quality care, "but there is little evidence that this is so." In fact, she commented that the for-profit agencies offered a broader range of services seven days a week, 24 hours a day. With the sudden growth in the number of proprietary home health agencies in recent years, this recurring quality care theme of inferior service is still commonly heard. Additionally, the trend toward joint ventures and a restructuring of voluntary agencies to include a mixture of nonprofit and profit-making subdivisions clouds the interrelationship of quality and profiteering. Furthermore, the entrance of hospitals into the home health care business, seeking to replace lost revenue from the Medicare PPS/DRG restricted reimbursements, adds another layer of complexity to the issue of quality of homecare services.

It is difficult to classify these themes as being pluses or minuses in the consideration of quality care. On the one hand, a certain professionalism is added by the entrance of organizations with experience in quality care assurance. On the other hand, the emphasis on management and business principles may tend to deliver services in accord with the dollar value received. Where does this leave the consumer?

Rights of Patients

Patients' rights have been advocated in the health care industry generally. A "Bill of Rights" was endorsed by the AHA in the early 1970s, and other organizations have issued similar doctrines. Essentially, the patient is supposed to be treated courteously; given information, know the names of those caring for him or her; get the bill explained; have choices regarding treatment; and informed consent procedures are to be followed. Homecare agencies and professional organizations have come up with similar patients' rights documents. One home health agency (Home Health Homemaker Services GHI 1979) lists 15 points in its patients' bill of rights, including considerate and respectful treatment; confidentiality of records; access to the treatment plan; reports of progress; full informed consent; right to refuse treatment; bills explained; no discrimination; and workers' respect for you, your premises, and your property. A proprietary agency, Quality Care, (1981) distributed a "Patient Policy" that resembles an insurance policy, but with stronger wording to appeal to the public. The list includes professional service by highly qualified personnel; full protection through employee insurance; professional care management and supervision; competent handling of all administrative matters; complete assistance with health insurance; and problems resolved 24 hours a day, seven days a week. Within 72 hours of an assignment, the firm states that a patient care supervisor, a registered nurse, visits to prepare a plan and coordinate all care.

In a discussion on defining patients' rights, McAllister, Black, Griffin, et al. (1986) spoke about the initial decision to enter or not enter into homecare, the use of homecare brochures marketed to inpatients, closed circuit hospital TV for information, and training of patients. It was also noted that patients' rights could be seriously affected by the fact that Medicare and Medicaid will cut costs if they can.

Proposed federal quality care legislation (House Select Committee on Aging 1985; *Home Health Journal* 1986a) calls for consumers to take a more active role in reviewing quality care matters; this could certainly enhance their rights. Furthermore, the Joint Commission on Accreditation of Hospitals (JCAH) (1983a; 1986) standards for home health care and hospice care both have criteria relating to patients and their families being given specific rights.

"Assuring the rights of patients" is common terminology in the literature and in a variety of documents. All of the material says the proper thing, whether it be in a hard sell advertising approach or a soft sell tone. Regardless of the wording, the rights of patients are still only on paper. Simply stating that the homecare agency is going to provide high quality care does not actually make it so. Voluntary and regulatory mechanisms, governmental or private, appear to do more to achieve the quality care objectives.

Standards, Norms, and Criteria for Quality Care

Whether the quality care mechanisms are voluntary or governmental, accreditation, licensure, certification, certificate of need, and other avenues start out with standards that provide the unifying factor. As defined in *A Discursive Dictionary of Health Care* (House Subcommittee on Health and the Environment 1976, 155):

> *Standards*: Generally a measure set by competent authority as the rule for measuring quantity or quality. Conformity with standards is usually a condition of licensure, accreditation, or payment for services. Standards may be defined in relation to: the actual or predicted effects of care; the performance or credentials of professional personnel; and the physical plant, governance and administration of facilities and programs. In peer review programs, standards are professionally developed expressions of the range of acceptable variation from a norm or criterion.
> Two additional related definitions follow:
> *Norm(s)*: Numerical or statistical measure(s) of usual observed performance ... A norm can be used as a standard but does not necessarily serve as one. Both norm and standard imply single proper values rather than a range
> (House Subcommittee on Health and the Environment 1976, 109).
>
> *Criteria*: Predetermined elements of health care against which the necessity, appropriateness or quality of services may be compared ... Often used synonymously with guidelines
> (House Subcommittee on Health and the Environment 1976, 41).

In the introduction to the accreditation manual, JCAH (1986) states that their standards are characteristically:

- Valid--Relating to the quality of care or services rendered.

- Optimal--Reflecting the highest state of the art within available resources.

- Achievable--Compliance has been demonstrated in an existing facility.

- Measureable--Capable of being measured for compliance goals.

As professionals decide upon the ingredients of quality care, standards are constantly in a process of updating and revision. Information is gathered from professional associations in the field, from subject matter experts, from governmental agencies concerned with the area, from individual practitioners, from trade associations, from research reported in the literature, and from consumer groups.

It is possible that standards set by consensus of diverse parties may be watered down to the lowest common denominator. It is also conceivable that standards may be interpreted differently and be inconsistent in regulating the quality of care (Trager 1980, 15). Nevertheless, working toward standards that are clearly defined, measureable and enforceable is a suitable goal and a mainstay of quality of care activities. The Health Industry Manufacturers Association (1985) commented to the FDA that home use in-vitro diagnostics should have performance parameters for sensitivity, specificity, precision, and accuracy. Chrystal (1985) told how to make the National Intravenous Therapy Association standards work for practitioners. Hospice Association of America (1986) sponsored a JCAH seminar on hospice standards for accreditation and noted that several members of its Board of Directors worked on the standards. In these examples and in general, delivery of the highest quality care is the aim and purpose of setting standards.

Homecare Accreditation

With the preparation of standards, norms and criteria, an accreditation process can be undertaken. As a quality control mechanism, accreditation has been used in the health care system for some time, particularly with institutions. A National League for Nursing (NLN) brochure lists the following benefits of accreditation:

- Stimulates growth through self-evaluation.

- Determines quality services and quality management strategies according to nationally accepted standards.

- Gives competitive edge for marketing an agency to consumers.

- Attracts third-party payers and contracts with HMOs and PPOs.

- Helps recruit and retain staff and attract students for field experience.

- Serves as a risk management tool to safeguard an agency.

Holzemer (1985), also from the NLN, explained how to "make accreditation work for you" in benefits to the clients, the agency, students, and agency personnel. Potential dollar savings are estimated for each of the categories.

Accreditation Defined

An expanded definition of accreditation appears in A Discursive Dictionary of Health Care (House Subcommittee on Health and the Environment 1976, 6):

> *Accreditation*: The process by which an agency or organization evaluates and recognizes a program of study or an institution as meeting certain predetermined standards. The recognition is called accreditation. Standards are usually defined in terms of: physical plant, governing body, administration, medical and other staff, and scope and organization of services. Accreditation is usually given by a private organization created for the purpose of assuring the public of the quality of the accredited . . . Accreditation may either be permanent once obtained or for a specific period of time. Unlike a license, accreditation is not a condition of lawful practice but is intended as an indication of high quality practice, although where payment is effectively conditioned on accreditation, it may have the same effect.

Accreditation granting organizations are most often composed of professionals who are familiar with the types of programs under review. Consumer participation is not routine for many accrediting bodies and reports are not readily available to the public. In some instances, governmental and private reimbursement programs may require accreditation before allowing the specific institution or program to render care to individuals covered by the program. In certain situations, governmental bodies recognize accreditation in lieu of their own evaluations as a condition for licensure. This is called "deemed status." JCAH accreditation may serve as deemed status for Medicare certification; Pennsylvania gives deemed status to Medicare certification for state licensure. Therefore, accreditation can be instrumental in a variety of ways to improve the quality of care in any system.

Existing Homecare Accreditation Organizations

Because of the diversity of the homecare field, there is not a single agency that accredits all participants. Among the organizations, the JCAH accredits homecare and hospice services; the NLN accredits homecare and community health programs; the National Home Caring Council (NHCC) accredits homemaker-home health aide services; the Council on Accreditation of Services for Families and Children (COA) focuses on social and mental health agencies; and Volunteer - the National Center (VNC) works in the field of volunteerism. All these organizations are voluntary bodies with national reputations. However, each agency has its own type of constituency and expertise. While there may be some overlap, none of the groups can claim to represent all the concerns of the others.

JCAH Homecare Accreditation. In the completely revamped JCAH (1986, 47) accreditation manual for hospitals, there is an eight-page section on homecare services that allows the JCAH to accredit units that are affiliated with hospitals. This section lists five standards and the required characteristics of each standard covering the specification of objectives and scope of services, administrative and medical direction, policies and procedures, documentation, and quality assurance activities. Each standard and characteristic can be rated from one (substantial compliance) to five (noncompliance) with emphasis called to those central to accreditation with an asterisk.

Standard 1 calls for the objectives and scope of services to be specified and documented. Furthermore, the written documents can be distributed to patients, the public, professionals, and other concerned parties. Homecare programs should meet all federal, state, and local regulations, and/or licensure/certification requirements. Programs must provide professional nursing and one other therapeutic service. Homecare programs should be organized to assure effective coordination of all patient care services. Representatives of the community should be involved in the determination of needed services. There must be written guidelines defining patient eligibility for admission to homecare; procedures/services to be provided in the home; circumstances when patients are to be discharged or terminated from homecare; and conditions when patients are transferred within or outside of the hospital.

Each homecare patient shall be under a physician's care and receive an initial evaluation from a physician or registered nurse. Professional coordination of all homecare services is the hospital's responsibility, while a physician or registered nurse supervises all activities in the home. When services are secured from another agency on an hourly or per visit basis, there should be a written agreement. Specifics in the agreement should cover the services to be provided, the supervision, the preparation of a patient care plan, progress notes, case conferences, reimbursement, and the term of the contract.

Standard 2 opts for administrative and medical direction of a sufficient number of qualified personnel to deliver homecare and to meet the objectives of the program. Qualifications for the homecare director are detailed with the authority, duties, and responsibilities to be spelled out in writing. Importantly, this standard notes that homecare personnel should have the same qualifications as hospital employees providing comparable services. In addition to paid staff, volunteers are to be adequately trained and supervised with their duties also specified in writing. Staff and volunteers should be involved in relevant educational programs, including inservice and orientation. "The medical staff shall assure that the quality of care provided to homecare patients is comparable to that provided to inpatients, ambulatory patients, and emergency care patients."

Standard 3 posits that homecare programs shall be guided by appropriate written policies and procedures. This translates into sound administrative management procedure. Policies and procedures are to be reviewed annually with at least one physician and one registered nurse participating, as well as individuals representing the homecare services. Financial operations and personnel policies should be consistent with overall hospital policy.

Standard 4 advises that administrative and professional activities should be documented. Each patient should have a written care plan detailing: all pertinent diagnoses; prognosis with long- and short-term treatment objectives; types and frequency of services to be provided along with medications, equipment, transportation, etc.; functional limitations; permitted activities; required safety measures; and the sociopsychological needs of the patient.

Clinical medical records for each homecare patient are to be maintained in a professional manner enabling program evaluation. Data in the records should include the name of the attending physician, the name of the family member responsible for the patient at home, the suitability of the patient's home, signed and dated progress notes for each home visit, copies of all summary reports, and a discharge report. Critical to quality care, this standard calls for a written summary to be sent to the attending physician at least every 60 days and for that report to be part of the patient's record.

Standard 5 states: "As part of the hospital's quality assurance program, the quality and appropriateness of homecare services are monitored and evaluated, and identified problems are resolved." Using a planned process and agreed-upon objective criteria, the homecare program is monitored and evaluated. All major clinical functions are subject to the process, including the collection and assessment of relevant program information. When problems are identified, action is taken and evaluated for effectiveness. Findings from this evaluation process are documented and reported. As part of the hospital's annual reappraisal of the overall quality assurance program, homecare is also included to measure the effectiveness of the monitoring, evaluation, and problem-solving activities. When outside sources provide homecare services, the hospital's chief executive officer is responsible for planning and implementing a monitoring, evaluation, and problem-solving system.

In essence, the JCAH accreditation tends to apply the same standards to homecare services as to the rest of the hospital's services. Pointedly, Dr. Bluestone, originator of the pioneer Montefiore homecare program in 1947, stated at that time that a hospital with 500 inpatient beds and 50 homecare patients is a hospital with 550 beds (Ryder 1967, 2).

There is a close relationship to the Medicare Conditions of Participation that home health agencies must meet to be a part of the Medicare program. JCAH standards may include more physician involvement, use of hospital committees, a bit more recordkeeping, and standards for the use of volunteers, along with training and written responsibilities for them.

After the initiation of the Medicare PPS/DRG plan, more hospitals began to provide homecare services and showed tremendous growth in becoming Medicare certified agencies. Since many hospitals entered into arrangements with existing home health agencies, the JCAH acquired experience in accreditating homecare provided by nonhospital-based community agencies. More than 2,000 hospital-affiliated homecare services have been accreditated by the JCAH and it is likely that eligibility for JCAH homecare accreditation will expand to be similar to JCAH hospice accreditation.

JCAH Hospice Accreditation. After a three-year study (Joint Commission on Accreditation of Hospitals 1985) involving representatives from the major relevant organizations, JCAH developed standards for voluntary hospice accreditation (1983a) and a self-assessment and survey guide (1983b). Standards emphasize the patient and family as the unit of care; interdisciplinary team services--at least physician, nursing, psychological, social work, spiritual and bereavement services--with attention to professional stress, inservice, and continuing education; continuity of care; physical and psychosocial symptom management; homecare with a registered nurse available 24 hours a day, 7 days a week with emergency care and homemakers-home health aides; and the availability of inpatient care as needed. In addition, the JCAH accreditation process addresses the usual program elements of governing body responsibilities; management and administration with written policies; medical records; utilization review;

and quality assurance activities. Services can be delivered by employees or volunteers with written contracts or guidelines as appropriate.

Affeldt (1984) noted that JCAH began surveying hospice programs in January 1984. Hospices based in hospitals, long-term care facilities, and psychiatric facilities, as well as home health agencies and independent community hospice programs can opt for JCAH accreditation. "Interestingly, the independently operated programs had the largest number of registered nurses, psychosocial support staff, and home health aides and technicians per patient" noted in JCAH's *Hospice Project Report* (*Hospitals* 1985). Hospice accreditation is given for three years, and the JCAH survey costs $850 per surveyor day, with it taking an average of one day for hospital-based programs (Affeldt 1984). Using the self-assessment guide and the same 1 to 5 rating system as the JCAH hospital manual, compliance with the standards is based upon the documentation, statements from designated hospice program personnel, answers to questions, on-site observations, and information from the public.

Tehan (1985) considered the hospice accreditation process and noted the changes resulting from reimbursement practices. An issue was raised concerning the dulling of creativity and innovation via the accreditation process. However, Amenta (1985) commented that the JCAH does not presuppose any particular hospice organizational model as being better than any other. "There are no utilization quotas, time limits on care of any type, or caveats vis-a-vis contracting for components of care . . . Their purpose is to define and evaluate optimal hospice service in order to turn what began as a philosophy into the concrete ingredients of humanistic care."

National League for Nursing Accreditation. NLN operates an accreditation program for homecare and community health agencies. "Accreditation is available to all organizations that offer nursing and other health services to people outside hospitals, extended care facilities, and nursing homes" (National League for Nursing 1985a, 11). In its approach and ability to consider various types of agencies, the NLN is more flexible than the JCAH. In addition, the NLN uses a broader scope of health care orientation that appeals to the nursing-dominated homecare industry.

Four steps are involved in the accreditation policies and procedure: a self-study report by the homecare provider; an on-site visit; a professional review panel; and a Board of Review (National League for Nursing 1985a, 12). In 1984, the cost for an NLN accreditation was $4,500 for a five-year cycle, with per diem visitor fees set at $225 per visitor per day. Once the homecare agency is accredited, a brief interim report is required three years later; the process is repeated at the fifth year.

An accreditation criteria, standards, and substantiating evidences manual (National League for Nursing 1985b) is used by the homecare agency to prepare the self-study report. There are five standards dealing with strategic planning and marketing, organization and administration, program, staff, and overall program evaluation. In addition, there are 24 criteria with numerous subsections. Each standard illustrates the type of evidence to be collected for documentation in the self-study.

Strategic planning and marketing deals with the homecare agency's programs and services, and development of a strategic multiyear plan for future community/provider needs. Criteria call for a community assessment and a plan for the use of resources. Requested evidence includes demographic data, community status indicators, minutes of meetings, and copies of plans and revisions.

Organization and administration covers the role and responsibility of the governing body, the administrative relationships, the functions of the executive, the delegation of authority, fiscal management, contractual agreements, and the evaluation of policies and procedures. Examples of documentation requested include copies of bylaws, minutes of governing boards, organizational charts, curriculum vitae for top personnel, job descriptions, explanations of the budgetary process, insurance coverage, contracts, and a written evaluation of the organization and management with recommendations.

In the program accreditation section, the homecare agency is asked to justify the relation between programs and the agency's purpose. Criteria deal with the management information system, the objectives in the multiyear plan, service records for patients, the education of students in the health professions, and the evaluation of its programs. Evidence to be gathered includes flow sheets with objectives, priorities for each program, active and inactive client records, contracts with educational institutions, and a plan for program evaluation including utilization and peer review.

Staffing patterns, practice, and policies are reviewed in the next standard section. Criteria call for job descriptions, written personnel policies, supervision and consultation with staff, and staff development. Documentation requires assignment rosters, union contracts, personnel records, written supervisory plans, performance evaluations, promotion and reassignment policies, inservice training reports, and evidence of staff involvement in procedures and policies.

Overall mission evaluation standard states that, "The provider is accountable to the community for the quality of its care." Criteria deal with the existence of a structure and plan for evaluation and the resultant setting of goals after the process. Evidence to be collected includes the written systematic formal evaluation plan, annual reports, and an explanation of how the annual evaluation alters the strategic plan and marketing activities.

All told, the explicit standards, criteria, and evidence requested in the self-study require the homecare agency to laboriously gather a sizable volume of data. Much of the material is oriented toward the mechanics of the agency's operation with the underlying tenet that the quality of the administration is related to the quality of care delivered to the community. Of course, while involving its own staff, other allied professionals, and many other community groups and individuals, the agency is forced into a critical self-analysis of its policies and programs.

A list of accredited home health agencies and community nursing services is published regularly and circulated. As of June 1986, almost 90 organizations in some 30 states were identified as being NLN accredited. This listing is used as a guide for prospective consumers seeking excellent, professionally qualified homecare agencies.

Achieving "deemed status" is one of NLN's goals so that the NLN accreditation will automatically gain Medicare certification for the homecare agency.

National HomeCaring Council Accreditation. Formerly called the National Council for Homemaker-Home Health Aides Services, the National HomeCaring Council (NHCC) sets standards, guidelines, and accredits agencies in a manner similar to the JCAH and the NLN. Basically, the NHCC accreditation seeks to qualify homemaker-home health aide agencies that are efficient and effective, and which provide safeguards to protect the people served. About 135 agencies are accredited; some states require accreditation for specific federal program reimbursement: North Carolina, Title III; Maine and Missouri, Title XX; New Jersey and Colorado, 2176 Medicaid waivers.

Basic national standards for homemaker-home health aide services are divided into four areas: structure, staffing, service, and community (National HomeCaring Council 1981a). Eleven standards and interpretations for each one are also available (National HomeCaring Council 1981b). These standards are practical and appropriate for primarily nonmedical agencies with a community focus. Standards tend to emphasize financial responsibility, the logistics of supervision and services, and nondiscrimination. Partially because of the wide range of possible services, the standards do not get too specific about the actual services themselves.

Structure standards deal with legal authorization, governance, nondiscrimination, and responsible fiscal management. In the governance standard, there is a caution about possible conflicts of interest by affiliated board and advisory committee members. Consumer representation is also called.

Staffing standards cover personnel management and training for every homemaker-home health aide. There are explanations that detail the recruitment, selection, retention, and termination of aides. Written personnel policies, job descriptions for staff and volunteers, and a wage scale for each job are also in the standards. When tasks are performed by students and volunteers, agency staff supervises them.

Service standards spell out directions for written eligibility criteria and referral to other resources. Two essential components of the service provided to every individual and/or family served include: service of a supervised homemaker-home health aide, and service of professional persons responsible for case management functions.

Three items dealing with community are included in the final NHCC standard: need for an ongoing community assessment of health and welfare needs and plans to meet them; need for an ongoing interpretation of the service to the community; and an evaluation of all aspects of the service. Board and staff are urged to actively participate in planning and coordination groups in the community. Interpretation to the public includes annual reports, statistics, and mass media materials. Input from consumers is recommended during the evaluation process.

Again, there is more similarity than difference among the JCAH, the NLN and the NHCC accreditation processes, despite their distinctly disparate target agencies. Evidently, organizations and individuals involved in homecare activities have like beliefs about the critical elements of high quality homecare.

Council on Accreditation of Services for Families and Children. The Council on Accreditation of Services for Families and Children (COA) focuses on accrediting social service and mental health agencies providing care to families, children, and other individuals. Accreditation includes a self-study, on-site evaluation, review of and comment on the accreditation report, an appeals process, public identification of accredited agencies, and monitoring to ensure continued compliance. About 500 agencies are accredited. A four-year evaluation cycle is involved, with a cost of about $4,000 per agency plus the travel costs of surveyors, except for the five funding organizations who do not pay additional costs: Association of Jewish Family and Children's Agencies, Child Welfare League of America, Family Service America; Lutheran Social Service System, and National Conference of Catholic Charities.

Provisions of accreditation (Council on Accreditation of Services for Families and Children 1985) are divided into two major parts: generic provisions and 22 specific service area provisions.

Generic standards must be met by every agency and deal with governance, administration, personnel, facilities, equipment, and the agency's internal evaluation. Interestingly, the COA dispensed with separate considerations for volunteers and paid staff since they believe that whether or not one is paid should not be a critical factor in determining the quality of care.

Service provisions scrutinize care specific to specialized areas such as community mental health, foster care, homecare, social development, older age activities, youth-related services, and family counseling. This enables distinct standards to be set for each specialty to be investigated. It is apparent that many of these services use numerous volunteers and that extends the scope of accreditation. Provisions for each of the 22 specific areas are comprehensive and arrived at in consultation with concerned organizations, group participation, and consensus. For example, the NHCC assisted with the development of standards for homemaker-home health aide agency types. COA does not accredit units within agencies, such as the homemaker portion of a homecare program.

Volunteer -- The National Center Accreditation. This organization sets standards for volunteer agencies designed to make the volunteer contribution in America more efficient and effective. Almost 500 agencies are accredited.

Standards are in two parts: organization and administration, and program components (Volunteer -- The National Center 1978). Organization and administration standards deal with the agency's framework, paid and unpaid staff, facilities, financial management, and budget. Since volunteers may be handicapped, the standards call for accessibility for the disabled.

Program components cover resource information, recordkeeping, job descriptions, recruitment, interviewing, selection and placement, follow-up, orientation and training, supervision, evaluation, motivation, and career development. Standards are precise and straightforward with easy application to a variety of organizations. This process has the advantage of promoting accountability without requiring the burdensome documentation and reporting that may be beyond the ability of many volunteer agencies.

Accreditation in the Future

While accreditation will undoubtedly be with us in the future, its value may change. With the specter of cost containment overshadowing all aspects of the health care delivery system, providers may have to restructure their activities drastically and skimp on quality of care. The standards may also reflect the lowering of care levels. Is adequate quality care good enough? Does care have to be optimal? These are not idle questions in some parts of the world where such choices are routinely made. Therefore, additional mechanisms designed to promote high quality care such as licensure, certification (including Medicare conditions of participation), certificate of need, quality assurance activities, and personnel standards require examination.

Licensure

In the absence of federal regulations, the states assume responsibility for the regulation of professionals and/or institutions, often through licensing laws. By 1985, about 60 percent of the states had statutory and regulatory authority over home health agencies and about 30 percent licensed hospices (Exhibit 8-1 lists the localities requiring licenses). However, the total number of states is in constant flux as new licensing bills are introduced and/or repealed. According to *The Discursive Dictionary of Health Care* (House Subcommittee on Health and the Environment 1976, 91), licensure is defined as follows:

> *Licensure*: A permission granted to an individual or organization by competent authority, usually public, to engage in a practice, occupation or activity otherwise unlawful. Licensure is the process by which the license is granted. Since a license is needed to begin lawful practice, it is usually granted on the basis of examination and/or proof of education rather than measures of performance. License when given is usually permanent but may be conditioned on annual payments of a fee, proof of continuing education, or proof of competence. Common grounds for revocation of a license include incompetence, commission of a crime (whether or not related to the licensed practice), or moral turpitude. Possession of a medical license from one state may or may not suffice to obtain a license from another. There is no national licensure system for health professionals, although requirements are often so nearly standardized as to constitute a national system.

Generally, states establish agencies composed of a majority of professionals to set the guidelines for licensure and to resolve complaints. In theory, licensure protects the public from unqualified practitioners, provides the legal basis for practice, and assures reimbursement from third-party payers (Blum and Robbins 1985). However, a distinction must be made between actually assuring the quality of care and the act of promoting or contributing to quality care. Licensure in itself does not necessarily promote quality. Individuals can meet the educational and/or experience requirements and still not provide high quality care. Licensure does, however, allow the state the means to revoke the privilege and thereby prevent an agency, institution, or individual from continuing lawfully in a provider role. Critics of state licensure laws contend that some states merely use the legislation as a fundraising device rather than as a quality control regulator.

Hospices are licensed in 15 states: Colorado, Connecticut, Delaware, Florida, Illinois, Maryland, Michigan, Montana, New Mexico, New York, Rhode Island, South Carolina, Virginia, and West Virginia (Blum and Robbins 1985). There is no one state model hospice licensing law. Critics argue that licensing hospices now could stifle innovation and that federal regulations still need to be enacted; therefore, the hospice license is premature.

State licensing regulations generally display great disparity in the actual licensing procedures, including application, hearings, appeals, penalties, and fees. On the other hand, the greatest uniformity is observed in the

Exhibit 8-1 Status of State Licensure and Certificate-of Need Laws for Home Health Agencies

	Licensure		Certificate-of-Need	
	1984	1986	1984	1986
Alabama	N	N	Y*	Y
Alaska	N	N	I	I
Arizona	Y	N	N	I
Arkansas	N	N	Y	Y
California	Y	N	N	N
Colorado	N	Y	N	N
Connecticut	Y	Y	I	I
Delaware	N	Y	Y	Y
D.C.	N	N	Y	Y
Florida	N	Y	Y*	Y
Georgia	Y	Y	Y	N
Hawaii	Y	F	Y	Y
Idaho	P	N	N	N
Illinois	Y	N	N	N
Indiana	Y	Y	H	H
Iowa	N	N	I	I
Kansas	Y	N	N	N
Kentucky	Y	Y	Y	Y
Louisiana	Y	N	N	N
Maine	Y	N	Y	N
Maryland	F	F	Y	Y
Massachusetts	N	N	I	N
Michigan	N	Y	I	Y
Minnesota	N	N	N	I
Mississippi	Y	N	Y	N
Missouri	Y	N	N	I
Montana	Y	Y	Y	I
Nebraska	N	N	Y	N
Nevada	Y	Y	Y	Y
New Hampshire	N	N	P	Y
New Jersey	Y	N	Y	N
New Mexico	Y	Y	N	N
New York	Y	N	Y	N
North Carolina	Y	N	Y*	N
North Dakota	Y	N	Y	N
Ohio	R	N	I	I
Oklahoma	N	T	I	I
Oregon	Y	N	N	N
Pennsylvania	Y	N	H	N

Exhibit 8-1 continued

	Licensure		Certificate-of-Need	
	1984	1986	1984	1986
Puerto Rico	Y	Y	Y	Y
Rhode Island	Y	N	Y	N
South Carolina	Y	Y	Y	I
South Dakota	N	N	Y	I
Tennessee	Y	N	Y	N
Texas	F	Y	N	N
Utah	Y	N	Y	Y
Virginia	N	Y	Y	Y
Vermont	N	N	Y	Y
Washington	N	F-T	Y	F-T
West Virginia	N	Y	Y	Y
Wisconsin	Y	N	Y	N
Wyoming	N	N	N	N
Totals	Y = 28	Y = 16	Y = 26	Y = 16
	N = 20	N = 32	Y* = 3	N = 23
	P = 1	F = 3	N = 13	I = 11
	F = 2	T = 2	I = 7	H = 2
	R = 1		H = 2	F = 1
			P = 1	

Abbreviations:

F - Freestanding   T - Inpatient

H - Hospital   V - Voluntary

I - Institutional   Y - Yes

N - No   R - Registration bill only

P - Proprietary

* = Moratorium

Source: National Association for Home Care April 1986.

definition and duties of registered and practical nurse and in personnel policies and procedures.

Certification

Closely aligned with licensure is the process of certification. Importantly, one can practice without certification, but not without a license if required by state law. Certification is defined as follows:

> *Certification*: Process by which a governmental or nongovernmental agency or association evaluates and recognizes an individual, institution, or educational program as meeting predetermined standards. One so recognized is said to be certified. Essentially, the term is synonymous with accreditation, except that certification is usually applied to individuals and accreditation to institutions. Certification programs are generally nongovernmental and do not exclude the uncertified from practice, as do licensure programs (House Subcommittee on Health and the Environment 1976, 26).

Certification processes vary considerably among professional organizations engaging in the activity. Some groups investigate thoroughly while others do a perfunctory job before granting certification. In some associations, the only requirement may be the number of years on the job and have nothing to do with competency. Obviously, certification is no guarantee that the certified professional will deliver high quality care.

As far as consumers are concerned, certification may be a bit of a mystery. People do not know exactly what certification involves, except that certified providers may charge more for their services.

Certified via Medicare Conditions of Participation

To participate in the Medicare program and to be reimbursed, home health agencies must meet the Conditions of Participation detailed in sub-part L of the regulations (*Federal Register* 1973). Requirements "define areas of responsibility, authority, and operation of the home health agency, including but not limited to: governing body, administration, medical direction, quality assurance, supervision, qualifications of personnel, provision of services" (Weinstein 1985). An agency is said to be "certified" when it satisfies the Medicare conditions of participation. As of 1986, 5,964 home health agencies and 253 hospices were certified to participate in the Medicare program (Sandrick 1986a; Jones 1986).

Medicare Conditions of Participation carry considerable weight since the specifics are used as models by most of the states in establishing their own regulatory legislation. Therefore, a detailed examination is in order.

Firstly, the home health agency must satisfy the six specific requirements of section 1861(o) of the Social Security Act as follows:

(o) The term "home health agency" means a public agency or private organization, or subdivision of such an agency or organization which--

    (1) Is primarily engaged in providing skilled nursing services and other therapeutic services.

    (2) Has policies, established by a group of professional personnel (associated with the agency or organization), including one or more physicians and one or more registered professional nurses, to govern the services (referred to in paragraph 1) which it provides, and provides for supervision of such services by a physician or registered professional nurse.

    (3) Maintains clinical records on all patients.

    (4) In the case of an agency or organization in any State in which State or applicable local law provides for the licensing of agencies or organizations of this nature.

    (A) is licensed pursuant to such law, or (B) is approved, by the agency of such State or locality responsible for licensing agencies or organizations of this nature, as meeting the standards established for such licensing;

    (5) Has in effect an overall plan and budget that meets the requirements of sub-section (z); and

    (6) Meets such other conditions of participation as the Secretary may find necessary in the interest of the health and safety of individuals who are furnished services by such agency or organization; except that such term shall not include a private organization which is not a nonprofit organization exempt from Federal income taxation under section 501 of the Internal Revenue Code of 1954 (or a subdivision of such organization unless it is licensed pursuant to State law and it meets such additional standards and requirements as may be prescribed in regulations; and except that for purposes of Part A such term shall not include any agency or organization which is primarily for the care and treatment of mental diseases.

In addition, the Conditions of Participation cover the following:

- Definitions of program aspects, such as coordination and subcontracting.

- Organization, services, and administration.

- Acceptance of patients, written plan of treatment, and supervision.

- Standards and duties of service professionals, including physician, nurse, occupational therapist and occupational therapy assistant, physical therapist and physical therapy assistant, social worker and social work assistant, speech pathologist and audiologist, practical and vocational nurse, and home health aide.

- Establishment and maintenance of clinical records.

- Evaluation of the agency's total program.

Deadlines are included in the Conditions of Participation for certain actions to occur as follows:

- A written summary report for each patient is sent to the attending physician at least every 60 days (Section 405.1221).

- The total plan of treatment is reviewed by the attending physician and home health agency personnel as often as the severity of the patient's condition requires, but at least once every 60 days (Section 405.1223).

- The registered nurse, or appropriate professional staff member, if other services are provided, makes a supervisory visit to the patient's residence at least every two weeks, either when the aide is present to observe and assist, or when the aide is absent, to assess relationships and determine whether goals are being met (Section 405.1227).

- Clinical notes are written the day service is rendered and incorporated no less often than weekly; copies of summary reports sent to the physician; and a discharge summary is prepared (Section 405.1228).

- The home health agency has written policies requiring an overall evaluation of the agency's total program at least once a year by the group of professional personnel (or a committee of this group), home health agency staff, and consumers, or by professional people outside the agency working in conjunction with consumers (Section 405.1229).

- There is a continuing review of clinical records for each 60-day period that a patient receives home health services to determine adequacy of the plan of treatment and appropriateness of continuation of care (Section 405.1229).

It has been suggested that the Medicare Conditions of Participation serve as the basic structure upon which to build a quality assurance program for homecare programs. In fact, this is what happens as programs other than Medicare tend to use the existing Conditions of Participation as guidelines for a minimum set of quality care recommendations.

Regulation via Certificate of Need

Under the National Health Planning and Resources Development Act (P.L. 93-641), the Certificate-of-Need (CON) mechanism was created to control the expenditure of large dollar amounts for facilities, equipment, and services deemed unnecessary. Using federal dollar amounts as guidelines, the 200+ Health Systems Agencies required providers to apply for a CON before initiating the purchase and changes. A definition follows: *Certificate-of-Need:* A granting of permission by the state to operate a home health agency in a specific area, provided the applicant proves the need for the agency in terms of the need criteria established in the law or regulations.

If a state has both a licensure and CON requirement, the CON requirement must be met before the agency can get its license.

In some states the CON requirement is a separate law from the licensure requirement. In others, the CON requirement is in the licensure law itself (Collier 1984; Exhibit 8-1 gives localities requiring both).

There is disagreement over the relation between home health agencies and the need for a CON to enter into the field. Some critics view CON as a barrier to the entrance of new home health agencies in the market (Weinstein 1985). Collier (1984) states that "neither the federal CON program nor Section 1122 explicitly subject home health agencies or the rendering of homecare services to review." State governors, via Section 1122, can enter into agreement with HHS to assure health planning guidelines. In addition, the House Committee on Interstate and Foreign Commerce in a report (1979, 76) on the health planning amendments noted that "the Committee specifically considered and rejected a proposal to include home health services in the minimum requirements for a satisfactory Certificate-of-Need program."

Arguments continue over the need for a CON, since home health agencies generally do not require significant dollar expenditures for facilities or equipment. Anderson and Kass (1986, 105) estimate fixed costs at about $15,000 per year. Furthermore, as Pettey (1985) illustrates, trade associations believe that the states exceed their statutory authority and discriminate in favor of currently certified home health agencies. Nevertheless, according to the critics, the states have interpreted the CON requirements differently; more than 30 states have adopted varying types of CONs for home health agencies, while about 30 have CON regulations for hospices (Collier 1984).

A report of the Federal Trade Commission (Molotsky 1986) investigated CON regulation of entry into the home health care field from an economic viewpoint. Anderson and Kass (1986, 12) found that costs were about 2 percent higher where there is CON regulation. That percentage translated into a total added cost increase of approximately $46 million in 1984, due to the absence of competition. In a strong conclusion, the authors stated: "We found no evidence that CON regulation contributes to lower costs for the provision of home health care services. If anything, CON regulation appears to be associated with higher costs. Further, a CON program for home health firms involves administrative costs. Perhaps more importantly, by retarding or stopping entry of new firms, CON regulation of home health markets may be denying consumers the benefits of innovative or low cost services that could lower the cost or improve the quality of health care. There is no reason for not allowing the market to function unencumbered by these regulations" (Anderson and Kass 1986, 107).

Interestingly, Salkever (1978) also came to the same conclusion some time ago--regulation would not really do the job of curbing costs in the long run. Around the same time, Havinghurst (1977) opted for consumer initiatives to control the market; Ruchlin (1977) looked at public utility status, nonprofit control, and market regulation; and McClure (1978) posited that consumer choice and provider competition could produce superior cost performance, distribution, and quality. Hyman (1977) considered health regulation, CON, and Section 1122, and also opted for a hiatus before imposing constricting regulations.

Quality Assurance Programs

Joint Commission and Quality Assurance

In the JCAH (1986,205) accreditation manual there is a separate section on quality assurance wherein the four standards and required characteristics spell out what to look for in a quality assurance program. JCAH starts with the requirement that, "There is an ongoing quality assurance program designed to objectively and systematically monitor and evaluate the quality and appropriateness of patient care, pursue opportunities to improve patient care, and resolve identified problems."

Beginning with the governing body, the JCAH calls for the involvement of all staff in monthly meetings to review components such as surgery, medical records, blood use, drug use, and pharmacy operations. Infection control, utilization review, and accidents would be reviewed on a facility-wide basis. Additional data to be secured from vital statistics, diagnostic testing reports, financial data, patient and staff surveys, insurance company data, and other peer review activities would be added to the quality assurance reviews. Williams, Gaumer, and Cella (1984,73) point out the quality assurances that are also required by the Medicare Conditions of Participation, including professional advisory groups, clinical record review, appropriateness review, and annual evaluation. Deficiencies are to be reported to the governing body along with reports on progress and outcomes of efforts to resolve problems.

Quality assurance is mandated as part of the JCAH (1983a) manual for hospice accreditation in a similar fashion.

Internal and External Review

Two types of quality assurance are commonly used: internal review and external review (Hughes 1982; Williams, Gaumer, and Cella 1984, 73). Internal review includes items such as the audit and advisory committees, and refers to the organizational procedures that the agency is required to initiate, administer, and maintain on an ongoing basis. External review refers to the fiscal intermediaries and/or the state licensing agency's methods of reviewing compliance with conditions of participation or licensure. Major external mechanisms relating to quality of care involve the fiscal intermediary's review of reimbursement claims, the state agency's surveyor audits recompliance with licensure requirements and federal mandates, and the federal HCFA surveyor audits of clinical records for compliance with Medicare Conditions of Participation.

Drawbacks to Quality Assurance

There may be serious drawbacks to the methods used to assure the quality of homecare, including the following (Hughes 1982):

- A lack of regional or national norms to which homecare utilization patterns can be compared.

- An absence of normative data on appropriate outcomes of homecare service for specific patient populations such as the terminally ill vs. the acute vs. the chronically ill.

- The lack of any direct observation of patients by external reviewers.

- The linking of state licensure to Medicare Conditions of Participation.

Homecare System Characteristics

Public funding of homecare services is probably responsible for a major impetus to engage in quality assurance activities. Words such as "appropriate," "adequate," "effective," and "efficient" appear frequently in governmental guidelines. These terms are not easily measured, and criteria are needed. Six characteristics of a health care system were identified in a health planning research project funded by the federal government: acceptability, accessibility, availability, continuity of care, cost, and quality of care. Exhibit 8-2 defines the terms; the interrelationships between each of the characteristics are apparent, as well as the totality of quality of care. These six elements apply equally as well to the homecare system (Spiegel and Hyman 1979,359) as a measurement of quality assurance:

- Are homecare services *acceptable* to groups with varied sociocultural backgrounds?

Exhibit 8-2 Characteristics of the Health Care System, Definitions

Acceptability. An individual's (or group's) overall assessment of the available medical care. The individual appraises such factors as the convenience, cost, quality, results and provider attitudes in determining the acceptability of health services.

Accessibility. An individual's (or group's) ability to obtain or use services, given the fact that they are available. It may be measured either in terms of use, which is the definitive verification of access, or in terms of the existence or absence of barriers and obstacles to use.

Availability. A measure of the supply of health services, as correlated with need and distribution, and an indication of the resources able to provide it.

Continuity of Care. A measure of the degree of effective coordination of effort in providing services, regardless of whether care is provided within one setting or within multiple settings. Actual need, preventive care, and single as opposed to continuing treatment are ancillary considerations.

Cost. The expenses incurred in providing or in receiving a service or good. Expenses should be distinguished from charges, which are the prices assigned or the amount billed for a service. Although charges might or might not be the same as costs, or based on them, they are frequently used as a measure of cost.

Quality of Care. A measure of the degree to which health services delivered to a patient, regardless of by whom or in what setting, approximate satisfactory delivery of services as determined by health professionals. Quality is frequently described as having three dimensions: (1) quality of input resources (certification and/or training or providers — both manpower and facilities), (2) quality of the process of service, delivery (use of appropriate procedure for a given condition), and (3) quality of outcome of service use (actual improvement in condition or reduction of harmful effects).

Source: Department of Health, Education and Welfare. Bureau of Health Planning and Resources Development. 1976. *Draft guidelines concerning the development of health systems plans and annual implementation plans.* Washington, DC (17 June) pp 13 - 14.

- Is *access* to homecare equitable, easy, and affordable to all?

- Are homecare services *available* within the neighborhood?

- Is the *cost* of homecare reasonable while still maintaining *continuity of care*?

- Is the *quality* of homecare up to the standards set by the experts?

Using the definitions in Exhibit 8-2 and the type of questions listed above, home health agencies can gain some insight into the quality of their programs.

State regulatory mechanisms usually focus upon seven system characteristics related to the quality of homecare. Most legislators and regulators concentrate their efforts on the area that is least amenable to manipulation through regulation--the assurance of quality service. This situation arises because drafters of legislation have little knowledge of the business of homecare, and they also rely upon the Medicare Conditions of Participation to achieve the other standards and criteria. Quality assurance issues related to the homecare system involved the optimal mix of services and the credentials of providers; the services supplied under contracts with outside firms, along with the supervision and control of such services; responsibility of providers, along with the day-to-day supervision and the overall direction of the attending physician in the homecare environment; ability of the home health agency to meet the needs of the patient/client including attention to "dumping" and insurance coverage; coordination of an adequate treatment plan, including the maintenance of medical and social services and the periodic review; keeping of administrative and clinical records, including the type of data to collect and how long to keep such data; and the evaluation of the homecare system, including consumer input.

Pennsylvania Assembly Quality Assurance Project

A two-year quality assurance project was conducted by the Pennsylvania Assembly of Home Health Agencies (Berkoben 1976). More than 30 agencies with varying sponsorship participated in the effort to design a patient care audit system that would allow for quality care measurements. Audit criteria were developed for 12 diseases/conditions: chronic obstructive lung disease, congestive heart disease, hip fracture, mental illness, post-cataract surgery, cerebrovascular accident, diabetes mellitus, arthritis, cardiovascular disease, cancer of the colon, care of the adult patient, and maternal and child health care. Exhibit 8-3 presents the quality assurance criteria developed for the care of patients with diabetes mellitus.

Investigators found that documentation was a major deficiency in that the criteria did not contain enough information. Audits also revealed that equipment was not always on hand as needed. Recommendations to correct deficiencies suggested stronger health teaching, standardization of data systems, coordination between acute care facilities and homecare programs, and establishing the number of annual audits required. According to the researchers, "The results of the Quality Assurance Project have demonstrated that a structured evaluation system for home health care can provide direction for improving services" (Berkoben 1976,6).

Problem Oriented Medical Record

POMR (Problem Oriented Medical Record) is used in the inpatient facility and starts with a complete listing of the patient's problems. Progress notes then classify problems according to SOAP: (subjective data; objective data; assessment; and plan). Parzick and Nolan (1978) described such a system at work in a home health agency in Homestead, Pennsylvania. Eighteen advantages were listed by the authors, including the focus on patient care, the use of the data for quality care, the clear audit trail, the ease of computerization, and the requirement for analytical thought. Disadvantages included the extra time to collect data, added staff orientation, monitoring to prevent errors, possibility of overlooking patient strengths, and the reorientation of staff after using POMR. Weighing the pluses and minuses, the authors conclude that, "Because the care plans are much more sophisticated, POMR doesn't save time . . . But it's all worthwhile when you see the benefits derived by the patients."

Patient Appraisal

Patient Appraisal (PA) is a review of the physical, psychosocial, and socioeconomic aspects of the quality of an individual's care. In this context, PA is a prerequisite for the appropriate selection of homecare services needed for a patient. A patient care management (PCM) system incorporates the elements of PA, care planning (CP), and care evaluation (CE). To carry out the PCM system, the federal government sponsored the development of the PACE II instrument: Patient Appraisal, Care planning and Evaluation (Warhola 1980,34). This quality assurance instrument focuses on the patient/client and the use of multidimensional information through the collection of admission data, medical data, impairment record, functional capacity, patient care data, and discharge data.

Appropriateness of care based on such assessments can form the basis for determining community needs for homecare services.

Exhibit 8-3 Criteria to Assess Quality of Home Health Care Rendered to Patients with Diabetes Mellitus, on Insulin

Criteria	Standards %	Exceptions	Instructions and Definitions for Data Retrieval
Outcomes			
1. Controlled blood glucose	100	1A. None	1. Controlled blood glucose = 80-120 mg/100 ml, or range approved by physician.
2. Stabilized urine glucose	100	2A. None	2. Stabilized urine glucose = negative to 1+, or level approved by physician.
3. Patient (pt.) status understanding of disease	100	3A. None	3. Pt or significant other (SO) states understanding of disease process following teaching program.
4. Pt. demonstrates independent insulin administration	100	4A. Insulin administration responsibility by SO	4. Pt or SO states prescribed insulin dosage; demonstrates preparation and care of equipment, injection method, injection site rotation.
5. Pt. states diabetic diet and follow-through	100	5A. Diabetic diet not prescribed	5. Pt states understanding of diabetic diet. Follow-through documented in diet history..
6. Pt. states signs and symptons (S&S) of hyperglycemia and importance of medical attention if they occur	100	6A. None	6. S&S of hypoglycemia = sweating; cold, clammy skin; nervousness; trembling; headache; weakness; dizziness; nausea and vomiting; semiconsciousness.
7. Pt. states S&S of hyperglycemia and importance of medical attention if they occur	100	7A. None	7. S&S of hypoerlycemia = increased sugare in urine (3+ or 4+), excessive urination, excessive thirst, fruity breath, mental confusion.
8. Pt. demonstrates skin and foot care to prevent complications	100	8A. None	8. Skin and foot care = skin surfaces kept clean and dry properly fitted shoes and stockings worn; exposure to extreme temperatures avoided while washing and bathing; a septic first aid treatment given for cuts and skin irritations; toenails, including ingrown nails, cut to avoid soft tissue injury.

Exhibit 8-3, continued

Criteria	Standards %	Exceptions	Instructions and Definitions for Data Retrieval
Complications		Critical Management	
9. Pt. demonstrates correct technique of urine testing	100	9A. None	9. Look for evidence that pt or SO demonstrated proper urine testing technique.
10. Pt. wears diabetic identification	100	10A. None	10. Identification = bracelet, card or pendant.
11. Hypoglycemia	0	11A. If pt conscious orange juice with 2 tsp. sugar given 11B. If pt unconscious, physician and emergency service notified immediately	11. For S&S of hypoglycemia, see instructions for criterion 6.
12. Hyperglycemia	0	12A. Physilain and emergency service notified immediately	12. For S&S of hyperglycemia, see instructions for criterion 7.
13. Peripheral infections	0	13A. Physician notified 13B. Skin and nail care, dietary intake, attention to skin abrasions and cuts reviewed	13. S&S of peripheral infections = skin redness; heat, tenderness, swelling, or pain in peripheral areas; localized abscess, drainage at wound site.

Source: Berboken, R.M. 1976. *Quality assurance in home health care.* Camp Hill, PA: Pennsylvania Assembly of Home Health Agencies, p. 8.

Structure, Process, and Outcome Measures of Quality Care

Developed by Donabedian (1966), the use of structure, process, and outcome quality of care measurements has withstood the test of time. Exhibit 8-4 identifies examples of the items in each classification. Most of the research into the quality of care has concerned itself with the process of care: Did the providers do everything that was appropriate? In recent years, there has been interest in linking the process with the outcomes of care. Applying this quality assurance technique to homecare, the technical elements may not be as critical as in acute care situations. However, the upsurge in high technology homecare may change that, although the caring aspects of homecare will probably still be dominant. Measuring the art of caring could result in quality assurance data indicating minor health status outcome variations.

Definitions in *The Discursive Dictionary of Health Care* will help to clarify the use of structure, process, and outcome in homecare quality assurance efforts:

> *Input measure (Structure):* A measure of the quality of services based on the number, type, and quality of resources used in the production of the services. Medical services are often evaluated by measuring the education and training level of the provider, the reputation and accreditation of the institution, and the number of dollars spent as proxy measures for the quality of the services. Input measures are generally recognized as inferior to process and outcome measures because they are indirect measures of quality and do not consider the actual results or outcomes of services. They are often used nonetheless because people are accustomed to their use and they are easily obtained (House Subcommittee on Health and the Environment 1976,83).

> *Process Measure:* An indicator of the quality of medical care used to assess the activities of the health manpower and programs in the management of patients. Process measures document the process of care used for various populations or diagnoses. They do not necessarily measure the results of care, although they measure the use of diagnostic and treatment methods which are thought or proven to be effective. Generally, such measures indicate the degree of conformity with standards established by peer groups or with expectations formulated by leaders in the profession (House Subcommittee on Health and the Environment 1976,129).

> *Outcome measure:* A measure of the quality of medical care in which the standard of judgment is the attainment of a specified end result or outcome. The outcome of medical care is measured with such

Exhibit 8-4 Examples of Components of a Structure, Process, Outcome Evaluation Measurement

Structure Components	Process Components	Outcome Components
Facilities	Provider/Patient encounters	Mortality
Equipment	Health care system process	Morbidity
Organization patterns	Desirable health practices	Disability
Funding	Technical aspects of care	Individual physical and social functioning
Staffing	"Art" aspects of care	Provider satisfaction
Personnel qualifications		Consumer satisfaction
Personnel experience		Community satisfaction
Environmental quality		Wellness level
Risk factors		Tests and vital signs relative to norms
(Resources)	(Curing process)	(Health Status)

Source: Adapted from Donabedian, A. 1966. Evaluating the quality of medical care. *Milbank Memorial Fund Quarterly, Part 2* 44 (Suppl.): 166-206.

parameters as improved health, lowered mortality and morbidity, and improvement in abnormal states.

Any disease has a "natural history" which medical care seeks to alter. To measure the effectiveness of a particular medical action in altering a disease's natural history is to carry out an outcome measure. Such measures are the only valid way to measure the quality of medical care. To carry out cost benefit analyses of medical care, such measures are necessary. However, they are difficult to devise and have not often been done in comparing medical settings (House Subcommittee on Health and the Environment 1976,116).

Application of the structure/process/outcome quality assurance model to homecare would be beneficial in a number of ways. Firstly, an accepted health care system technique can be used that is readily understood in the field. Next, the methodology has a solid research base to build upon for experimental designs. Thirdly, the emerging emphasis upon outcome measures may provide a better fit for homecare measures of quality care.

A major difficulty still lies with the ability to develop instruments to measure changes in functional capability that are accurate, reliable, and valid. This is not an easy task since medical experts have the same problem relating cause and effect in therapeutic actions with more readily defined disease states. In homecare situations, as in medical care generally, a patient's health status, knowledge, feelings, and behavior are influenced by many factors besides his/her treatment. Gould (1985) reports on the application of the structure/process/outcome to home health care nursing with a four-part format: a nursing diagnostic statement; patient-centered outcome goals; flow sheet to document teaching and objectives achievement; and implementation of nursing processes. Examples of diagnoses, outcome measures, flow charts, and process standards are included in the article.

Building upon the large body of available research using the structure/process/outcome, and examples such as Gould (1985), homecare can demonstrate quality assurance applications.

Utilization Review

Simply put, utilization review (UR) looks at the appropriate use of resources required for specific diseases/conditions. A definition from *The Discursive Dictionary of Health Care* expands upon the meaning:

> *Utilization Review:* Evaluation of the necessity, appropriateness, and efficiency of the use of medical services, procedures, and facilities. In a hospital, this includes review of the appropriateness of admission, services ordered and provided, length of stay, and discharge practices, both on a concurrent and retrospective basis. Utilization review can be

done by a utilization review committee, peer review group, public agency, or a Professional Review Organization (PRO) (House Subcommittee on Health and the Environment 1976,165).

Under the federal legislation creating PROs, there is no mandate that the agency review homecare agencies. However, there is federal legislation pending that does require the PRO to evaluate community and homecare organizations. In addition, a PRO may choose to review homecare services by including those agencies in the areawide examinations of the appropriateness of the existing health care delivery system.

In the JCAH (1986,205) accreditation manual there is a separate section on quality assurance. Essentially, the standard calls upon the facility to review the appropriate allocation of resources through UR in an ongoing quality assurance program.

Kleffel and Wilson (1975) identified three areas that homecare agencies must resolve relative to UR: a need for a uniform database; a need to develop explicit criteria with norms, standards, and parameters; and a need for effective, efficient UR activities.

Minimum uniform data for homecare documentation must be specified and used by all agencies to allow for meaningful comparisons. In a booklet on UR for home health agencies, Kleffel (1973) gives precise examples of the data required in charts and forms. Data relate to patient characteristics, diagnostic groupings, visits by discipline and by outcomes, patients' special diets and appliances/equipment, discharge disposition, and medications administered. Even though the booklet was first prepared in 1972, the material is still valuable for homecare agencies concerned with UR for quality control.

Criteria, norms, standard, and parameters for homecare clients pose serious problems for multiple diagnoses. Nevertheless, objective UR would require that there be such criteria. Lessons can be adapted from the work of the PROs as similar criteria are developed for inpatients and others. Both internal and external quality care reviews are dependent upon checking patient records against professionally acceptable criteria.

UR has also moved into professionalism with the establishment of the American College of Utilization Review Physicians (ACURP) in 1973 and with certification from the American Board of Quality Assurance and Utilization Review Physicians in 1978. Certification examinations test the applicant's knowledge of UR, quality assurance, cost containment, and risk management. A major activity of the ACURP centers on helping hospital administrators meet JCAH standards. In addition, the ACURP works to include material in medical school curriculums on the topic of UR.

UR and all of the other quality assurance programs depend upon accurate and reliable data for implementation. Therefore, medical records in homecare have a pivotal role in any quality care activity.

Medical Records--Key to Quality Care

Jacob (1985) discusses the impact of medical records documentation in home health care and cites five rationales: to provide a legal record for the delivery of quality care; to reimburse for services rendered; to allow for coordination of services; to provide for continuity of care; and to enhance professional and institutional credibility. Noting that the PPS/DRG payment plan will ultimately affect homecare agencies, Stevens and Kirk (1985) review the role of the health record practitioner in public health nursing and home health agencies. A team approach is described in a local VNA with an emphasis on identifying interactions and understanding programs. Using examples of forms and types of data to record, Wilde (1985) comments that "developing a clinical record system for a home health agency with many programs requires patience, flexibility, nontraditional thinking, creativity, and system planning skills."

Regarding the legal issues, Connaway (1985) focused on documentation required of home health care nurses in a two-part article. Ten legal guidelines were identified: write legibly; use ballpoint pen only; don't leave blank lines; sign and date notes; never erase; label addendums; never allow anyone to enter notes and sign for you; use common abbreviations only; document nursing process and patient's reactions; and document communication between team members. Special issues for homecare nurses involve supervision at a distance; several agencies sharing the care of a patient; physician orders via telephone; documentation of family intervention and environmental factors; and the use of part-time personnel. In addition to the legal aspects, the quality of care implications are also quite clear in this legal advice.

Miller (1985a) reports on a project to develop medical record documentation materials for homecare organizations. She found that agencies providing skilled/intermittent care seem to document quite thoroughly. However, "Routine documentation of health status items appears to be lacking." Because many agencies do not provide data for the inpatient record, coordination between inpatient and homecare settings may suffer. In addition, Miller suggests using a problem oriented medical record, securing informed consent, keeping records in the home to improve coordination, and writing patient care evaluations. Finally, she lists a number of administrative details to consider, arguing that "there is little professional medical record support in home health agencies . . . some improvements in home health record management are needed." Toward that end, Miller (1986) used the data from the project to produce *Documentation for Home Health Care: A Record Management Handbook*. This handbook seeks to provide a medical record system to assure high quality homecare. Topics cover field tested model record forms, a recommended uniform minimum data set, quality assurance guidelines, model confidentiality policies, ICD-9-CM coding guidelines, management guides, and review guidelines, along with documentation for Medicare reimbursement.

Calling for improvement in hospice medical record documentation, Miller (1985b) also reviewed that area. "Very little formal quality assessment is done in hospices." She found that many hospices do not code a patient's diagnoses and problems, and don't maintain indexes. "It is time for medical record professionals to become involved in hospice medical record management." Translating the task into words, Miller (1984) authored a handbook for documentation in hospices.

Giving attention to medical record documentation in homecare, *Home Health Journal* publishes a regular feature on the subject in each issue. For example, Engelbrecht detailed skilled care recording (1986a), what Medicare won't pay for (1986b), and documenting physical therapy services (1986c) in recent issues.

An axiom among medical records professionals states that if "something isn't documented, it probably didn't happen." It should be apparent that poor records result in inferior quality of care. With concern for assuring high quality care and for securing proper reimbursement, appropriate medical record documentation in homecare organizations is an essential.

Personnel Standards and Quality Care

Several generic quality of care concepts apply to all homecare personnel: establishing who should authorize homecare; supervision of personnel; and the basic and continuing education of staff.

Arguments become quite heated when the issue of authorization of homecare services to be reimbursed via federal and other programs arises. Basically, the dispute centers over whether physicians or registered nurses should authorize homecare services. In fact, testimony at public hearings (Department of Health, Education and Welfare 1977, 58) indicated that many nurses already did the patient assessment and telephoned the physician with recommendations which were usually approved. Physicians were criticized for their lack of involvement, although some witnesses did argue for more such involvement with the nurse carrying out the plans. However, legal mandates in most states require the physician to authorize the homecare services. There may be breaks in that provision as some states do allow other health professionals to extend their functions into areas such as writing prescriptions. In the interim, physicians and nurses tend to cooperate despite the fact that the nurse may be more intimately involved in the total homecare treatment plan. Legal mandates will have to be met to assure reimbursement and meet any conditions of participation.

Supervision of paraprofessionals is critical to maintaining quality homecare services. Simple geographic logistics hamper adequate supervision and add unproductive travel time to the care picture. In addition, who should provide the supervision?--physician? registered nurse? Again the practicalities of the situation dictate that the physician is going to provide little on-site supervision. Most medical supervision will be at a distance based on phoned reports, medical records, and perhaps an occasional home visit. Registered nurses appear to be the major supervisors of the ancillary personnel rendering care, with perhaps the specialty professional overseeing his/her area of concern. Since most homecare is rendered by nurses and home health aides, it is apparent that supervision will probably remain in nursing hands with medical agreement. Furthermore, Beard (1984) pointed out the supervisory problems with the use of "independent contractors" not under the direct supervision of the employing home health agency. Within this work situation, homecare experts do argue for greater physician involvement in the frequent monitoring of the patient's condition, and if that requires supervision, so be it.

Basic and continuing education and training, especially in specialty areas, is a recognized need as homecare expands into high technology care. Geriatrics, cancer care, emergency medical techniques, infusion therapies, respiratory therapy, and discharge planning are a few of the areas. Kaye (1985) talked about setting educational standards for gerontological homecare personnel. A federal government group (Department of Health and Human Services 1981) produced a two-part manual for educating nurses about hospice care. A text, *A Model Curriculum and Teaching Guide for the Instruction of the Homemaker-Home Health Aide*, was prepared by a government-sponsored group (Department of Health and Human Services 1981). Accreditation standards usually spell out requirements for a variety of professionals and paraprofessionals, as well as for volunteers. For those homecare workers attuned to acute care settings, a medical/social model is advocated in continuing education efforts.

Division of labor among a wide variety of homecare workers does not make educational efforts any easier. Many people are providing care who have differing educational levels and various skills. Furthermore, the status of homecare workers is dubious, and many do not receive the appropriate recognition (Fine 1984). A former federal Assistant Secretary for Health, Dr. Philip R. Lee (1975,311), commented on the value of ancillary workers: " . . . nontraditional workers, such as community health aides, may be able to contribute more to helping patients solve health-related problems than can the highly trained professional."

Butler (1981) urged the inclusion of the nursing home into the professional education system with student placements similar to the teaching hospital concept. Homecare is included as an outreach program of the facility in this model. Many health professionals graduate their educational programs without ever having been on a home visit or in a nursing home.

In the final analysis, the quality of homecare depends upon the skill of the caregiver. Anything that can be done to upgrade the ability of providers to render higher quality care should be a prime target for those concerned with assuring quality homecare.

Physicians and Quality Homecare

In response to requests for information, the AMA (1981) published a *Physician Guide to Home Health Care*. Sections of the 38-page booklet deal with such topics as using homecare services, insurance coverage, payment for services, and physician leadership in homecare.

To obtain information about services in their own localities, physicians are advised to consult their hospitals' homecare units or discharge offices, state and local health departments, local health planning agencies, local medical societies, insurance companies, and homecare associations. In addition, physicians are directed to the classified pages of the local telephone book.

To evaluate the quality of homecare service, the guide suggests asking initially if the agency meets the Medicare Conditions of Participation. Then, inquiries should follow about state licensing, if mandated, JCAH accreditation, if hospital-based, NLN accreditation, if community-based, and NHHC accreditation, if a homemaker-home health aide agency. This advice covers the major approval mechanisms for a home health agency. However, the AMA guide also suggests that physicians secure the agency's literature and make personal visits to the administrator and staff to help with their appraisals of the potential quality of care.

A sample physician homecare treatment plan in the appendix of the AMA book illustrates sections on skilled nursing care, occupational therapy, progress notes, and addenda to the treatment plan. Frequency of visits and specific treatment modalities are indicated in the medical plan.

Stressing the pivotal role of physicians in assuring quality care, the AMA guide says that, "Appropriate physician participation and leadership is indispensible to the delivery of high quality home health care. Care that patients receive must be prescribed by a physician. When there is insufficient participation, the quality of care may suffer." Interestingly, Sandrick (1986c) found that the number of procedures being performed by physicians served as an indicator of professional proficiency and for consideration of hospital privileges. There appeared to be a link between doing too few procedures and increased mortality and morbidity; professional competence increased with usage.

With the impact of the PPS/DRG payment plan, Lavin (1985) tells physicians that they will have to love homecare in the future. This refers to the movement toward earlier hospital discharge and the need for care at home or in the community. Advice similar to the AMA guide suggests ways for physicians to evaluate home health agencies. There is some disagreement over whether or not physicians should have their own nurses participate in rendering homecare services to patients. On one side, a homecare expert feels that the local physician and nurse don't have the expertise or the time. On the contrary, physicians claim that their orders are not followed and homecare nurse coordinators overstep their authority in patient care. In *Patient Care,* a journal for practicing physicians, Borders (1986) recommends that physicians become more involved in discharge planning to attend to the homecare needs of their patients.

At a conference more than 20 years ago, Chapin (1966) listed seven broad responsibilities for physicians involved in homecare:

1. Being aware of when to use coordinated homecare for patients.

2. Referring to available services known to be quality care.

3. Supervising as leader of the homecare team.

4. Maintaining patient records and exchanging data with other members of the homecare team for comprehensive files.

5. Being available for consultation and discussions with others.

6. Discharge planning, including termination of services.

7. Participating in advisory activities in relation to the hospital, medical society, or other groups.

In support of the contention that the dedication of the physician is the focal point in achieving high quality homecare service, Dr. Morris Alex (1966, 7) described the qualifications of such dedication:

> Not only must he be thoroughly qualified, but he must have warmth, understanding, a feeling for people, sensitivity, empathy, and ability to understand chronic illness and its impact upon people and families. He should have some understanding of his own reactions to people and above all, must have the ability to work with other professional groups. In a word, if you will consider that the homecare physician is practicing "medicine with a heart," then you have the essence of the function of the doctor.

Win or Lose with Quality Care

In an interview, Richard P. Kusserow (*Hospitals* 1986a), Inspector General of HHS, was asked about the impact of PPS/DRG upon the quality of health care delivered in the U.S. His response was that "the quality of health care is improving" under PPS/DRG. Presumably, the quality of homecare is included in that comment.

High quality care is a saleable commodity. "Homecare is an extremely competitive industry, and having an edge such as NLN accreditation can attract business from health maintenance organizations, preferred provider organizations, and other groups managing corporate personnel health care policies" according to Kathy Janz, the director of Stanford University Hospital's Home Care Program in Palo Alto, California (Ready 1986). Obviously, accreditation, licensure, and certification from other reputable associations or governmental agencies could also be used to attract patients in competitive situations.

A cover story in *Hospitals* (Sandrick 1986b) asked, "Will [quality] make or break your hospital?" Clayton McWhorter, president of Hospital Corporation of America, was quoted: "I'm convinced that quality will be the key factor that we're going to be talking about--the quality of our services and the way we document and measure that quality." In agreement, Daniel Bourque, executive director of the National Committee for Quality Health Care, said that "quality is becoming a competitive factor for hospitals." Four practical reasons for hospitals and other health care services to deal with quality assurance issues were identified: quality care is no longer a shield against budget cuts; providers cannot hide behind quality that is too difficult to measure; economic incentives to provide quality care are diffusing; and patients/consumers want value for their dollars as well as comparison information on how well providers are doing. This can be done by removing the cloak of confidentiality from statistical data on mortality and morbidity and other measures of quality.

Commercial companies also utilize quality words to sell their services even without the stamp of approval of sanctioning bodies. One brochure notes that the high tech home infusion therapy programs are "maintaining the highest standards of professional medical care . . . reassuring professional quality care for patients . . . " (Abott Home Care 1985). It is apparent that like great art, quality of care may be in the eye of the beholder, since many intangibles affect an individual's determination of quality of care.

Additionally, Sandrick (1986b) noted that one of the biggest problems was that there was no single definition of the quality of care. A quality definition should cover objective as well as subjective evaluations and the quality of social interactions as well as the quality of management.

At an AMA convention (*Hospitals* 1986b), the assembled physicians took a stab at defining the quality of care:

Treatment that improves patients' physical and emotional status as quickly as possible; promotes health and early treatment; involves patients in decision making; is given by practitioners sensitive to illness-related anxiety; is based on accepted medical principles; uses technology and other resources effectively; and is sufficiently documented in medical records.

That definition does imply the inclusion of accreditation, licensure, certification, and the other standards, norms, and criteria considered vital to high quality homecare service.

In an attempt to provide standards for home health agencies, Reisman and DeLong (1983) developed a quality assurance primer and visit screening guidelines. This primer includes methodologies and approaches for an annual program evaluation. Evaluation consists of a review of overall policies and administration, as well as a clinical record review. A suggested program evaluation model requires a systematic description and measurement of each program variable detailing resources, activities, and objectives. There are four sections in the evaluation instrument: organization and administration; professional services; statistical/fiscal information; and clinical record review. This evaluation model is intended for program personnel who are familiar with the philosophy and objectives of the home health agency. However, the evaluation can be used by an outside evaluator who can assess the homecare program objectively and compare the results to trends and nationally accepted standards.

Griffith (1986) summed up the quality of care predicament: "As the homecare industry grows, responsible homecare agencies must work to ensure that all individuals receive the highest quality service possible, while also working to remain competitive in a booming marketplace."

References

Abbott Home Care. 1985. *High-tech home infusion therapy programs.* North Chicago (July).

Affeldt, J. E. 1984. Questions addressed regarding new hospice program. *Hospitals* 58(2):110.

Alex, M. 1966. *The physician speaks on home care.* Washington, DC: Government Printing Office. Pub. No. (PHS) 1654.

Allgaier, J. A. 1980. Home care needs physicians who care. *The Hospital Medical Staff* 9(5):2-11.

Altman, L. K. 1982. Health quality and costs: a delicate balance. *New York Times* (30 March).

Amenta, M. O'R. 1985. Hospice in the U.S. *Nursing Clinics of North America* 20(2):269-279.

American Association of Retired Persons.

1984. *A handbook about care in the home.* Washington, DC.

American Medical Association. 1981. *Physician guide to home health care.* Chicago (July).

Anderson, K. B., and D. I. Kass. 1986. *Certificate of need regulation of entry into home health care.* Washington, DC: Federal Trade Commission (Jan.).

Beard, J. G. 1984. Testimony on Older Americans Act before Subcommittee on Aging. Washington, DC: American Federation of Home Health Agencies, Inc. (31 Jan.).

Berkoben, R. M. 1976. *Quality assurance in home health care.* Camp Hill, PA: Pennsylvania Assembly of Home Health Agencies.

Blum, J. D., and D. A. Robbins. 1985. Considerations in hospice licensure in *Hospice programs and public policy* edited by P. R. Torrens. Chicago: American Hospital Publishing, Inc.

Borders, C. R. 1986. Avoiding poor outcomes in home care. *Patient Care* 20(3):139-150.

Brazil, P. 1986. Cost effective care is better care. *Hastings Center Report* 16(1):7-8.

Brodsky, H. 1979. The role and evaluation of profit making in the health care industry. Presentation at annual meeting of the American Public Health Association, New York.

Butler, R. N. 1981. The teaching nursing home. *Journal of the American Medical Association* 245:1435-1437.

Chapin, S. E. 1966. The professional community in home care in *The physician speaks on home care.* Washington, DC: Government Printing Office. Pub. No. (PHS) 1654.

Chrystal, C. 1985. Making the NITA standards work for you. *National Intravenous Therapy Association* 8(5):363-364.

Collier, G. 1984. Certificate of need requirements for home health services. *Caring* 3(5):19-27.

Congressional Budget Office. 1977. *Long term care report.* Washington, DC: Government Printing Office (18 Feb).

Connaway, N. I. 1985. The legalities of home care. *Home Healthcare Nurse Part I* 3(5):6-8. *Part II* 3(6):44-46.

Council on Accreditation of Services for Families and Children, Inc. 1985. *Provisions for Accreditation.* New York.

Department of Health and Human Services. 1981. *Hospice education program for nurses. Volume I: participant manual. Volume II: facilitator manual.* Washington, DC: Government Printing Office. Pub. No. HRA 81-27 (June).

Department of Health and Human Services. Bureau of Community Services. 1980. *A model curriculum and teaching guide for the instruction of homemaker-home health aides.* Washington, DC: Government Printing Office. Pub. No. HSA 80-5508.

Department of Health, Education and Welfare. 1977. *Home health care. Report on the regional public hearings. Sept. 20-Oct. 1, 1976.* Washington, DC: Government Printing Office. Pub. No. 76-135.

Dolan, K. R. 1986. Medicare home service is shrinking (Letter to editor). *New York Times* (5 Feb.).

Donabedian, A. 1966. Evaluating the quality of medical care. *Milbank Memorial Fund Quarterly, Part 2.* 44(Supplement):166-206.

Egdahl, R. H., and C. H. Taft. 1986. Financial incentives to physicians. *New England Journal of Medicine* 315(1):59-61.

Engelbrecht, L. 1986a. Document! *Home Health Journal* 7(3):11.

Engelbrecht, L. 1986b. What not to document! *Home Health Journal* 7(6):8.

Engelbrecht, L. 1986c. Documenting physical therapy services. *Home Health Journal* 7(7):8-9.

Federal Register. 1973. Subpart L. Conditions of participation; home health agencies. Washington, DC: Government Printing Office (16 July).

Federal Register. 1983. Medicare program: hospice care. 48(243):56008-56036 (16 Dec.).

Fine, D. R. 1984. The home as workplace: prejudice and inequity in home health care. Position paper prepared for VNA of San Francisco (Jan.).

General Accounting Office. 1979. *Hospice care - a growing concept in the U.S.* Washington, DC: Government Printing Office. Pub. No. HRD 79-50.

Gould, E. J. 1985. Standardized home health nursing care plans: a quality assurance tool. *Quality Review Bulletin* 11(11):334-338.

Griffith, D. 1986. Blending key ingredients to assure quality in home health care. *Nursing and Health Care* 301-302.

Hagedorn, H. J., K. J. Beck, S. F. Neubert, et al. 1976. *A working manual of simple program evaluation techniques for community mental health centers.* Washington, DC: Government Printing Office. Pub. No. (ADM) 76-404.

Hargreaves, W. A., C. C. Atkinson, and J. E. Sorenson. 1977. *Resource materials for community health program evaluation.* Washington, DC: Government

Printing Office. Pub. No. (ADM) 77-328.

Havinghurst, C. C. 1977. Health care cost containment regulation: prospects and alternatives. *American Journal of Law and Medicine* 3(3):309-322.

Health Industry Manufacturers Association. 1985. Home use in-vitro diagnostics. Washington, DC (25 Nov.).

Henry, T. 1986. Industry reels from latest attack. *Home Health Journal* 7(6):1,11,16.

Holzemer, S. P. 1985. Make accreditation work for you. *Home Health Journal* 6(4):15-16.

Home Health Journal. 1986a. Quality assurance act could "watch" HHAs. 7(3):4,8.

Home Health Journal. 1986b. '87 federal budget proposes cutback on homecare service. 7(3):8.

Home Health Homemaker Services GHI. 1979. Patients' bill of rights. New York.

Home Health Services and Staffing Association. 1981. *Home health and certificate of need. A position paper.* Washington, DC (Jan.).

Hospice Association of America. 1986. Hospice association to sponsor standards seminar. Washington, DC (25 Feb.).

Hospital Week. 1984. Only 21 hospices apply for Medicare certification under HHS' new rules. 20(2):2.

Hospitals. 1985. More than 1,500 hospice programs are operating in U.S.: JCAH study. 59(14):70.

Hospitals. 1986a. Inspector general lauds quality of care under PPS. 60(10):78-79.

Hospitals. 1986b. Docs take stab at defining quality of care. 60(13):18.

House Committee on Interstate and Foreign Commerce. 1979. Report on 1979 Amendments to the federal planning legislation. Washington, DC: Government Printing Office (15 May).

House Select Committee on Aging. 1985. *Health care cost containment: are America's aged protected?* Washington, DC: Government Printing Office. Comm. Pub. No. 99-522.

House Subcommittee on Health and the Environment. 1976. *A discursive diction-*ary *of health care.* Washington, DC: Government Printing Office (Feb.).

Hughes, S. L. 1982. Home health monitoring. Ensuring quality in homecare services. *Hospitals* 56(21):74-80.

Hyman, H. H. 1977. *Health regulation, certificate of need and 1122.* Rockville, MD: Aspen Systems Corporation.

Jacob, S. R. 1985. The impact of documentation in home health care. *Home Healthcare Nurse* 3(5):16-20.

Joint Commission on Accreditation of Hospitals. 1983a. *Hospice standards manual.* Chicago.

Joint Commission on Accreditation of Hospitals. 1983b. *Hospice self-assessment and survey guide.* Chicago.

Joint Commission on Accreditation of Hospitals. 1985. *The hospice project report.* Chicago.

Joint Commission on Accreditation of Hospitals. 1986. *Accreditation manual for hospitals.* Chicago, IL.

Jones, P. July 17, 1986. Personal communication. Hospice Association of America, Washington, DC.

Kaye, L. W. 1985. Setting educational standards for gerontological home care personnel. *Home Health Care Services Quarterly* 6(1):85-99.

Kleffel, D. 1973. *A utilization review program for home health agencies.* Washington, DC: Government Printing Office. Pub. No. HSM 72-6502 (May).

Kleffel, D., and E. Wilson. 1975. *Evaluation handbook for home health agencies.* Washington, DC: Government Printing Office. Pub. No. HSA 76-3003.

Lavin, J. H. 1985. You'd better learn to love home care. *Medical Economics* (29 April).

Lee, P. R. 1975. Quoted in *Humanizing health care,* edited by J. Howard and A. Strauss. New York: John Wiley and Sons.

McAllister, J. C., III, B. L. Black, R. E. Griffin, et al. 1986. Controversial issues in home health care: a roundtable discussion. *American Journal of Hospital Pharmacy* 43(4):933-946.

McClure, W. 1978. *On broadening the definition and removing regulatory bar-*

riers to a competitive health care system. Excelsior, MN: Interstudy.

Miller, S. C. 1984. *A medical record handbook for hospice programs.* Chicago: American Medical Record Association.

Miller, S. C. 1985a. Home care project survey data Part I and Part II. *Journal of American Medical Record Association* 56(11):21-24 and 56(12):25-28.

Miller, S. C. 1985b. Hospice medical record documentation and management: opportunity for improvement. *Topics in Health Record Management* 5(3):13-23.

Miller, S. C. 1986. *Documentation for home health care: a record management handbook.* Chicago: American Medical Record Association.

Molotsky, I. 1986. Laws cost car buyers, study finds. *New York Times* (14 March).

National Home Caring Council. 1981a. *Basic national standards for homemaker-home health aide services.* New York.

National Home Caring Council. 1981b. *Interpretation of standards.* New York.

National League for Nursing. 1985a. *Policies and procedures for the NLN accreditation program for home care and community health.* New York. Pub. No. 21-1612.

National League for Nursing. 1985b. *Accreditation program for home care and community health.* New York. Pub. No. 21-1306.

Parzick, J., and M. Nolan. 1978. POMR at work in a home health agency. *Family and Community Health* 1(1):101-113.

Pettey, S. M. 1985. Comments on New York State proposed regulations on home health agencies and hospices. Home Health Services and Staffing Association. Washington, DC (13 Sept.).

Quality Care. 1981. *Patient policy.* Rockville Centre, NY.

Ready, V. 1986. NLN accreditation gives agencies close ties with nursing community. *Hospital Home Health.* 64-65.

Reisman, L. J., and D. J. DeLong. 1983. *Quality assurance primer.* Memphis, TN: Healthcare Concepts, Inc.

Ruchlin, H. S. 1977. A new strategy for regulating long term care facilities. *Journal of Health Politics, Policy and Law* 2:190-211.

Ryder, C. F. 1967. Changing patterns in home care. Washington, DC: Government Printing Office. Pub. No. PHS 1657 (June).

Salkever, D. S. 1978. Will regulation control health care costs? *Bulletin of the New York Academy of Medicine* 54:73-83.

Sandrick, K. 1986a. Home care: cutting health care's safety net. *Hospitals* 60(10):48-52.

Sandrick, K. 1986b. Quality: will it make or break your hospital? *Hospitals* 60(13):54-58.

Sandrick, K. 1986c. Physician volume: tying privileges to procedures. *Hospitals* 60(13):56.

Simmons, K. 1986. Caring for elderly: challenge for now and 21st century medicine. *Journal of the American Medical Association* 255:3057-3058.

Spiegel, A. D. 1979. *The Medicaid experience.* Rockville, MD: Aspen Systems Corporation.

Spiegel, A. D., and B. Backhaut. 1980. *Curing and caring. A review of the factors affecting the quality and acceptability of health care.* Jamaica, NY: SP Medical and Scientific Books.

Spiegel, A. D., and H. H. Hyman. 1979. *Basic health planning methods.* Rockville, MD: Aspen Systems Corporation.

Spiegel, A. D., and S. Podair. 1975. *Medicaid: lessons for national health insurance.* Rockville, MD: Aspen Systems Corporation.

Spiegel, A. D., and S. Podair. 1981. *Rehabilitating people with disabilities into the mainstream of society.* Park Ridge, NJ: Noyes Medical Books.

Stevens, L., and C. R. Kirk. 1985. The role of the health record practitioner in public health nursing and home health care agencies. *Topics in Health Record Management* 5(3):61-64.

Stewart, J. 1979. *Home health care.* St. Louis: C. V. Mosby Company.

Tehan, C. 1985. Considerations in hospice accreditation in *Hospice programs and public policy* edited by P. R. Torrens. Chicago: American Hospital Publishing, Inc.

Torrens, P. R. 1985. *Hospice programs and public policy.* Chicago: American Hospital Publishing, Inc.

Trager, B. 1980. Home health care and national health policy. *Home Health Care Services Quarterly* 1(2):1-103.

Volunteer - The National Center. 1978. *Standards and guidelines for the field of volunteerism.* Arlington, VA.

Warhola, C. F. R. 1980. *Planning for home health services. A resource handbook.* Washington, DC: Government Printing Office. Pub. No. HRA 80-14017

(Aug.).

Weinstein, S. M. 1985. Regulations governing home care programs. *National Intravenous Therapy Association* 8(5):361-362.

Wilde, D. J. 1985. Home health agencies with multiple programs: flexibility is key for clinical records. *Topics in Health Record Management* 5(3):1-12.

Williams, J. L., G. Gaumer, and M. A. Cella. 1984. *Home health services: an industry in transition.* Cambridge, MA: Abt Associates, Inc. (3 May).

Chapter 9

Variety of Homecare Workers
Professionals and Others

There can be no doubt that professionals, organizations, and individuals involved in homecare believe that their activities are appropriate, humane, and cost-effective, and promote access to health and social services needed by the community.

Professional organizations accredit educational training programs for their specialties, accredit institutions, and manage existing certification programs within their area of expertise. A wide variety of continuing education activities are usually offered by professional organizations to maintain the skills of their memberships. Most professional organizations also have a code of ethics--written professional standards and procedures for monitoring the criteria. Some engage in political lobbying to influence legislation favorable to their members. All of these activities and others are part and parcel of the routine of professional groups. Professionals belonging to such groups usually ascribe to the policies and practices and work on committees, task forces, and the like on a voluntary basis to promote the welfare of the profession.

Within the homecare system, the list of active professionals is quite varied: physicians, registered nurses, public health nurses, practical and vocational nurses, nursing aides, homemaker-home health aides, physical therapists, speech and audiology therapists, social workers, and occupational therapists. In addition, dietary and nutritional personnel, pharmacists, dentists, volunteers, and family members are part of the homecare team. Most homecare workers are licensed, certified, or otherwise qualified to render care. In order of the percentage of home health agencies offering services, the frequency starts with 100 percent for nursing and follows with homemaker-home health aide, physical therapy, speech therapy, medical social service, and occupational therapy. Physicians are not included because a medical order is required before a home health agency initiates services.

As with all groups, homecare workers are concerned with professional and nonprofessional functions, provider reputation, certification, prescribing authorization, independent provider status, reimbursement, and protection of their own domain.

With such a mixed grouping of professionals, paraprofessionals, volunteers, and family members, it is obvious that homecare personnel have to be diplomats as well.

283

Physicians

Although most home health agencies don't have physicians on staff, services cannot be delivered without the written order of the attending physician (Schwartz 1980). In addition, the physician is still the leader of the team insofar as the patient is concerned, and the AMA advocates that role for doctors (American Medical Association 1981).

Most physicians support the concept of homecare. Yet, many do not use it partly because of unfamiliarity with the capability of the services, and also because of displeasure with reimbursement for patient care or case management. Koren (1986) also commented that "third-party payers must recognize the time and thought necessary to develop good plans for homecare, and they must make adequate provision for reimbursement."

Dr. Frank Randolph, a member of the California Medical Association's long-term care committee, expressed a common attitude: "I'm for homecare, and most doctors seem to be for it. But I sense a lot of concern about when it's (homecare) indicated, the lack of outcome studies, and the fact that private business is becoming so heavily involved that it's sometimes hard to tell whether it's the patient or the homecare agency who's benefiting" (*Home Health Journal* 1986).

Dan Thomas of Health Insurance Association of America (HIAA) noted a common complaint from insurers about homecare benefits. Although the policy covered the homecare benefit, attending physicians frequently do not prescribe homecare, or patients see the service as a second-class approach to care. "We need more education on the part of health professionals, patients and insurers . . . It's time for physicians to have confidence in their patients' being at home . . . physicians must feel confident that prescribing homecare will not place them at increased risk of being sued for malpractice" (*Hospitals* 1984).

Edwardson (1985) investigated attitudes of attending physicians toward a nurse-directed homecare program for terminally ill children in Minneapolis, Minnesota. She wanted to know what factors pediatric oncologists considered when making the choice between home or hospital care. Physicians tended to make referrals based on a judgment of the family's technical and emotional ability to provide homecare. There was a high level of agreement on the chief benefits of homecare; "a belief that the child and family would be happier and that the family would have greater involvement and find greater meaning in the event."

From a marketing viewpoint, de Ulibarri (1986) suggested ways to get physicians involved in homecare. She seeks to match the doctor's life cycle, from practice preparation through practice decline, to a need to use homecare for patients. Involving physicians in homecare provides an opportunity for communications and persuasion, according to the author.

Despite the rapid growth of homecare, Koren (1986) notes the contradiction that a majority of physicians know little about the field. She attributes the lack of awareness to "general isolation of the medical profession from homecare" and urges physicians to acquaint themselves with homecare services and to provide medical input to "protect patients from becoming pawns of market forces and fiscal policy directives." Rationales for this situation include the extreme diversity and complexity of homecare service programs and providers with their increasing sophistication and intensity, and the historical quirk of homecare arriving on the scene in 1947 when the practice of physician house calls was waning in favor of improved technological care in the hospital.

"Home health agencies in general are not unhappy about the current lack of involvement by the medical profession, arguing that agencies have considerable trouble even obtaining physicians' signatures on orders, let alone getting actual, detailed plans for care." Koren also reported that at a national convention of the National Association for Home Care (NAHC) "ripples of laughter swept the auditorium at the mention of physician participation."

With the opposite poles of strongly expressed medical support for homecare and the actual experience of indifference, what is the physician's role?

Role of the Physician

Writing in a state medical society journal, Weller (1978) listed six elements of the physician's role in homecare: knowing what homecare is available in the area; understanding the mechanics of referral to homecare services; coordinating homecare in the community; maintaining the reports and keeping clinical records on each patient; helping establish coordinator positions to manage each patient; and being aware of reimbursement alternatives for payment. That listing was reinforced by the AMA (1981) guidebook for physicians, among others.

Commenting that homecare will soon become a significant part of the physician's practice, a number of articles in *Patient Care* (Borders 1985a, 1985b, 1985c) sought to assist practitioners in the transition. Even while one article noted that patients feel better and may improve at home, it was also stated that "training, experience and remuneration may influence physicians to avoid homecare" (Borders 1985a). Physicians are urged to hone their office interviewing techniques to question patients about their ability to perform activities of daily living to identify patients at risk of institutionalization. However, doctors are cautioned that patients who fear institutionalization may not answer questions truthfully. The suggestion is made that physicians can follow patients between visits, or those in the community at large, through a senior-visiting-senior program. This activity could evolve from the physician's involvement with a senior center or as an outgrowth of community activities.

Another article (Borders 1985b) focused on the physician's role in helping patients to avoid institutionalization. It is suggested that the physician do an immediate assessment of a patient's ability to manage at home after a debilitating event. Housecalls are advocated when the patient has a non-emergent problem and cannot get out of bed. Patient and family education at home should be undertaken, with physicians providing their own protocols or revising material provided by the homecare agency. Attention should also be given to family caregivers and their problems, including burnout and the need for respite care. Mutual support groups should be used if available in the locality. Homecare follow-up by the attending physician is recommended as part of the integral treatment plan. This can be achieved through progress reports and telephone calls from the homecare workers attending to the patient.

Preparation for posthospital homecare can be started in the facility with a patient and family education program (Borders 1985c). Activities include preoperative and postoperative teaching packets, focus sessions for office nurses, specific disease/condition teaching materials including the nursing record, and disease/condition specific discharge materials. Cooperative care, similar to parents learning how to care for their hospitalized child, could be initiated to prepare the patient and family for the transition to care at home after discharge.

Illustrating the universality of the physician's role in homecare, Freer, Almind, Gray, et al. (1985) devoted 28 pages to a discussion of the contribution of the primary care doctor to the medical care of the elderly in the community in a supplement to the *Danish Medical Bulletin*.

It is evident that there are mixed signals regarding what is verbalized as the physician's role and what that role is in actual practice in the community. Critics argue that the translation of high sounding words into action will not take place until the medical education of physicians integrates homecare into the process of becoming a physician.

Medical Education

Some time ago, an editorial in *Geriatrics* (Nash 1974) commented that the main problem in the use of homecare was the education of physicians. Butler (1981) enumerated the features of medical education for a teaching nursing home. With homecare substituted for nursing home, these same elements fit:

- Create a homecare unit in professional schools.

- Add homecare to the required curriculum for physicians and allied professionals.

- Rotate students through homecare services.

- Add grand homecare rounds in various disciplines.

- Share facilities, labs, and other services with homecare programs.

- Institute preservice and inservice training for all homecare workers.

- Set up outreach programs with homecare programs in hospitals and other facilities.

George Washington University Medical Center established the Case Assessment/Case Management (CA/CM) project to maintain the frail elderly at home in cooperation with two other medical centers and many local support groups (Koshes 1984). Using an interdisciplinary team that includes medical students, the team arranges for coordinated homecare services. "For the medical student involved, the experience is an invaluable opportunity to learn multidisciplinary care for the elderly and the value of being part of a care team." Medical students reported four benefits from the program: gaining knowledge about medical, social, and emotional aspects of aging; coming to terms with their own aging after being uncomfortable about working with the elderly; having an opportunity to work with the "well elderly" rather than with only severely impaired patients; and having a chance to function in the team efforts.

Tideiksaar, Libow, and Chalmers (1985) described a program at Mount Sinai School of Medicine that mandated housecalls to older patients as part of a fourth-year clerkship in geriatrics. In cooperation with the Jewish Home and Hospital for the Aged, medical students made homecare visits along with other team members. During orientation, the students were instructed to observe the neighborhood, and physical/functional/safety characteristics of the home, the other people in the home and their interactions, and to inquire about the impact of medical and psychological illness upon the patient's life. Overwhelmingly, the medical students evaluated the homecare visits positively, saying that the experience should be part of a medical student's education, and stressing the importance of the nurse in homecare. Most of the medical students have never made a homecare visit prior to the clerkship. These medical educators concluded that "Little doubt remains about the importance and effectiveness of the homecare house call experience for medical students." Similar positive experiences were reported in a mandatory homecare teaching program for fourth-year medical students at Boston University School of Medicine (McCahan, Bissonnette, and DiRusso 1983).

A survey by Barry and Ham (1985) reported that more than 80 percent of U.S. medical schools provide some geriatric education for their students, mainly in the acute hospital or nursing home. About 40 percent of the schools use the patient's home as the educational site.

What's Ahead

About 500,000 physicians are licensed by the states to practice medicine. Federal studies estimate a surplus of physicians in a number of specialty areas. Yet, despite the host of professional associations that exist and the various certification programs, no specialty group really takes homecare into its domain. However, the medical leadership role in homecare is evident in law and by tradition. A major issue relates to motivating physician involvement. Some contend that physician inertia may be more of a barrier than outright resistance, but the end result is the same: physicians don't use homecare as often as possible. With the coming together of a projected physician surplus, the cost containment push for earlier discharges and the growth of hospital-based homecare units, it is possible that physician attitudes toward the use of homecare may change. Importantly, physician involvement in homecare has to be settled before much else can happen in homecare programs.

Nursing

Under the Medicare Conditions of Participation, all of the almost 6,000 home health agencies must provide skilled nursing care and at least one other service. In addition to services provided by a registered nurse, care is also given by licensed practical and vocational nurses and nurses' aides. Estimates of the personnel employed in rendering nursing care may be as high as three million. Obviously, most of the nursing staff work in facilities and not in homecare programs. Traditionally, most homecare nursing services came from VNAs, public health departments, and voluntary health organizations. Martin (1984) noted that now "everyone wants a piece of the home health care pie." She expressed concern that community nursing roles and responsibilities would be diluted or overlooked in the rush to get into the homecare act by hospitals, proprietary agencies, nursing homes, and others.

Nursing Responsibilities

Lash (1980) spelled out the role of the community health nurse clearly: "Whether the nurse acts as a change agent, caregiver, teacher, coordinator, facilitator, advocate or counselor, he or she should act *with* (author's emphasis) the client and with objectives that are meaningful to the client." Expanding that a bit, Anderson and Brown (1981) talk about nursing care for cancer patients in the community. "As nurses, we have a responsibility to act as catalysts of communication between the physician, patient, family, and significant others. It is within this framework of interface between the patient and the health care team that our accountability as cancer nurses is defined." In view of the fact that every homecare agency employs nurses, any other disease/condition could be substituted for "cancer" and the comment would still hold true.

Christopher (1986) identifies three needs in homecare for the elderly: meeting the health needs; making the home safe; and putting the patient and family in touch with community services. A chart in the article lists the community resource and the type of aid provided by each, such as home health aides, support groups, friendly visitors, and telephone reassurance. She calls for homecare nurses to focus on personal care related to ADL, medications, respiration and circulation, nutrition, sensory changes, mobility, finances, love and belonging, self-esteem, and spiritual needs.

In calling home health nursing a rediscovered concept, not a new concept, Belair (1986) discussed career aspects. She said, "Home health nursing offers autonomy, flexibility, and the opportunity to work one-to-one with patients and families from a range of socioeconomic groups. The nurse must be independent, creative, resourceful, and demonstrate the ability to accept responsibility." Responsibility was identified as the key to home health nursing. Nurses in homecare programs obviously play a vital role in the success or failure of any treatment plan. To define the responsibilities, the American Nurses Association (ANA) published community health nursing practice standards (1985) and a conceptual model of community health nursing (1980).

Nursing Education

"A baccalaureate in nursing best prepares a nurse for entry into community health nursing, although agencies may hire graduates of associate degree and diploma programs" (Belair 1986). Crowley and Standerfer (1985) agree, and opt for incorporating home health care into the baccalaureate nursing program. Senior nurses intervene with families at discharge and develop their own homecare caseloads from referrals from the head nurse or from rounds. Students contract with the families with a written identification of the family's major concerns, long- and short-range objectives, student and family responsibilities, and the specific information on treatment details. Nursing students keep logs and prepare reports. Response from attending physicians has been enthusiastic, and the benefits to the families and nursing students are manifold.

Also in relation to nurses learning about family needs, Hirst and Metcalf (1986) state that families continue to provide support to family members even after the impaired family member is institutionalized. Nurses must be educated to do a family learning needs assessment to allow the nurse to work with and teach the family. Family assessment involves discovering the family's knowledge level, their educational desires, the stressors in the family situation, and the readiness to learn.

Cruz, Jacobs, and Wood (1986) surveyed 237 home health agencies in Los Angeles to look at the educational needs of home health nurses. They found that two-thirds of the nurses had less than two years of experience in homecare, and the majority had associate degrees or diplomas in nursing. Only 42 percent of the 325 nurses responding had public health nursing certificates. In a training program, Littlejohn (1980) found that new nursing staff learned the difference between working in an institution and in homecare activities. Immediately, the nurses realized that there is more independent decision-making in homecare by the nurses. In addition, the trainees identified educational learning related to planning day-to-day work activities, length of home visits including travel time and paper work, how long it takes to admit a patient, how to set priorities and expectations, when to discharge a patient, and simply what's important and what's not.

In a review of homecare literature, McCorkle and Germino (1984) found that "the most critical direct care function that the nurse performs is *an ongoing assessment* (author's emphasis) of the person in his own environment in relation to the people who are important to him." They included this ongoing assessment knowledge among items that nurses need to know about homecare. Other required knowledge related to the conceptual framework for homecare, utilization of services, scope of practice, direct and indirect services, and accountability. "Nurses in various settings have a responsibility to become knowledgeable about the resources in the community and teach patients and other professionals about their benefits." In addition, the authors also project the need for nurses educated in homecare subspecialties.

A commonly identified nursing specialty is geriatric nurse practitioner (GNP) (Capezuti 1985). With the elderly population growing, with the desire to remain at home evident, and with the PPS/DRG system discharging older patients sicker and earlier, the GNP is an adjunct to vital homecare services. Capezuti emphasizes that the GNP is not a replacement for the community health nurse, but a supplement to care.

There are about 35 training programs for GNPs in the U.S., up from 15 in 1980 (Mountain State Health Corporation 1985). "At the heart of graduate education in geriatric nursing is the belief that older people must be given the resources to determine their own destiny" (Capezuti 1985). In a survey, Capezuti reported that homecare is an integral part of the curriculum of GNP programs but the results were mixed regarding the amount of time devoted to actual home visits. Classroom offerings included social gerontology, health assessment, clinical decision-making, health care system analysis, and the usual nursing courses.

Exhibiting an interest in geriatric nursing, almost 350 GNPs and 1,751 gerontological nurses were certified by the ANA as of April 1984 (Fickeissen 1985).

A survey of general practitioners in London by Haines and Bookoff (1986) inquired about terminal care at home to gain the attending physician's perspective. Another nursing specialty area emerged, as 75 percent of the almost 200 physicians stated that more nursing home support in terminal care was needed.

In 1983, the University of Michigan School of Nursing began the first organized program to prepare nursing administrators and managers for roles in home health agencies (*Home Health Journal* 1984). Curriculum content focuses on principles of marketing, quality assurance, staffing, personnel management, program evaluation, and the arts of negotiation and delegation. A home health care concentration features extensive supervised clinical experience for practical applications.

Trend to Independent Practice

As with other professions, community nursing is exhibiting movement toward independent practice. Keating (1985) described the formation of a for-profit, independent nursing corporation. Direct nursing services and consultation are provided by the agency. Usual management aspects covered include the process of incorporation, legal issues, financial considerations, structure and management, and contracting with clients. Similarly, the Nursing Dynamics Corporation evolved from research into a functioning independent nursing service agency (Kelly and Crossman 1985). This agency provides adult day health programs, inhome services, caregiver support, research, consultation, and continuing education.

LPN and LVN

Licensed practical and vocational nurses play an important role in homecare programs. Under the supervision of a physician or registered nurse, the LPN/LVN is expected to use appropriate and safe nursing techniques in drainage, irrigation, catheterization, routine medication, taking vital signs, and in preparing clinical and progress notes. States license these homecare professionals upon graduation from approved educational facilities and on passing a state board examination. A typical organization, the National Federation of Licensed Practical Nurses, represents the profession.

Considering the level of care required for homecare patients and the abilities of the LPN/LVN, it is apparent that many homecare clients could be adequately served by these professionals.

As with other professions wherein there are varying levels of competence, there are always efforts to upgrade or downgrade one of the other professionals. Psychiatrists argue with psychologists, orthopedists with podiatrists, and registered nurses with LPNs and LVNs. In response to an NLN proposal for broader liberal arts coverage in nursing curriculums, the National Association for Practical Nurse Education commented (*American Medical News* 1982) that, "First and foremost we support excellence in medical care, not only by physicians but also for nurses. I fail to see how clinical skills can be significantly affected by a lack of increased knowledge of English literature or a greater understanding of the causes of World War I."

Again, these disagreements reflect the changing faces of professional education. At times, the pendulum swings toward the emphasis on sticking to the clinical skills to be used at the bedside. At other times, the movement is toward a broader-based professional education that includes liberal arts. Theories abound on what content makes the better practitioner, but there are no definitive answers.

Aides and Orderlies

Nursing aides, usually women, assist registered and practical nurses by performing less skilled tasks in the care of patients. Many of their functions are detailed in a text used to educate individuals to deliver home nursing care *Home Nursing Care for the Elderly* (Hogstel 1985).

Orderlies and attendants, usually men, assist by carrying out a variety of duties, mainly for male patients. Tasks requiring physical strength for ill patients fall within their domain. In addition, orderlies and attendants are more prominent in the care of the mentally ill and mentally retarded.

Although definite educational requirements for nursing aides and orderlies may be nebulous, most homecare agencies do provide some type of orientation and training program, usually taught by a registered nurse. However, training programs vary greatly in their intensity and length.

Home Health Aide

In a review of homemaker-home health aides in the U.S., Trager (1973) commented that the aide lends the presence of an intact, warm, healthy personality in contact with a sick or threatened family. Aides provide the clients with safety, security, and familiarity. Trager felt that those functions made the homemaker-home health aide service different from other services and not a substitute for them.

Different Titles

A number of different titles are used to identify people doing aide tasks, such as homemaker, attendant, child care worker, day care worker, chore worker, personal care aide, community aide, visiting housekeeper, family aide, and teaching homemaker. Differences have been listed among the titles, but the lines are not always that clear. It appears that homemaker-home health aide (H-HHA) covers much of the functional territory and is more frequently used. Hall (1986) defines the role of the paraprofessional in homecare and touches on capabilities and functions of these personnel.

In Europe, the term "home helps" has been used for some time and is similar to H-HHA. Norway, Sweden, and the Netherlands have the largest number of home helps. Much further down the listing are Finland, Belgium, France, Switzerland, and Great Britain. While the U.S. is not last in using aides, there is still quite a distance to go before reaching the level of the Scandinavian countries (Little 1981).

Tasks

Major duties of a homemaker include meal preparation, light housekeeping, laundry, marketing and errands, money management, child care, teaching, and personal care. Not included are washing windows or walls, scrubbing floors, moving heavy furniture, cleaning closets, and climbing to high places.

An H-HHA's tasks include personal care skills (bathing, eating, dressing, grooming); simple treatments and procedures (taking temperature, pulse and respiration, giving enemas, irrigating Foley catheters and changing colostomy bags); planning and preparing nutritious meals; and assisting with self-administered medications. H-HHAs do have considerable latitude. Burns and Ciaccia (1985) discuss their changing roles, while Raff (1985) even notes the use of H-HHAs in perinatal care of high risk infants.

Both jobs involve keeping records, attending meetings, and participating in educational programs. Both types of employees are expected to be able to work with people of all ages, races, cultural groups, or lifestyles during times of illness, family stress, or both. These homecare workers require maturity, good judgment, dependability, initiative, and flexibility. They have to care for people. Indeed, such care can be found across this nation: in Alaska (Eboch 1986); in Iowa (Howell 1986); in central New York (O'Leary 1986); and in North Dakota (Sanderson 1986).

Worker Traits of H-HHAs

Trager (1973) listed seven essential characteristics of applicants for H-HHA jobs:

- Ability to perform effectively in a wide variety of situations.
- Capacity to accept behavior under stress.
- Possession of a high degree of organization and stability.
- Physical stamina.
- Capacity for careful observation and differentiation among regular and uncommon occurrences.
- Capacity to accept and follow instructions.
- Capacity for a strong identification with the goals of the agency.

H-HHAs work under the auspices of a number of homecare agencies: VNA, family service agency, welfare department, public health department, religious agency, or independent organization. Each homecare agency appears to develop its own outlook and style of rendering service.

Profile of a Typical H-HHA

Typically, H-HHAs are middle-aged, almost all women, experienced as unpaid homemakers, able to read and write, and with compatible personalities. Owing to that type of background, "Most apparent is the continuing lack of acceptance of homemakers beyond the role of auxiliary staff" (Stempler and Stempler 1981). Professionals tend to regard the homemaker as not "professionally educated." Within that ideological rigidity, the homemaker is unable to operate as a full-fledged member of the homecare team. Fine (1986) also made a point about the lack of status given to homecare workers, particularly those in the aide groupings.

Clients may not agree with the lowered status of H-HHAs and probably consider the H-HHA to be more professional than otherwise. After all, the client is paying for services from a certified home health agency, and the H-HHA is the official representative of that agency. Certainly, clients do not appear to regard H-HHAs as servants. Most clients seem to be able to detect a definite improvement in the quality and quantity of homecare because of the aide's contributions.

A Model Curriculum

To attack the problem of educational knowledge required of H-HHAs, a multidisciplinary working group convened and developed a 529-page model curriculum and teaching guide (Department of Health and Human Services 1980). This book includes content material as well as suggestions for teaching the material to students. Instructions to the home health agency suggest the formation of a committee on education as well as a budget, and the appointment of a training coordinator. All told, the curriculum calls for 60 classroom and laboratory hours plus 15 hours of field practice.

Five sections and appendices are in the book. Section one tells what H-HHA service is, the role of the aide on the homecare team, and how a homecare agency operates. Section two deals with how to work with children, older adults, the ill, the disabled, the mentally ill, and the terminally ill. Generic parts covered communications and understanding basic human needs. Section three details home management skills and knowledge including a clean environment, food and nutrition, and managing time, money, and energy. Section four goes into the personal care area covering body systems, body functions, disease prevention, bed care, ambulatory care, medications, rehabilitation, emergency care, and mother and baby care. Section five illustrates the application of the practicum, the field practice. Appendix one contains special teaching/learning modules on cancer, the circulatory system, developmental disabilities, and mental illnesses/diseases. Appendix two reprints the national standards for H-HHAs, and includes a sample practicum, a sample agreement for field practice, and documentation of a practicum experience.

In content and in teaching examples, this curriculum guidebook is a tremendous asset to any homecare agency employing H-HHAs. Personnel can really be trained in conformance with the tenets of highly qualified experts. This model curriculum is included in the NHCC standards as the basic training document.

Personnel Issues

In recent history, the American health care system stressed the use of the institutional facility rather than any other alternative, such as homecare. Therefore, the combined thrust of professional clinical care decisions and third-party payer reimbursement awards created a barrier to utilization of homemaker-home health aides. That situation is further aggravated by the lack of a clear policy regarding homecare on any governmental level. Rationales for an absence of policy include costs and standards. Policymakers fear that liberal approval of reimbursement for H-HHAs would cause the demand for homecare services to increase tremendously and inflate expenditures. Additionally, the issue of acceptable standards of care is bothersome to policymakers despite advances in that area: NHCC links training and accreditation (Robinson 1986) and Connecticut similarly connects training and certification (Mercier 1986). Particularly troublesome is the use of independent self-contracting H-HHAs. These workers make their own deals with home health agencies or directly with clients, and supervision and accountability may be spotty at best.

Regulation has been a consistent part of the H-HHA problem as efforts aim to control abuses and assure quality care. On the other hand, there are those who opt for a decentralized, competitive marketplace to resolve the issues and achieve parity with the health care delivery system.

Future of H-HHAs

Based on the past history of the use of H-HHAs, it is obvious that the pool of H-HHAs will grow. Hall (1981) cites three solid reasons for the projection:

- Public opinion backs the use of homecare and opposes alternatives that are too costly, too inhumane, and too ineffective.

- Members of Congress hear from their constituents that they favor homecare rather than institutionalization.

- Populations at risk are increasing in number.

In addition, the "quicker and sicker" syndrome of patients needing care at home because of the PPS/DRG payment plan will increase the demand for H-HHAs.

Furthermore, the H-HHA can combine the health and personal aspects of care and deliver efficient and effective homecare rather than requiring two workers: a home health aide and a homemaker.

Currently, the H-HHA is second only to the required nursing service that all home health agencies are mandated to supply. There is no reason to doubt that the future will continue to have H-HHA services offered by more than 90 percent of homecare agencies.

Physical Therapist

Physical therapy (PT) was first classified as a profession in the *Dictionary of Occupational Titles* (1977): Physical therapists (PTs) are licensed in all states and graduate from schools with curriculums approved by the American Physical Therapy Association (APTA), an AMA group, or both. Schools are implementing master's degree programs for entry level into the profession. Pagliarulo (1986) links accreditation to the move to master's degree entry level and to self-improvement. However, it was noted that some educators regard accreditation as a "threat and a nuisance."

PTs are concerned with the restoration of function and prevention of disability following disease, injury, or loss of a body part. To achieve this goal, PTs use modalities such as therapeutic exercise, heat, cold, electricity, ultrasound, traction and massage, along with assistive, supportive, and prosthetic devices. Treatment programs aim to restore function, relieve pain, and prevent disability while patients reach the maximum performance level within the limits of their capabilities.

Physical therapy assistants (PTAs) meet similar licensing requirements when mandated and graduate from a two-year approved PTA program. PTAs function under supervision of a PT carrying out directed activities in rehabilitating patients.

In evaluating severely disabled patients who are about to be sent home, Lamont and Langford (1980) posed some critical questions for PTs: "Have you ever wondered, when working in a hospital, what really happened to patients when they were discharged home, still probably far from 100 percent fit, perhaps with a permanent disability, often incapable of doing their own shopping, cooking, and daily chores? How do these people cope, and do they actually receive the services they need?"

Considering the reported impact of the PPS/DRG scheme upon patients, the situation becomes even more critical. However, Edelstein (1984) felt that the revised Medicare reimbursement rates for PT services would not have a significant effect upon PTs. Nevertheless, some hospitals are moving toward setting up their existing PT units as separate services. This "unbundling" of the PT service from those included in the hospital's package may allow the facility to charge for care unrestricted by the PPS/DRG limitations. Possibly, the PT unit could be established as a distinct corporate entity or as part of an entity.

Patient Referrals

Physicians generally refer patients to PTs for treatment. There are varying sides to the problem of whether or not physicians make adequate referrals for physical therapy. In this case, adequate could refer to the prescription specifics or to not actually making a referral when the patient could be helped.

With the surge of HMOs establishing health care centers throughout the U.S., McDonnel (1986) reported on PTs coping with the referral problem. A dramatic decrease in medical referrals to PTs occurred in Albuquerque, New Mexico, and Denver, Colorado, as the HMOs set up shop. Upon investigation, PTs learned that the HMO tended to limit referrals and to reduce the use of PT services. It seems there was a set dollar pool for outside PT services, and physicians could share in the savings if the funds were not expended. Local PT groups worked with the HMOs to alleviate this referral situation.

On the other hand, commercial companies urge physicians to set up their own PT services--POPTS (physician-owned physical therapy services). Considering the low investment and high returns, physicians can increase their referrals to PTs.

Image of Physical Therapist

Some assert that referrals to PTs are not made because the PT is not seen as a professional. Luna-Massey and Smyle (1982) compared the professional image of the physical therapist with that of the physician. Consumers of PT services rated both on five criteria: motivation; representative organization; specialized education; evaluation skills; and autonomy of judgment. Overall, the consumers indicated no significant difference between the professional image of the PT and the physician. Most disagreement related to autonomy of judgment. Consumers do "accept and recognize physical therapists as professionals."

Stereotyping was investigated by Parker and Chan (1986) as they asked 53 PTs and 53 occupational therapists (OTs) to characterize themselves and each other. Using a Health Team Stereotype Scale, results showed that PTs viewed themselves more positively than the OTs. PTs attributed positive adjectives to themselves such as sociable and friendly, while the OTs disagreed. In addition, the PTs viewed the OTs less favorably.

In a study of reputational assessment, Dean and Davies (1986) found that physical therapy was moving from a practice orientation to a scientific orientation. Therefore, the reputation of PTs writing about their research in professional journals was higher. "We conclude that, with the increased emphasis on research in physical therapy, a stronger relationship will develop between subjective and objective measures of the professional impact of contributors on the profession."

Quality Assurance

A model assessment center for professional development and evaluation was developed by the Missouri PT Association (Deusinger, Sindelar, and Stritter 1986). Self-assessment of competency is made using multimethod testing: paper and pen; audiovisual; case study; laboratory; chart evaluation; patient simulation; and in basket testing. PTs receive feedback on how they did and are urged to take steps to alleviate any deficiencies while fostering professional growth.

Competency statements in 11 categories were rated by 176 practicing PTs in Quebec, Canada (Aston-McCrimmon 1986). These practitioners looked at the 224 competency statements in terms of the level of importance in clinical practice and self-evaluation of their own level for each skill. High importance was attributed to eight competency groups: the plan of treatment; interpersonal relations; theoretical knowledge; personal qualities; ethics and attitudes; professional growth; and administrative skills. Low overall importance rankings occurred in the remaining three competency categories: treatment skills and implementation; societal awareness; and research skills. Investigators were surprised by the low rating given to treatment skills and reasoned that the scores reflected the PTs' preferred treatment techniques, their clients, and the clinical environment. While caution was urged in using the data, the results could indicate a change in educational offerings at the undergraduate and graduate programs.

Bohannon and LeVeau (1986) examined the PTs' use of research findings. They found that "PT clinicians may not be applying many of the research findings that are relevant to their practice." To increase the use of research, it was suggested that PT students be prepared to be research consumers; that researchers be helped to communicate effectively, increasing the availability of information; and that clinicians be tutored in the use of research.

Adequate Personnel

A survey of 13 states revealed that 70 percent of PTs work in nursing homes and hospitals (Wilson, Langwell, Deane, et al. 1982). Even though the percentage may be reduced as PPS/DRG takes hold, it is likely that most PTs will continue to work in facilities. As with other professionals, PTs prefer to work in urban/suburban areas within easy traveling distance of opportunities for professional exchange and cultural activities. Motivating professionals to move into underserved areas is a constant problem.

The demand for physical therapy services still outstrips the supply of trained and qualified personnel.

Occupational Therapist

Consumers sometimes find it difficult to distinguish between OTs and PTs. In fact, some health care professionals have the same difficulty. Both, consumers and professionals, may be unaware of the distinct functions of each professional group.

OT Functions

Generally, the OT is "helping the patient to see himself as a *doer* in his own home" (author's emphasis) (Holdeman 1962). Occupational therapy is concerned with an individual's capacity to perform those daily tasks essential to a productive and satisfying life. Through the use of activities selected for their appropriateness to the individual's developmental, restorative, or health needs, the OT evaluates learning and performance abilities crucial to independent and health functioning. Home and daily family role demands, work and play needs, and social/community factors that impede or contribute to health form the perspectives of occupational therapy practice.

In a document prepared for the American Occupational Therapy Association (AOTA) Commission on Practice, Marshall and Kerr (1981) developed guidelines for the role of OTs in home health care. This document covers the philosophical base of occupational therapy, the history, screening, evaluation, and treatment. Six treatment areas are identified: activities of daily living; sensorimotor skills; cognitive skills; psychosocial skills; therapeutic adaptations; and prevention. Within the framework of the therapy situation, family participation is encouraged. In conclusion, "The AOTA contends that there is a need to extend occupational therapy services to the individual in the home and community environment."

OT Training

OTs are graduates of schools approved by the AMA and the AOTA. Licenses are required in a number of states, and there is a national certification program. Those meeting the certification requirements become OTRs (occupational therapist registered). In addition, some occupational therapy assistants (OTAs) meet approved educational mandates and may be certified as COTA (certified occupational therapy assistants) after examination.

Most OTs work in facilities, although there has been a spurt in the percentage of OTs and COTAs listing home health agencies as their primary source of employment (Steinhauer 1984). In fact, the *American Journal of Occupational Therapy* devoted the entire November 1984 issue to the theme of home health care (Viseltear 1984).

Royeen (1986) advocates the master's degree as the standard for entry level into the field. If that move is not made, it is argued that OT will be relegated to the technician level and eventually be phased out of the university and college curriculums. Also concerned about the entry level question, Yerxa and Sharrott (1986) suggest a study to seek consensus. They claim that occupational therapy lacks agreement on the theory base, the technical tools, the contribution to society, the ethical stance, and the relation to medicine. Liberal arts is proposed as the foundation for a "new breed" of OT educated to think critically.

Uniqueness of OT Homecare

OTs have to be on-the-spot problem-solvers in the home. Often clients must learn to iron, to cook, and to wash dishes sitting down, a position totally unnatural for most people. Every home becomes its own separate clinic where the OT uses only the tools and materials brought along or improvises with what is available. On top of all that, the OT is most exposed to the emotional interactions of the family. Levine (1984) listed nine unique constraints on the homebound OT delivery model:

1. Participating in a working team that is frequently led by a nurse.

2. Working independently without day-to-day supervision.

3. Delivering services in a home environment.

4. Working with minimal supplies and equipment.

5. Making decisions that must be consistent with the patient's and caretaker's value systems.

6. Changing one's therapeutic milieu with every patient.

7. Offering uninterrupted one-to-one therapy to the patient and the caretaker.

8. Interacting with the patient's social groups.

9. Using documentation to justify retroactive payment for services.

Levine also presented a case study to demonstrate the "pervasive influence of culture on the patient's volitional, habituation, and performance subsystems."

To assist OTs with the unique aspects of therapy in the home, the AOTA prepared the following information packets: Adapted Clothing; Adapted Equipment/Rehab Engineering; Architectural Barriers/OTs Consulting to Architects; Geriatrics; Handicapped Homemaker; Home Health; and Nursing Homes/Long-Term Care.

Standards of Practice

As with most other professional groups, the AOTA has a Code of Ethics. In addition, the AOTA (1978) sets standards for OT services in homecare. Note the time factors in the specific items:

- Referrals with a timetable for responses.

- Evaluation of the client's performance, including orientation of the family and an assessment.

- Preparation and documentation of a program plan seven working days after the referral.

- Implementation of the program plan.

- Preparation and documentation of an occupational therapy discharge plan.

- Re-evaluation of the client after discharge.

- Systematic review of the quality of care, including outcomes using appropriate criteria.

Menzel and Teegarden (1982) described a tripartite model of quality assurance in Iowa that included traditional quality assurance activities, professional education, and credentialing. In this case, the model coordinated peer review, the state OT association, and the professional standards review organization.

Continuing education is another standard technique used by professional groups to maintain their members' performance levels. Occupational therapy schools and organizations routinely offer programs in skills, techniques, and general information.

In operational terms, Trossman (1984) dealt with administrative and professional standards for the OT in home health care. Areas covered included contractual relations, referral systems, third-party reimbursement, documentation, equipment, and ethics. Specific and practical details are comprehensively reviewed in the day-to-day activity of providing OT services to people at home while meeting regulations and guidelines.

Medicare and OT

Medicare regulations originally required that OT services could be prescribed only in addition to another of the qualifying skilled services and had to end when the other ended. For a time, from July 1, 1980 to December 1, 1981, the Omnibus Reconciliation Act of 1980 (P.L.96-499) made OT a qualifying skill capable of being ordered and reimbursed under the same conditions of clinical eligibility. However, the 1981 Omnibus Reconciliation Act reversed that in a section entitled, "Elimination of Occupational Therapy as a Basis for Initial Entitlement to Home Health Services." For additional insight, Mallon (1981) reviews the history of that short Medicare flip-flop. Currently, the need for occupational therapy alone does not qualify an individual for Medicare coverage.

McRae (1984) reviews clinical and professional consideration of the OT in a Medicare-certified home health agency. She includes the effect of Medicare regulations on occupational therapy screening, evaluation, treatment, and discharge. Her study indicates that the majority of patients referred to OT have more than one treatable diagnosis; and patients receive an average of 7.25 home visits, ranging from 4.70 to 12.08. Furthermore, 79 percent of the patients treated by OTs are able to remain safely at home either independently or with assistance. "OTs working within Medicare guidelines for a home health agency have limitations on the types and amounts of services that they can provide." For example, regulations require OTs to discharge patients who fail to show continued progress toward written goals within a reasonable time, do not comply with the rehabilitation program, or who have achieved maximum potential.

Medicare reimbursement for homecare by an OT is conditioned to the regulations. "Reimbursement is denied when skilled care or patient progress is not documented" (DePaoli and Zenk-Jones 1984). With that in mind, indications for charting are suggested by the authors. They state that, "Medicare intermediaries are looking for significant practical improvement; therefore, words such as *plateau, maintain, or stable,* or phrases such as *patient still* . . .indicate less than significant gains and should be avoided." This means that the OT has to acquire writing skills to attune chart entries to the Medicare guidelines for reimbursement.

Future Concerns

Issues that have been raised about future professional concerns of occupational therapists include the following: recertification; specialization; locus of employment in facilities, in the community, and in the home; type and content of educational programs; reimbursement in a prospective payment system; impact of various legislation such as rehabilitation bills; and the adequate supply of OT personnel. Steinhauer (1984) identifies issues specific to homecare as the need to secure the skilled Medicare status again; the impact of the cost containment thrust of the PPS/DRG payment plan; the gaps in the Medicare program that hinder OT contributions to total patient rehabilitation; and the tendency of third-party payers to imitate governmental practices, thereby also inhibiting OT patient care.

As with the other professions, it is likely that occupational therapy will also be affected by the fallout from the Medicare PPS/DRG program. Exactly how and in what manner remains to be determined.

Medical Social Work

Social workers stress individual self-determination, privacy, and the ability to control one's own life. Because of these basic premises, homecare is the modality of choice for medical social work. A cornerstone of social work practice in the U.S. has been the provision of services in the home (Pumphrey and Pumphrey 1961,20). Fawcett (1961) also recalled that "the home visit was a usual procedure in all social work undertakings and during the formative years of our profession, but fell into disfavor a few decades ago." Part of that disfavor was linked to the belief that the home visit was a nonprofessional function.

Social workers usually have a master's degree from an institution accredited by the Council on Social Work Education. Some states have licensing requirements and/or registration laws. In addition, the National Association of Social Workers administers a certification program to allow members to enter the Academy of Certified Social Workers (ACSW). There is also a Social Work Assistant category similar to positions of that type in other professions.

Caroff and Mailick (1985) reported an overall accelerating trend toward the inclusion of health concentrations in graduate schools of social work. Of 72 schools responding to a survey, 42 (58 percent) had health concentrations. Major groupings of courses included direct practice in health and mental health settings, policy and planning, and psychosocial aspects of health and illness.

Tangible or Intangible Services?

Compared to the tangible services offered by nurses and others, medical social work is talk oriented. Understandably, patients may respond better to the "laying on of hands" than to verbalizing.

Auerbach, Bann, Davis, et al. (1984) concentrated on the role of the social worker in home health care. They characterized three separate but related components: direct service to the patient; consultation service to other staff members; and being a vital part of a community resource system. Additionally, the social worker in homecare can identify missing but needed community resources, can coordinate services for patients, manage cases, and develop and review policy. "As an effective team member, the social worker can be a counselor, enabler, advocate, planner, negotiator, and educator."

Special Areas

Dobrof (1984) focused upon gerontological social work in home health care relating theory to practice. That book covers social work activities in day care programs, volunteer visitors, mutual help groups, case management, foster care, and in relations with the hospital social worker. Obviously, with the older population increasing, the book is aimed at social workers in planning, delivery, and evaluation of services to chronically impaired, noninstitutional elderly in the community.

Another rapidly growing homecare service in which social workers are involved is hospice care. Anderson, Neal-McCollum, and Spann (1985) detail the role of the social worker with attention to psychosocial assessment factors in working with the family. Alleviation of caregiver guilt is an area where the social worker can assist the family with an emotionally distressing problem. In addition, the social worker aids the family with finding funding, with filling out insurance forms, and with interpersonal relations between family members.

Respite care and family functioning in families with retarded children was the subject of a study of the social worker's impact (Halpern 1985). Based on the data, social workers should get more information on family support systems, sources of stress, family perceptions of stress, behavioral status of the patient, and engage in outreach to make families aware of services. Results indicated that "families needing respite care seek it out." Social workers can apply their specialized skills to help the families who are inhibited from securing respite care.

Planning and Policy

Epstein (1980) argues that the special values of social work allow its planners to put forth unique solutions in long-term care. Social workers are trained to analyze the problems, define the alternatives, and aid in selecting the appropriate option; all within the preferences and values of social work. In the transition from hospital to home, Sharp and Sivak (1985) believe that social workers can find creative solutions. They can make arrangements with multiple agencies and various vendors while counseling the patient and family. It is suggested that social workers should research the psychosocial consequences of the increasing sophistication of medical care in the home. The homecare social worker should be attuned to the issues of mobility, high technology, and the changing role of women.

Relative to planning and policy, social workers can consider the effectiveness and cost of homecare in an information synthesis prepared by Hedrick and Inui (1986). Taking the lead in planning, social workers can integrate information of this nature into their decision-making.

In homecare programs, social workers contribute to continuity of care since they are trained to seek out services to meet the needs of clients. These efforts result in a coordinated attack on the multiple problems of people requiring homecare services.

Communication Services

Use of a speech pathologist and/or audiologist by home health agencies has been expanding. These personnel are primarily concerned with disorders in the production, reception, and perception of speech and language. After assisting in identifying persons with disorders, they determine the etiology, history, and severity of specific disorders through interviews and special tests. Optimal treatment is facilitated through speech, hearing, and language remedial procedures, counseling and guidance using rehabilitation techniques and devices as necessary. In addition, appropriate referrals are made for medical or other professional attention. Larkins (1986) reviews the delivery of speech-language and audiology services in the home and also comments on the involvement of the family, the interdisciplinary nature of the services, quality assurance and documentation.

Speech therapy services are provided only by or under supervision of a qualified speech pathologist or audiologist. A Certificate of Clinical Competence in either or both areas is awarded by the American Speech and Hearing Association (ASHA) after the applicant meets the educational and experience requirements. Educational programs at a master's degree level are accredited by the American Board of Examiners in Speech Pathology and Audiology. As of May 1986, there were about 150 accredited master's level educational programs and eight in the process of securing approval (*ASHA* 1986a). State licenses are required to practice in more than 50 percent of the states. Almost an entire issue of *ASHA* (1986b) focused on licensure, detailing characteristics of state licensing laws, the relation of licensure to third-party reimbursement, the role of the National Council of State Boards of Examiners, and the harm to the public from unlicensed practitioners.

As of January 1986, there were 44,425 professionals with certificates of clinical competence: 35,828 in speech-language pathology; 5,359 in audiology; and 1,238 with dual certificates (Hyman 1986). Standards, educational requirements, national examinations, procedures, and appeals for competency certificates are reviewed regularly (*ASHA* 1986c).

Utilization of Personnel

Speech-language pathology services are reasonably available in home health agencies, while audiology services do not appear to be used extensively. Considering the relation to illness in the population, it is unlikely that a need does not exist, but that there are other reasons for the lack of widespread use of these services. Rationales include limited referrals from physicians and nurses, exclusion from insurance coverage for homecare services, and the use of part-time speech-language pathologists and audiologists. Homecare agencies often employ personnel who moonlight from their full-time jobs at institutions.

It has been suggested (Hester 1981) that the status of services in the home setting could be improved with the following actions: perform routine speech-language evaluations on all stroke patients; educate other homecare professionals to create awareness of the services and to stimulate referrals; initiate a public awareness educational campaign emphasizing the communication services and their availability in homecare programs; integrate homecare experiences into the curriculums of the communication services schools; secure adequate reimbursement from third-party payers, governmental and private; and lobby for legislative action liberalizing services and reimbursement procedures. Additionally, and in typical professional fashion, an ASHA Task Force on Classification Systems developed a draft on procedures and estimates of length and frequency of home visits for communication services to present to the Health Care Financing Administration (*ASHA* 1986d).

Ethics and Business

As with most professional groups, ASHA has a Code of Ethics that deals with the welfare of clients, standards, the provision of accurate information, objectivity, honoring responsibilities, and the dignity of the profession. An annotated bibliography on ethics and professionalism appeared in *ASHA* (1986e). Areas covered included hearing aid dispensing policy, ethical standards of other professional and trade associations, business related ethics, and current issues in ethics and professionalism.

"A significant proportion of the ASHA membership is interested in the business aspects of speech-language pathology and audiology practice" (*ASHA* 1986e). Continuing the annotated bibliography in the business and marketing section, articles delved into dispensing systems, purchasing and starting a business, legal aspects, marketing and advertising, management, insurance, time allocation, and reimbursement.

Pharmacist

Pharmacists have been involved with drug therapy problems of patients in a home setting for some time. With the advent of the PPS/DRG reimbursement plan, the activities of pharmacists in homecare activities have intensified. An entire issue of *Topics in Hospital Pharmacy Management* (1984) dealt with a wide variety of subjects, most resulting from the need to provide pharmaceutical services to discharged patients who were leaving the hospital. High technology homecare in which pharmacists play a major role include infusion procedures such as home parenteral nutrition (Dzierba, Mirtallo, Grauer, et al. 1984), parenteral chemotherapy (Bishop 1984), and antibiotic therapy (*Drug Intelligence and Clinical Pharmacy* 1985). In addition, pharmacists moved into the durable medical equipment area as well. Henry (1986) reported on a chain of drug stores opening total capability centers to supply homecare services. With the rush into the homecare business becoming a stampede, the *National Association of Retail Druggists Journal* (1985) stated that as the "home health care competition intensifies, pharmacists can beat 'em ... or join 'em."

Role of the Pharmacist

Reflecting the prior concern limited mainly to drug problems, pharmacists concentrated on making sure that the patient's prescriptions were provided in the home setting with safety and efficacy. They participated in inservice training, in consultations with other professionals, and made home visits as required (Katzoff 1980). Commenting on the significant change in role, Pierpaoli and McAllister (1984) list the more intensely patient-focused pharmacy services as including "parenteral hyperalimentation, enteral feeding, antibiotic therapy, cancer chemotherapy, and drug-related hospice care services. Other pharmacists have, for some time, provided an array of vendor or leasing services for durable medical equipment, surgical supplies, etc." Eckel (1984) tells us that, "Today's hospital pharmacy director cannot ignore the home health care market" as he/she details operational procedures for pharmacists involved in homecare.

Interestingly, pharmacist involvement in home parenteral nutrition was reported upon by Karnack, Gallina, and Jeffrey (1981) some time ago. It was noted that the pharmacist prepares the solution in bulk, prepares a teaching manual for patients receiving this therapy, and monitors the patient. Total parenteral nutrition is a popular homecare service supplied by commercial firms, such as Abbott and Baxter Travenol, using their own hired professionals and supplies.

Reimbursement Impact

Curtiss (1986) detailed the recent developments in federal reimbursement for home health care and pinpointed relations to the pharmacist. He covered Medicare, Medicaid, HCFA rules and regulations, durable medical equipment, and legislative initiatives. A major issue in reimbursement relates to whether or not the services of a pharmacist can be reimbursed as a direct cost. If not, the home health agency must figure out how to incorporate the expense into overhead or use creative accounting techniques. Within cost containment procedures, Eckel (1984) says that pharmacists need to consider product and supply standardization, competitive bidding, and "home-mix" programs "whereby patients are taught to mix and self-administer drugs within the home."

Independent Prescribing Authority

A few states allow pharmacists to select and dispense alternate drug entities independently. Although limited, pharmacists have been able to authorize refills in the physician's absence, adjust pediatric dosages, prescribe limited quantities of antitussive, antihistamine, and decongestant drugs, and monitor blood pressure and compliance by hypertensive patients. When the issue of engaging in medical practice without a license arises, arguments are made that a number of states allow PAs and nurse practitioners to prescribe (Carrell 1982).

Should pharmacists gain the prescribing authority, there could be a dramatic expansion of their homecare services. If both nurses and pharmacists are able to prescribe, home health agencies could significantly change their delivery styles.

"It is clear that pharmacists should conceptually extend their mission to include responsible involvement in the total drug use control process for the home health care patient" (Pierpaoli and McAllister 1984).

Dietitian and Nutritionist

Diabetes, hypertension, circulatory problems, cardiac disease, and other chronic ailments all have a relation to diet and nutrition. Often, the individuals have never really had sound dietary advice and expert assistance with their problems. Homecare, probably in the kitchen itself, is the appropriate place to discuss food.

Quite some time ago, the American Dietetic Association (ADA) (1968) prepared guidelines for dietitians and nutritionists in homecare services. Suski (1981a) described home visits for dietitians and home consultation for the terminally ill (Suski 1981b).

Typical Tasks

Dietary procedures may start before discharge from the facility with meetings with patient and family to explain the diet and determine if any devices are needed for feeding. Even though most patients follow a normal diet, guidance is still necessary. After discharge, patients can be visited at home to survey the kitchen, explain food budgeting, meal preparation, and food handling techniques. Depending upon the complexity of the diet and the family's capability, additional home visits are planned. Usually, a long-term nutritional plan is placed in the patient's folder for the use of all homecare team members.

Other typical tasks relate to "meals on wheels" programs that deliver nutritious meals to homebound individuals, preparing food for hot lunches at centers for senior citizens, school lunch programs, and public education activities.

Again, reflecting the movement of high technology into the home, dietitians and nutritionists are involved with total parenteral nutrition and other infusion feeding therapies. Rohde and Bruan (1986) prepared a practitioners guide on enteral/parenteral nutrition for the ADA. Yet, a survey of

300 clinical dietitians by Jones, Bonner, and Stitt (1986) revealed that more than 50 percent responded that they did not have adequate educational preparation to assume all the responsibilities on the nutrition support team. It was suggested that there be an emphasis on specialized educational programs to ensure dietitians a leadership role in enteral and parenteral nutrition.

Dietitian

Dietitians apply principles of nutrition and management in planning and directing food service programs, mainly in institutions. However, there are dietitians who work in the community, guiding and instructing people on their eating habits and food selection.

An ADA affiliate, the Commission on Evaluation of Dietetic Education, accredits educational programs and internships. After meeting educational requirements and passing an examination, the title of registered dietitian (RD) can be gained. Less than one-third of the states license or certify nutrition professionals, although there is legislative movement to pursue mandatory licensure in many others (Owen, Hughes, and Scialabba 1986).

"Dietetic education is in a process of transition" (Owen and Rinke 1986). That transition is being forced by the concentration on costs, the demographics of the nation, and the need to be flexible and responsive to the changes in the health care delivery system. Owen and Rinke (1986) seek to increase the depth of knowledge in dietetic education as follows: create a broader base, particularly in arts and humanities; emphasize management and business; stress communications and networking; focus on new technology; and provide greater depth in scientific knowledge of nutrition. Overall, the dietetic education is to zero in on conceptual and creative thinking to "enhance our self-image." Creativity was identified as the key to attaining excellence in a rapidly changing world (Rinke 1986). Critical skills of creative thinking and innovative behavior for ADA leadership was part of the growth and change. Educators are urged to stimulate creativity in students, and ADA members should learn to expand their creative horizons.

Nutritionist

Nutritionists are concerned with the maintenance and improvement of health throughout the life cycle. Activities include planning and conducting programs on food and nutrition for individuals and groups. They work in health and welfare agencies, in institutional settings, and in private industry. Public health nutritionists concern themselves with community nutrition needs, dietary control of disease, and the prevention of disease through nutrition.

Usually, academic training at the undergraduate and graduate level is required. Public health nutritionists usually secure an advanced degree supplemented with courses in behavioral sciences as applied to public health. Kaufman (1986) projects that to meet the future, public health nutritionists need to use community assessment skills, apply epidemiology techniques, and engage their program planning abilities. Graduate education should incorporate the rapid changes in demographics, health delivery systems, communication technology, and consumer demands. In addition, Kaufman called upon the nutritionist to be an advocate.

What's Ahead

Public health nutritionists are moderately satisfied overall with their work activities, mainly from their satisfaction with the kind of work done (Sims and Khan 1986). Another attraction is the multiplicity of roles while delivering services to people living in communities. However, Parks and Moody (1986) cited marketing as a survival tool for dietetic professionals in the 1990s. They indicated the competition from other professionals: dentists educate their patients about nutrition and dental care; pharmacists engage in nutritional supplement business and IV nutritional support; physicians offer nutritional services for a fee; chiropractors do likewise; and a host of commercial firms push low-sodium food, no-sodium food, caffeine-free soda, salad bars, weight loss clinics, health spas, and fitness centers. To survive, the authors state that the dietitian must be prepared to leave the hospital and meet consumer lifestyle changes. They call attention to the new opportunity in homecare programs. Parks and Moody direct dietitians to look to economics, social sciences, and marketing for survival. "Dietitians need to become leaders in providing nutrition care, not merely the adjuntants of doctors."

Public policy and legislation is another part of the ADA strategy and it opened an office in Washington, D.C. in 1986 (Owen, Hughes, and Scialabba 1986). Priorities included attention to food labeling, PPS studies of reimbursement, documentation of nutrition services, and cost-effectiveness briefings for Congress. Survival plans include attention to careful use of data, improvement of data collection along with analysis and monitoring, development of broad-based coalitions, and the achievement of modest piecemeal objectives while negotiating through the legislative process.

Dental Care

When people cannot get to a dentist's office, dental care is often neglected. Beck and Hunt (1985) looked at the oral health status and problems of special patients in the U.S. Preparation of hygienists to work in nontraditional settings with special populations also included homecare activities (Cohen, LaBelle, and Singer 1985). More than a decade of service to disabled and elderly people by the National Foundation of Dentistry for the Handicapped was covered by Coffee (1985). Warren (1980) discussed the treatment of the handicapped in the home, but he felt that care in the office was necessary. With grant funding, Dr. Monroe Elkin provided dental care in the homes of elderly people in New Jersey (American Association of Retired Persons 1981). Despite these examples, dental care delivered in the home is not common.

As a retired dentist, Jarmon (1980) said that the in-home service he delivered was suitable for him, but not for a practicing dentist. He summed it up: "Homebound care is a unique service requiring organization, fortitude, compromise, and a willingness to perform under trying circumstances. The goal is to make the patients comfortable, sometimes improving their appearance, their chewing ability, and improving oral and denture hygiene."

Technology moves to the forefront again, as Olsen, Weiss, and Carlson (1985) describe the use of fiber optics in dentistry for the homebound.

Volunteers

A social worker requested a male companion for a patient in the Montefiore Hospital homecare program in 1962 and initiated an activity for volunteers. From that experience, Goldstein and Benedikt (1964) isolated two key factors in successful volunteer placement in homecare situations: matching personalities and orientation. However, Goldstein and Benedikt did not anticipate that the homecare volunteer program would ever involve great numbers of people. Since the patient is likely to be alone in the home, there must be a matching of personalities for compatibility. Similar hobbies, cultural background, ages, and other factors also help to assure successful placement.

Most people realize that volunteers span the generations and include high school students, college students, graduates doing internships, middle-aged individuals, and older persons. Volunteers can also be professionals or persons having various skills.

Program Examples

Volunteers Organized In Community Elderly Services (VOICES) of Indiana helps people to remain safely in their homes (Mellinger and Hubbard 1985). Families are aided in filling out forms to acquire services, with maintenance chores, and with client and family education. A university gerontological center trains the volunteers and provides consultation.

A VNA and a hospital in Pennsylvania cooperated to teach volunteers to assist in homecare (Harris and Groshens 1985). Task training paid attention to psychosocial skills, cardiopulmonary resuscitation, transfer and feeding techniques, and observation on home visits. Both the volunteers and the patients evaluated the activity extremely positively.

A volunteer chore ministry in Seattle, a geriatric activity in San Francisco, and a mobile medicine clinic on wheels in Broward County, Florida, were all described as evidence of what happens when neighbors care (Leigh 1986). Appearing in a nationally circulated Sunday newspaper magazine section, this article called attention to the use of volunteers in home-related activities. In addition, there was a notice about securing a manual on how to start similar programs in other communities.

Typical Volunteer Tasks

The list of functions that volunteers perform can be long: reading to patients; being a companion; driving people on errands; marketing; babysitting for children of volunteers; performing clerical tasks; homemaking; directing patient care; doing home repairs; making friendly visits; educating patients; ensuring medication compliance; and doing a multitude of assorted, but important, odds and ends to help and comfort patients at home. Volunteers are particularly numerous in hospice programs. McDonnell (1986,41) and Hartshorn (1985) described the use of volunteers in a home health agency.

Obviously, the recruitment and training of volunteers is a critical part of the activity. Noting the Medicare mandate for the use of volunteers in hospice programs, Bunn (1985) called volunteers the backbone of the program. McDonnell (1986,61) indicated the comprehensive nature of training by listing topics that may be covered: history and philosophy of hospice; spiritual dimensions of hospice; dynamics of dying; coping mechanisms; bereavement process; dealing with anger and resistance; cancer diagnosis and treatment methods; and communication and creative listening skills.

Volunteers in homecare programs require emotional maturity, self-control, inner security, and an ability to empathize. Being a volunteer in a home situation without direct supervision or immediate aid necessitates a high degree of independent responsibility.

Family Members

Members of the family who care for ill and infirm parents and/or relatives at home could be classified as volunteers, since they are unpaid personnel. However, the relationship to the patient does make a difference. In today's material-oriented society, some cynics contend that families are abandoning their sick parents and relatives. Brody (1985) labels that contention a myth and claims that the provision of homecare to family/relatives is becoming "normative." Normal responsibilities of the family caregivers have been identified by Friedman (1986):

- Learn as much as possible about the patient's illness.

- Analyze the emotional, physical and medical needs of the patient and how they may change in the future.

- Assess how the patient is likely to deal with the problem.

- Foster maximum independence and involve the patient as much as possible in health care decisions.

- Recruit family, friends, and health care professionals to help meet the needs of the patient.

Importantly, Pless (1984) summed up three studies related to the oft-stated medical proposition that families are central to the practice of "good medicine." Results showed that family specialists and other primary care practitioners know relatively little about the structure or functioning of the families of patients they treat. Another sociological study (*New York Times* 1985) indicated that "families in general already give their elderly as much assistance as they are able." Additionally, the investigation said that efforts to shift more costs to the families may exhaust their resources and shift people to institutions. Cash value of services performed by families exceeded the combined costs of government and professional services.

In view of the normative family homecare status, the limited knowledge of attending physicians, and the range of family caregiver responsibilities, actions to establish public policies are critical.

Public Policy and Family Homecare

In a comprehensive review, Doty (1986) identified five public policy initiatives under discussion by Congress and others to stimulate family homecare for the impaired elderly:

1. Tax incentives to care for impaired family members at home.

2. Public funding for respite and other supportive services.

3. Cash grants to low income families to care for elderly relatives.

4. Rule changes allowing the elderly to retain their food stamps and supplemental security income (SSI) when they move in with family members.

5. Allow family members to work as paid helpers under programs paid for with government funds.

Doty analyzed existing research to answer three questions: Are American families becoming less able to provide homecare for elderly disabled relatives? What would be the impact of government support or incentives? What difference would the form of government assistance make on the situation.

Before answering the questions, specific factual information should be kept in mind. Only one in five of the disabled elderly are in nursing homes; "the remaining four-fifths are able to go on living in the community primarily because family and friends provide all or most of the assistance they require . . . three-quarters of all such noninstitutional paid care is privately financed by the elderly themselves and their relatives; only 26 percent is government financed."

Doty found little evidence that families are becoming, or in fact are, less willing to provide homecare. Government programs would impact mainly through the reduction of negative consequences such as emotional stress, fatigue, and the loss of personal time. Cash grants and tax and other incentives appear unlikely to motivate more homecare than families would have rendered otherwise. Financial reasons were rarely at issue in stimulating additional family homecaring. "The primary motivations for families to provide informal long-term care to an impaired elderly relative are a sense of family responsibility, affection for the individual and a desire to reciprocate past help given by the impaired elderly person."

Similarly, Burwell (1986) studied Medicaid program policies regarding family homecare as a substitute for institutional care. Options included paying family members as Medicaid providers, expanding federal tax incentives, and legally forcing children to contribute toward the care of their parents in government programs. He detailed the quite limited experiences with all three policy efforts as fodder for discussion and debate. His conclusion called for policymakers "to strive for a proper balance between the obligations of family and the obligations of government in meeting the long-term care needs of the elderly. Clearly, it is a shared obligation; neither government nor families have the requisite resources to meet the demand for care."

Homecare Problems for Family Members

Family caregivers are often unprepared to perform personal care or body contact tasks such as bathing, feeding, and toileting, and perceive those activities as a burden (Hooyman, Gonyea, and Montgomery 1985). On the other hand, impersonal tasks such as shopping, laundry, and housecleaning are not seen as such.

Jones and Vetter (1984) interviewed 1,066 elderly who identified 256 family caregivers who in turn were interviewed looking at psychological morbidity and distress. Psychological morbidity included measures of anxiety and depression, while distress was rated on a four-point scale from none to severe. Tasks included washing, dressing and undressing, toileting, bathing, medication, eating, and drinking. Results showed that 93 caregivers (36 percent) exhibited borderline and pathological anxiety, and 15 percent had borderline and pathological depression. Interestingly, daughters providing care revealed significantly more morbidity than spouses doing the same. Incontinence was a particularly distressing common problem. Eighteen percent of the caregivers considered themselves under a great or unbearable amount of stress. In addition, this study did not find the involvement of a large network of informal or formal caregivers. Home helps and "granny sitters" were suggested to relieve the problems of the family caregivers.

For children needing care at home, Miller, Fein, Howe, et al. (1985) discuss a program to "parent the parent." Paraprofessional home visitors work with parents to provide preventive and remedial services where children are at risk of abuse or neglect. In the Jones and Vetter (1985) study, 70 percent of the caregivers were not working and 29 gave up their jobs in order to care for the elderly person at home. However, investigations reveal that many full-time employees provide a great deal of homecare for family members who are ill or disabled.

Homecare While Working Full-time

Travelers Corporation in Hartford, Connecticut, surveyed 739 employees (Collins 1986) and found that 28 percent over the age of 30 reported spending an average of 10.2 hours a week caring for elderly relatives and friends over 55; 8 percent spent 35 hours weekly; and some employees reported as much as 80 hours a week. Caregivers were mainly women (71 percent) who cared for mothers (46 percent) and fathers (19 percent) or inlaws (16 percent). Surprisingly, 31 percent of the caregivers were in the 30-40 age group. While employees were not asked about work absences related to caregiving, the company executives felt it was possible that the stress affected productivity and time lost from the job. To help their employees find help and get information, Travelers considered lunch hour meetings, seminars, support groups, and educational videotapes. "If our people don't spend as much time worrying about these at-home issues, we'll get more productivity and loyalty." Later that year, Travelers Corporation held a "caregiving fair" in which 700 employees and 20 social agencies participated (Freudenheim 1986). Freudenheim (1986) also reported that other major companies were helping employees to care for their elderly parents and relatives at home. Westinghouse Defense Electronics, Mobil, Ciba-Geigy, and Con Edison held lunch hour seminars with local, state, and federal officials and experts to resolve difficulties for employees. Organizations such as Pathfinders/Eldercare in Scarsdale, New York, the Metropolitan Chicago Coalition on Aging, and the Caregivers Workplace Project of the AARP prepare guides and training programs for management and employee assistance. "Unanticipated lost time is the main problem," according to Dr. Leon J. Warsaw, executive director of the New York Business Group on Health. Some companies offer employees the opportunity to put aside up to $100 of nontaxable money to use for care of an elderly, dependent relative. However, the Internal Revenue Service restricts that benefit to cases where the ill person is a dependent, lives in the employee's home, and the employee would otherwise have to forego working.

Support Groups for Family Caregivers

In the workplace programs, support groups have been suggested to alleviate the stress on family caregivers. Mutual aid self-help (MASH) groups have existed for many years. Madara and Neigher (1986) suggest that hospitals and MASH groups offer opportunities and challenges to benefit the clients and the facilities. However, they note that there is sometimes resistance and tension from professionals who may feel a loss of professional control and have problems with autonomy of the patients.

In a study of families of Alzheimer's Disease victims, Scott, Roberto, and Hutton (1986) found "a desire expressed by many to have the opportunity to talk or share their problems with persons who had or were presently coping with the same type of situation." One caregiver even talked long distance to someone in a similar situation and received support in that fashion.

In a comparison study of a group support program for families caring for a relative with a dementing illness, Kahan, Kemp, Staples, et al. (1985) reported benefits for the group support program. While 22 subjects participated in an eight-session program, 18 control subjects did not. Data indicated significant differences in the support group on the change in family burden, levels of depression, and knowledge of dementia as a result of the sessions. "There was strong evidence to suggest that the acquisition of new knowledge was an important ingredient in reducing a caregiver's perception of burden and levels of depression."

Mutual support groups reaffirm the wisdom of the old axiom that posits that individuals benefit from knowing that they are not alone or unique with their particular problems. Groups focus on areas such as ileostomy and colostomy (QT, Inc.), heart surgery (Mended Hearts), bereavement (Widows Anonymous), and child abuse (Parents Anonymous), to name only a few.

Hospice and Family Caregiving

In a letter to the editor of a large newspaper, a husband and wife (Gibson and Gibson 1986) told about how they coped with providing homecare for a terminally ill mother/mother-in-law. They commented on the strong commitment required from the family and/or friends for support, and also the need to make the public aware of the available hospice services. Chekryn (1985) described nursing interventions to assist family members to support one another as they cared for a dying patient at home. Obviously, family caregivers in a hospice role could be experiencing severe emotional stress. Kane, Klein, Bernstein, et al. (1984) looked into the hospice role in alleviating the emotional stress of patients and their families. They found some positive effect on patient satisfaction and less anxiety for family and/or friend caregivers. Hospice care met the psychosocial needs of those providing care to the dying patient.

Findings of the National Hospice Study (Greer and Mor 1986; Greer, Mor, Morris, et al. 1986) showed that "the level of morbidity experienced by patient caretakers following patient death was less than anticipated." There was no increase in alcohol consumption or the use of medication for nervousness among family caregivers, although there were higher levels of stress and social disruption among the homecare hospice groups. This study compared hospice care at home, hospital hospice care, and conventional hospital care.

One of the constantly repeated needs of families caring for patients at home, in hospice, and other situations, is a desire for respite care.

Respite for Family Caregivers

South Miami Hospital offers weekend respite care to fill empty beds, as do licensed adult congregate residences in that state (Nordheimer 1986). However, families have to pay about $100 per night for such respite, and it is not covered by public or private medical insurance. Bader (1985) reviewed respite care research and concluded that it may be cost-effective to invest in such services. Attention to the physical, financial, and emotional well-being of family caregivers could be more advantageous than providing the required care when the caregivers themselves become patients. Recommendations address areas such as family/government partnership for care; increased support groups; adequate community resources for caregivers; allocations based on functional disability and not on a means test; and a concluding, "Appreciate the caregivers."

In a well-documented paper, Stone (1985) reviewed recent developments in respite care services for caregivers of the impaired elderly for the Aging Health Policy Center in Washington, DC. McFarland et al. (1985) described a typical respite program in TempCare, a 21-bed social model respite care program located in the convent wing of a parochial school in the Bronx, New York. Since its inception in 1979, TempCare served 503 people with 83 repeat users. Stays can vary from one to 30 days with three meals daily, housekeeping, personal care, and recreational activities. Costs are based on a charge of $32 per night, although a sliding fee scale is used.

Stone (1985) charts the duration of respite, the patient needs, and the paid/volunteer staff for various types of respite care: companion-homemaker; homemaker-home health aide; adult day care; residential care home; adult foster care; and nursing home. In addition, she lists information about 15 different state legislated respite programs.

Since respite care is being sought as a separate additional service, the report of the New York State Respite Demonstration Project (1985,40) stating a contrary opinion is of import: ". . . expansion of respite services in New York State is not likely if respite is viewed as a specific, distinct service and added to the already extensive list of distinct services. . . Rather, expansion of respite will occur in direct relationship to the state's ability to integrate respite into the array of existing services already available."

Regardless of whether respite care is a separate or integrated service, the AARP says that, "It's a demographic imperative and an absolute necessity to just sustain the family and to relieve the stress level for family caregivers" (Newald 1986).

Females, Families, and Homecare

Citing the significant role of women in long-term nursing care, Miller (1985) states that, "Whatever the model, the female influence is pervasive." If long-term home health care can work only with the cooperation of an involved family, then "the female influence cannot be underestimated." In fact, the executive vice president of the National Organization for Women (NOW), Lois G. Reckitt, says that "home health care for the chronically ill exploits women by driving them back into the home and out of the paid workforce" (Newald 1986). Donna Ambrogi of the Older Women's League adds that, "Women, and not men, are expected to quit their jobs and care for their spouses and fathers" (Newald 1986).

With a concentration on the feminist viewpoint, Feldblum (1985) examined the programs extensively, reviewing problems, and potentials of home health care for the elderly. Beginning with the principle that unpaid care provided by families is an essential part of the system and that 90 percent of the elderly receive homecare help from an informal network of family, friends, and neighbors, Feldblum moves into a discussion of the female caregiver. She cites a study that says "because of persistent sex role differences and greater female life expectancy, women are much more likely than men to assume responsibility for providing for direct care." A feminist paradox arises in homecare since the majority of people needing care will be women and it is likely that those providing services will also be women. Therefore, it is in the best interests of women to desire high quality care, and yet they may be dismayed at the discriminatory burden of homecare. Feldblum reports that social workers used persuasion appealing to a woman's maternal instincts and wifely commitments to make her feel responsible for providing homecare. Nevertheless, maternal instincts and responsible behavior aside, "We must come to terms with the changing roles of women in American society and we must shape our health care programs to respond to those changes. . . There is nothing inherent in women's psyches that makes them better than men at providing nurture and care." Feldblum notes that not all feminists would agree with that last assertion. Finally, Feldblum says that, "We need to work through the feminist movement . . . to change underlying attitudes regarding the separate and unequal roles of men and women in the province of caregiving."

Personnel in the Homecare Team

Working together as a team in homecare services may be an obvious truism. Yet, since people have taken the time and effort to write about the subject, there may be room for improvement. Is it realistic, for example, for the physician to be the team leader? Legally, physicians do have the responsibility, must prepare a written treatment plan, and review it periodically. In practice, experiences may accommodate the legal restraints in various shapes and forms. Perhaps systems engineers can resolve this health care delivery problem.

There can be no doubt that homecare programs need to use a team approach. Patients have a combination of diseases/conditions requiring the skills of a variety of professionals, as well as volunteers and family members. It would not be reasonable or logical to render care as independent entrepreneurs. A prime requisite of the team approach to homecare is the provision of a coordinator to assure continuity of care to the patient.

Future Homecare Personnel

Personnel involved in homecare services could change drastically as a result of the influence of the PPS/DRG program, the subsequent surge in high technology care, and in the use of sophisticated durable medical equipment. Much of the personnel could be affected by legislation and the regulations ensuing from it. If legislation permits professionals other than the physician to prescribe homecare, the entire team could be affected by a new type of leadership.

Regardless of the personnel changes, it is still likely that the organizations will have common elements of professional care: professional education and training; fieldwork placements and internships; continuing education and inservice training; accreditation, licensure, and certification of facilities and personnel; ethical considerations; legislative lobbying; research and evaluation; recruitment and integration of new homecare workers into the system.

All of these components are part of the descriptive material on the personnel involved in homecare. Since so many professionals, volunteers, and family members are engaged in homecare activities, it might be appropriate to consider a united homecare coalition to represent the entire team. Homecare trade associations usually take the lead in representing the entire industry.

References

Almind, G., C.B. Freer, J.A. Gray, et al. 1985. The contribution of the primary care doctor to the medical care of the elderly in the community. *Danish Medical Bulletin* 32 (Supplement No. 2):1-28.

American Association of Retired Persons. 1981. Dentist travels country roads to homebound elderly. *News Bulletin* (Sept.)

American Dietetic Association. 1968. Opportunities in home health services. Guidelines for dietitians and nutritionists. *Journal of the American Dietetic Association* 52(3):381.

American Medical Association. 1981. *Physician guide to home health care.* Chicago (July).

American Medical News. 1982. Practical nurse group is critical of NLN decision. Chicago (7 May).

American Nurses Association. 1980. *A conceptual model of community health nursing.* Kansas City, MO.

American Nurses Association. 1985. *Standards of or for community health nursing practice.* Kansas City, MO.

American Occupational Therapy Association. 1978. *Standards of practice for occupational therapy services in a home health program.* Rockville, MD (May)

American Speech and Hearing Association (ASHA). 1986a. Accredited speech-language pathology and audiology master's degree programs. 28(7):45-46.

American Speech and Hearing Association (ASHA). 1986b. Perspective on licensure. 28(6):

American Speech and Hearing Association (ASHA). 1986c. Proposed requirements for the certificate of clinical competence. 28(7):53-57.

American Speech and Hearing Association (ASHA). 1986d. ASHA responds to HCFA on HHAs. 28(2):19.

American Speech and Hearing Association (ASHA). 1986e. Business, marketing, ethics, and professionalism, an annotated bibliography. 28(3):27-35.

Anderson, A.K., L. Neal-McCollum, and C.H. Spann. 1985. The role of social work in hospice. *Caring* 4(2):21-23.

Anderson, J.L., and M.L. Brown. 1981. The cancer patient in the community: a nursing challenge. *Nursing Clinics of North America* 15(2):373-378.

Aston-McCrimmon, E. 1986. Analysis of the ratings of competencies used in physical therapy. *Physical Therapy* 66(6):954-960.

Auerbach, D., R. Bann, D. Davis, et al. 1984. The social worker in home health care. *Caring* 3(10):71-76.

Bader, J.E. 1985. Respite care: temporary relief for caregivers. *Home Health Care Services Quarterly* 10(2-3):39-52.

Barry, P.B., and R.J. Ham. 1985. Geriatric education: what the medical schools are doing now. *Journal of the American Geriatrics Society* 33(2):133-135.

Beck, J.D., and R.J. Hunt. 1985. Oral health status in the U.S.: problems of special patients. *Journal of Dental Education* 49(6):407-426.

Belair, P.S. 1986. Home health nursing: a rediscovered concept. *Imprint* 33(1):19-20.

Bishop, C.T. 1984. Home parenteral chemotherapy. *Topics in Hospital Pharmacy Management* 4(3):35-42.

Black, R.B., and D. Drachman. 1985. Hospital social workers and self-help groups. *Health and Social Work* 10(2):95-103.

Bohannon, R.W., and B.F. LeVeau. 1986. Clinician's use of research findings. *Physical Therapy* 66(1):45-50.

Borders, C.R. 1985a. Are you ready for the new home care? *Patient Care* 19(19):20-24.

Borders, C.R. 1985b. Home care: avoiding institutionalization. *Patient Care* 19(19):49-67.

Borders, C.R. 1985c. Preparing for posthospital home care. *Patient Care* 19(21):27-62.

Brody, E. 1985. Parent care as a normative family stress. *Gerontologist* 25:19-29.

Brody, J.E. 1986. Personal health column on home health care. *New York Times* (22 Jan.).

Bunn, E.G. 1985. Volunteers as the backbone. *Caring* 4(2):19-20.

Burns, S., and W. Ciaccia. 1985. Home health aides: the changing role, one agency's experience. *Home Healthcare Nurse* 3(1):35-37.

Burwell, B.O. 1986. *Shared obligations: public policy influences on family care for the elderly*. Washington, DC: Government Printing Office. Medicaid Program Evaluation Working Paper 2.1. HHS, HCFA, Office of Research and demonstrations.

Butler, R.N. 1981. The teaching nursing home. *Journal of the American Medical Association* 245:1435-1437.

Capezuti, E. 1985. Geriatric nurse practitioners: their education, experience, and future in home health care. *PRIDE Institute Journal of Long Term Home Health Care* 4(3):9-14.

Caroff, P., and M.D. Mailick. 1985. Health concentrations in schools of social work: the state of the art. *Health and Social Work* 10(1):5-14.

Carrell, S. 1982. Plan defeated, but pharmacists still seek ability to prescribe. *American Medical News* (14 May).

Chekryn, J. 1985. Support for the family of the dying patient. *Home Healthcare Nurse* 3(3):18-24.

Christopher, M.A. 1986. Home care for the elderly. *Nursing 86* 16(7):50-55.

Coffee, L. 1985. The National Foundation of Dentistry for the Handicapped. A decade of service to disabled and elderly people, and the dental profession. *Journal of the Indiana Dental Association* 64(1):9-12.

Cohen, L., A. LaBelle, and J. Singer. 1985. Educational preparation of hygienists working with special populations in nontraditional settings. *Journal of Dental Education* 49(8):592-595.

Cohen, S.N., and B. Egen. 1981. The social work home visit in a health care setting. *Social Work in Health Care* 6(4):55-67.

Collins, G. 1986. Many in work force care for elderly kin. *New York Times* (6 Jan.).

Crowley, C., and J. Standerfer. 1985. Incorporating home health care into the baccalaureate nursing program. *Family and Community Health* 8(2):81-86.

Cruz, F.A., A.M. Jacobs, and M.J. Wood. 1986. The educational needs of home health nurses. *Home Healthcare Nurse* 4(3):11-17.

Curtiss, F.R. 1986. Recent developments in federal reimbursement for home health care. *American Journal of Hospital Pharmacy* 43(1):132-139.

Dean, E., and J. Davies. 1986. Frequency of citation and reputational assessment of contributors in *Physical Therapy*. *Physical Therapy* 60(6)961-966.

DePaoli, T.A., and P. Zenk-Jones. 1984. Medicare reimbursement in home care. *American Journal of Occupational Therapy* 38(11):739-742.

Department of Health and Human Services. 1980. *A model curriculum and teaching guide for the instruction of the homemaker-home health aide*. Washington, DC: Government Printing Office. Pub. No. HSA-80-5508.

Department of Labor, Employment and Training Administration. 1977. *Dictionary of Occupational Titles, fourth edition*. Washington, DC: Government Printing Office.

de Ulibarri, M. 1986. Involving physicians in home care. *Home Healthcare Nurse* 4(1):11-14.

Deusinger, S.S., B. Sindelar, and F.T. Stritter. 1986. Assessment center. A model for professional development and evaluation. *Physical Therapy* 66(7):1119-1123.

Dobrof, R. 1984. *Gerontological social work in home health care*. New York: The Haworth Press.

Doty, P. 1986. Family care of the elderly: the role of public policy. *The Milbank Quarterly* 64(1):34-75.

Drug Intelligence and Clinical Pharmacy. 1985. Antibiotic cost-containment in the home health care environment. 19:278-296.

Dzierba, S.H., J.M. Mirtallo, D.W. Grauer, et al. 1984. Fiscal and clinical evaluation of home parenteral nutrition. *American Journal of Hospital Pharmacy* 41:285-291.

Eboch, S. 1986. Providing homemaker service in Alaska. *Caring* 5(4):56,58,68.

Eckel, F.M. 1984. the impact of home health care on hospital pharmacy. *Topics in Hospital Pharmacy Management* 4(3):80-85.

Edelstein, K. 1984. Medicare's home health rule and rates changed. *Progress Report* 13(9):7.

Edwardson, S.R. 1985. Physician acceptance of homecare for terminally ill children. *Health Services Research* 20(1):83-101.

Epstein, W.M. 1980. The social work planner in long-term home care. A case study of institutional geriatric care in the V.A. *Social Work in Health Care* 6(1):23-25.

Fawcett, E.A. 1961. A re-evaluation of the home visit in casework practice. *Social Casework* 42(9):439-455.

Feldblum, C.R. 1985. Home health care for the elderly: programs, problems, and potentials. *Harvard Journal on Legislation* 22(1):193-254.

Fickeissen, J.L. 1985. Getting certified. *American Journal of Nursing* 85(3):265-269.

Fine, D.R. 1986. The home as the workplace. Prejudice and inequity in home health care. *Caring* 5(4):12-19.

Freudenheim, M. 1986. Help in caring for the elderly. *New York Times* (1 July).

Friedman, J. 1986 *Home health care: a complete guide for patients and their families*. New York: W.W. Norton.

Gantt, A.B., and R.S. Green. 1985/86. Telling the diagnosis: implications for social work practice. *Social Work in Health Care* 11(2):101-110.

Gibson, R., and C. Gibson. 1986. The gentle hand of hospice care (letter). *Star-Ledger*, Newark, NJ (19 July).

Goldstein, S., and L. Benedikt. 1964. Use of volunteers on a health care program. *Hospital Management* 97:52-54.

Greer, D.S., and V. Mor. 1986. An overview of national hospice study findings. *Journal of Chronic Disease* 39(1):5-7.

Greer, D.S., V. Mor, J.N. Morris, et al. 1986. An alternative in terminal care: results of the national hospice study. *Journal of Chronic Disease* 39(1):9-26.

Haines, A., and A. Bookoff. 1986. Terminal care at home: perspective from general practice. *British Medical Journal* 292(6527):1051-1053.

Hall, H.D. 1981. Homemaker-home health aide services in *Handbook of the social services* edited by N. Gilbert and H.

Specht. Englewood Cliffs, NJ: Prentice-Hall, Inc.

Hall, H.D. 1986. The definition and role of the paraprofessional in home care. *Caring* 5(4):8-10.

Halpern, P.L. 1985. Respite care and family functioning in families with retarded children. *Health and Social Work* 10(2):138-150.

Harris, M., and B. Groshens. 1985. A cooperative volunteer training program. *Home Healthcare Nurse* 3(3):37-40.

Hartshorn, U.R. 1985. The use of volunteers in a home health agency. *Home Healthcare Nurse* 3(6):26-28.

Hedrick, S.C., and T.S. Inui. 1986. The effectiveness and cost of homecare: an information synthesis. *Health Services Research* 20(6 Pt.2):851-880.

Henry, T. 1986. Drug firm opens total capability centers. *Home Health Journal* 7(2):8,10.

Hester, E.J. 1981. The status of speech-language pathology in the home health setting. *ASHA* 23(3):155-162.

Hirst, S.P., and B.J. Metcalf. 1986. Learning needs of caregivers. *Journal of Gerontological Nursing* 12(4):24-28.

Hogstel, M.O. 1985. *Home nursing care for the elderly*. Bowie, MD: Brady Communications Co.

Holdeman, E.E. 1962. The role of the occupational therapist in the home care programs in *Dynamic living for the long-term patient*. Study course #3. World Federation of Occupational Therapists, Third International Congress.

Home Health Journal. 1984. University organizes 1st HHA administrator program. 5(5):7.

Home Health Journal. 1986. Physician support said based on familarity. 7(4):1.

Hooyman, N., J. Gonyea, and R. Montgomery. 1985. The impact of in-home services termination on family caregivers. *The Gerontologist* 25(2):141-145.

Hospitals. 1984. Insurers see cost benefits of home care. 58(5):46.

Howell, P.A. 1986. Homemaker-home health aide service in Iowa. *Caring* 5(4):46-48.

Hyman, C.S. 1986. The ASHA membership: how many? *ASHA* 28(3):25.

Jarmon, P. 1980. Dentistry for the homebound. An inbound patient. *N.Y. State Dental Journal* 46(5):276-278.

Jones, D.A., and N.J. Vetter. 1984. A survey of those who care for the elderly at home: their problems and their needs. *Social Science and Medicine* 19(5):511-514.

Jones, M.G., J.L. Bonner, and K.R.Stitt. 1986. Nutrition support service: role of the clinical dietitian. *Journal of the American Dietetic Association* 86(1):68-71.

Kahan, J., B. Kemp, F.R. Staples, et al. 1985. Decreasing the burden in families caring for a relative with a dementing illness. *Journal of the American Geriatrics Society* 33(10:664-670.

Kane, R.L., S.J. Klein, L. Bernstein, et al. 1984. Hospice role in alleviating the emotional stress of terminal patients and their families. *Medical Care* 23(3):189-197.

Karnack, C.M., J.N. Gallina, and L.P. Jeffrey. 1981. Pharmacist involvement in home parenteral nutrition programs. *American Journal of Hospital Pharmacy* 38(2):215-217.

Katzoff, J. 1980. A pharmacist in a home health agency. *American Pharmacy* 20(8):52-54.

Kaufman, M. 1986. Preparing public health nutritionists to meet the future. *Journal of the American Dietetic Association* 86(4):511-513.

Keating, S.B. 1985. The formation of an independent nursing corporation. Presentation at annual meeting of American Public Health Association, Washington, DC (Nov.).

Kelly, C.D., and L. Crossman. 1985. Nursing Dynamics Corporation: community health nursing in action. Presentation at annual meeting of American Public Health Association, Washington, DC (Nov.).

Koren, M.J. 1986. Home care - who cares? *New England Journal of Medicine* 314:917-920.

Koshes, R. 1984. Providing alternatives. *The New Physician* 33(3):14-15.

Lamont, P., and R. Langford. 1980. Community physiotherapy in a rural area. *PhysioTherapy* 66(1):8-10.

Larkins, P.G. 1986. The delivery of speech-language and audiology services in home care. *ASHA* 28(5):49-52.

Lash, M.E. 1980. Community health nursing in a minority setting. *Nursing Clinics of North America* 15(2):340-348.

Leigh, D. 1986. When a community cares. *Parade Magazine (13 July)*.

Levine, R.E. 1984. The cultural aspects of homecare delivery. *American Journal of Occupational Therapy* 38(11):734-738.

Little, V.C. 1981. A comparison of home health care for the elderly in the U.S. and Japan: a report of a cross national project. *Home Health Review* 4(1):21-28.

Littlejohn, C.E. 1980. What new staff learned and didn't learn. *Nursing Outlook* 28(1):23-25.

Luna-Massey, P., and L. Smyle. 1982. Attitudes of consumers of physical therapy in California toward the professional image of physical therapists. *Physical Therapy* 62(4):464-469.

Madara, E.S., and W.D. Neigher. 1986. Hospitals and self-help groups: opportunity and challenge. *Hospital Progress* 67(3):42-45.

Mallon, F.J. 1981. History of the occupational therapy Medicare amendments. *American Journal of Occupational Therapy* 35(4):231-235.

Marshall, E., and J. Kerr. 1981. *The role of the occupational therapist in home health care*. Rockville, MD: American Occupational Therapy Association.

Martin, P. 1984. Home health care - everyone wants a piece of the pie. *The Kansas Nurse* 59(1):4,19.

McCahan, J.F., A.M. Bissonnette, and B.A. DiRusso. 1983. A house call teaching program for fourth-year medical students. *Journal of Medical Education* 58(4):349-351.

McCorkle, R., and B. Germino. 1984. What nurses need to know about home care. *Oncology Nursing Forum* 11(6):63-69.

McDonnell, A. 1986. *Quality hospice care. Administration, organization, and models*. Owings Mills, MD: National Health Publishing.

McDonnel, J.M. 1986. Therapists exploring ways to cope with HMO growth. *Progress Report* 15(2):1,6,7.

McFarland, L.G., D. Howells, and B. Dill. 1985. Respite care. *Generations* 9(4):46-47.

McRae A. 1984. Occupational therapy in a Medicare-approved home health agency. *American Journal of Occupational Therapy* 38(11):721-725.

Mellinger, C.J., and R.W. Hubbard. 1985. Volunteer interventions in the home health care of the elderly. *Family and Community Health* 8(2):86-88.

Menzel, F.S., and K. Teegarden. 1982. Quality assurance: a tri-level model. *American Journal of Occupational Therapy* 35(5):312-316.

Mercier, H.K. 1986. Homemaker-home health aide service, training and certification in Connecticut. *Caring* 5(4):44-45.

Miller, D.B. 1985. Women and long-term nursing care. *Home Health Care Services Quarterly* 10(2-3):29-38.

Miller, K., E. Fein, G.W. Howe, et al. 1985. A parent aide program: record keeping, outcomes, and costs. *Child Welfare* 64(4):407-419.

Millman, D.S. 1986. Legal liabilities for the home health paraprofessional. *Caring* 5(4):25-27.

Mountain State Health Corporation. 1985. *Gerontological Nurse Practitioner Educational Directory*. Boise, ID.

Nash, D.T. 1974. Making use of home care services. *Geriatrics* 29:140-143.

National Association of Retail Druggists Journal. 1985. Home health care competition intensifies: pharmacists can beat "em... or join em." 107(6):22-32.

Newald, J. 1986. Women as caregivers face crisis at home. *Hospitals* 60(6):106.

New York State Department of Social Services. 1985. *Respite demonstration project: final report*. Albany, NY (Jan.).

New York Times. 1985. Study cites burdens on those who care for elderly relatives (15 Oct.).

Nordheimer, J. 1986. Florida burden: the aged retired. *New York Times* (14 July).

O'Donnell, K.P. 1984. Hospital-based home health care - gaining a competitive advantage where everyone benefits. *American Journal of Hospital Pharmacy* 41(1):147-148.

O'Leary, B.C. 1986. Home aides of Central New York. *Caring* 5(4):70,87.

Olsen, R.A., L.P. Weiss, and M.R. Carlson. 1985. Fiber optics in dentistry for the homebound. *Specialty Care Dentistry* 5(1):34-35.

Owen, A.L., B.A. Hughes, and M.A. Scialabba. 1986. Legislation and public policy: ADA's changing strategies. *Journal of the American Dietetic Association* 86(6):803-806.

Owen, A.L., and W.J. Rinke. 1986. Changes in dietetic education to maximize our contribution to society. *Journal of the American Dietetic Association* 86(3):375-377.

Pagliarulo, M.A. 1986. Accreditation. Its nature, process, and effective implementation. *Physical Therapy* 66(7):1114-1118.

Parker, H.J., and F. Chan. 1986. Stereotyping: physical and occupational therapists characterize themselves and each other. *Physical Therapy* 66(5):668-672.

Parks, S.C., and D.L. Moody. 1986. Marketing: a survival tool for dietetic professionals in the 1990's. *Journal of the American Dietetic Association* 86(1):33-36.

Pierpaoli, P.G., and J.C. McAllister, III. 1984. The evolution of home health care in hospital pharmacy. *Topics in Hospital Pharmacy Management* 4(3):1-8, 1984.

Pless, I.B. 1984. The family as a resource unit in health care: changing patterns. *Social Science in Medicine* 19(4):385-389.

Pumphrey, R.E., and M.W. Pumphrey. 1961. *The heritage of American social work.* New York: Columbia University Press.

Raff, B.S. 1985. The use of homemaker-home health aides in perinatal care of high risk infants. *Journal of Obstetric-Gynecology-Neonatal Nursing* 15(2):142-145.

Rinke, W.J. 1986. Creativity: a key to attaining excellence in a rapidly changing world. *Journal of the American Dietetic Association* 86(4):465-467.

Roach, J.P., and L.M. Cook. 1981. Physical

therapy assistant in a California home health agency. *Physical Therapy* 61(9):1281-1283.

Robinson, N. 1986. Standard setting and accreditation by the National Home Caring Council. *Caring* 5(4):34-39.

Rohde, C., and T. Bruan. 1986. *Manual on enteral/parenteral nutrition: a practitioner's guide.* Chicago, IL: American Dietetic Association.

Royeen, C.B. 1986. Entry level education in occupational therapy. *American Journal of Occupational Therapy* 40(6):425-427.

Sanderson, R.L. 1986. Homemaker-home health aide services in North Dakota. *Caring* 5(4):52,54.

Sankar, A. 1986. Out of the clinic into the home: control and patient-physician communication. *Social Science and Medicine* 22(9):973-982.

Schwartz, G.B. 1980. Physicians support home health care. *Hospitals* 54(4):52,56,65.

Scott, J.P., K.A. Roberto, and J.T. Hutton. 1986. Families of Alzheimer's victims. Family support to the caregivers. *Journal of American Geriatric Society* 34(5):348-354.

Sharp, J.W., and E.D. Sivak. 1985. The role of social work in contemporary home care planning. *Cleveland Clinic Quarterly* 52(3):355-358.

Sims, L.S., and J. Khan. 1986. Job satisfaction among public health nutrition personnel. *Journal of the American Dietetic Association* 86(3):334-339.

Steinhauer, M.J. 1984. Occupational therapy and home health care. *American Journal of Occupational Therapy* 38(11):715-716.

Stempler, B.L., and H. Stempler. 1981. Extending the client connections: using homemaker casework teams. *Social Casework* 62:149-156.

Stone, R. 1985. Recent developments in respite care services for caregivers of the impaired elderly. Washington, DC: HHS. Administration on Aging Grant No. 90AP003 Report (July).

Suski, N.S. 1981a. The dietitian makes home visits. *Journal of the American Dietetic Association* 79(3):311-312.

Suski, N.S. 1981b. Home consultation for the terminally ill. *Journal of the American Dietetic Association* 78(6):620-622.

Swoboda, R.J. 1984. Home health care: bane or boom for hospitals? *American Journal of Hospital Pharmacy* 41(1):149-151.

Tideiksaar, R., L.S. Libow, and M. Chalmers. 1985. Housecalls to older patients: the medical student experience. *PRIDE Institute Journal of Long-Term Home Health Care* 4(3):3-8.

Topics in Hospital Pharmacy Management. 1984. 4(3):1-85.

Trager, B. 1973. *Homemaker/home health aide services in the U.S.* Washington, DC: Government Printing Office (June).

Trossman, P.B. 1984. Administrative and professional issues for the occupational therapist in home health care.

American Journal of Occupational Therapy 38(11):726-733.

Viseltear, E. 1984. Home health care as a theme. *American Journal of Occupational Therapy* 38(11):5.

Warren, M.D. 1980. Planning the provision of dental treatment for handicapped persons living at home. *Public Health Reports* 94(1):30-39.

Weller, C. 1978. Home health care. *New York State Journal of Medicine* 78:1957-1961.

Wilson, S.D., K.M. Langwell, R.T. Deane, et al. 1982. Identification of physical therapy shortage areas. A study of thirteen states. *Physical Therapy* 62(3):315-323.

Yerxa, E.J., and G. Sharrott. 1986. Liberal arts: the foundation for occupational therapy. *American Journal of Occupational Therapy* 40(3):153-159.

Chapter 10

The Growth of Homecare

Growth Rationales

With a banner headline, DeCosta (1984) proclaimed: "Home Healthcare. It's Red Hot and Right Now." Tersely, that sums up the growth situation in the homecare industry. DeCosta added the rationale: "Home healthcare is growing by leaps and bounds--spurred by an aging population, pressure to contain soaring medical costs, and advances in medical technology." While Garland (1984) and Lenz (1985) agreed with the rationales, they also noted the impact of the PPS/DRG reimbursement plan with its potential for discharging patients "quicker and sicker" in need of more care at home. However, Lenz (1985), speaking for a homecare trade association, did add another reason--increasing public awareness of the availability of homecare services.

Awareness of Homecare

Awareness efforts are undertaken by consumer oriented publications, homecare trade associations, statewide associations of providers, and commercial marketing firms, among others.

A new magazine, *HomeCare Consumer,* advertised in a journal aimed at people engaged in health care publicity and promotion (*Medical Marketing and Media* 1986). The ad stated that the magazine is the first to address the needs of homecare patients with distribution by agencies that people look to for information.

An ongoing campaign to increase awareness of homecare is sponsored by the American Federation of Home Health Agencies (AFHHA) (*Home Health Agency Gazette* 1985) and other trade associations. AFHHA offers its members help in arranging mass media interviews and suggests urging the listening audience to contact their legislators to support homecare activities.

A series of five workshops in the New York area focused on the subject of licensed homecare agency development in day-to-day operations (New York State Association of Health Care Providers, Inc. 1986). A list of future seminar topics included how to capitalize on licensure using marketing and advertising.

Appealing to manufacturers of medical products, health insurers, proprietary health facilities operators, drug wholesalers, chain drugstores, national and regional distributors of medical products, health insurers, and homecare agencies and providers, a medical products and services market research firm announced the sixth annual conference on home/self health care (Frost & Sullivan 1986). Entitling the conference "Home/Self Healthcare--An Industry in Constant Flux," the brochure alerted attendees to the topics to be covered: new markets in self-care and self-diagnostics; reimbursement issues; marketing strategies; technology and new market opportunities; physician involvement; new techniques to reach consumers; and the coordination of products and services to achieve maximum synergism.

A publisher of health journals announced a new "Home Patient Care Series" comprised of 24 booklets with illustrations and easy-to-follow guides for technical care of patients at home (Cohen 1986). Topics covered include oxygen therapy, suctioning, incontinence care, bedsores, parenteral nutrition, colostomy care, urinary catheter care, feeding tubes and pumps, and injections.

Self-Testing at Home

Preventive aspects of homecare are usually overshadowed by the emphasis on services related to illness, similar to the situation where acute medical care dominates chronic and long-term care activities. Yet, dramatic growth is predicted for self-testing and monitoring in the homecare market (*Hospitals* 1985a). In vitro self-tests for diabetes, pregnancy, venereal disease, and strep throat are included in the projected $437 million by 1989, up from $142 million in 1984. Self-monitoring instruments include blood pressure gauges, electronic thermometers, apnea monitors, and ambulatory cardiac monitors in the predicted $327 million market by 1989, up from $206 million in 1984.

Consumer interest is prompted by increased education levels and health promotion activities in addition to "the demystification of the home health field" (*Hospitals* 1985a).

Market Research Forecasts

In the business/financial section of a large Sunday newspaper (Taylor 1984), a headline predicted "Big Growth Likely for Home Health Care." A burgeoning forth was expected over the next several decades.

"Expenditures for home/self-related health care delivery are estimated to have exceeded $11 billion in 1984 and are forecast to double to $22 billion in 1990. Products and services share this market at 40 percent and 60 percent respectively. Growth is averaging about 12 percent per year, representing one of the highest rates in the health care field" (Frost & Sullivan 1986; *Hospitals* 1984a). Equally optimistic predictions have come from other market research firms: FIND/SVP opts for 10.4 percent annual growth through 1995 and a $13.8 billion market by 1990 (*Rx Home Care* 1985; *Hospitals* 1985b); Predicasts projected a $24.8 billion market by 1995 (Edmonson 1985). Attention was called to the spurt in home infusion treatments, respiratory devices at home, continuous ambulatory peritoneal dialysis (CAPD) for patients, and the increased use of disposable incontinence products. McCormick (1986) called high-tech one of the fastest growing markets, noting that ten years ago the procedures would have been performed only in a hospital. Robotics in the future of homecare was also cited as a certainty.

Home health care for the elderly was called "a real comer," as Val Halamandaris of the National Association for Home Care (NAHC) predicted that by 1991 at least 50 percent of the hospitals will either develop or contract for home health services (Newald 1986). An earlier survey indicated that people in the health care business thought that home health agencies will be very successful competing with hospitals (about 50 percent) and hospices as well (about 25 percent) (Arthur Andersen & Co. 1984).

Inhibiting Growth Factors

On the down side, it was noted that policies and procedures of the Health Care Financing Administration (HCFA) restricted and curtailed homecare utilization (Rich 1985). In addition, Lenz (1985) testified before a Congressional committee on the dampening impact of new Medicare cost limits, elimination of the presumption of waiver of liability, and state licensure regulations on the growth of homecare services.

Using his own study data, an Ohio pharmacist, Jay Mirtallo, cautioned hospitals to look carefully before leaping into the homecare business (Douglas 1984). His investigation showed that hospitals needed 1,416 calendar days of home parenteral nutrition business to reach the breakeven point with the hospital supplying the solutions to the patients. After evaluation, Ohio State University Hospitals arranged for a commercial supplier to operate that homecare program.

Despite the growth in the number of homecare investors and the increase in consumers, Freudenheim (1985) warned about the squeezing of the profit margins by powerful forces, including the federal government, "turning the screws to limit what will be paid for." Medicare provides homecare benefits to almost two million beneficiaries, reimbursing for almost $3 billion worth of services (*Washington Report on Medicine & Health* 1985). A HCFA official, Dennis Siebert, warned about homecare expansion: "We are concerned that people who are being cared for by their families would turn to home health care if it became available . . . It could get out of hand" (Freudenheim 1985). Around 17,000 homecare providers compete for a piece of the action; the fragmented and chaotic situation has caused market analysts to become cautious, including those who made sanguine predictions in the not too distant past.

Marketing Homecare

With the competition in the homecare field and the projected growth, even if slightly diminished, the business concepts of marketing move to the forefront. Even though health care has not usually been associated with selling cars, TVs and other consumer products, the same methods and techniques are becoming more acceptable. Now, physicians and dentists advertise in newspapers, and on TV, and homecare providers do likewise.

Laxton (1985) commented that homecare providers may be uncomfortable seeing themselves as salespeople. The fast growing homecare industry has "very little marketing activity and virtually no formal marketing." As an inducement to get into the area, Smythe (1984) finds that, "Health care that makes house calls" is easily marketable. She identifies target audiences as people needing high technology services, high risk infants or handicapped children with chronic problems, those who need pain management at home, patients with ADL needs, and physicians who make the referrals to homecare services.

Harris (1983) referred to the "stampede to treat patients at home" because of soaring hospital fees. Writing in a sales and marketing management publication, his article was called, "House Calls With a Hard Sell." Types of companies getting into the hard sell homecare mode included rent-all retailers, retail drug chains, manufacturers of health care products, temporary personnel firms, individual hospitals, investor-owned facilities, and newly formed chains and multifacility operations. However, Ingram and Hensel (1985) let nonprofit homecare agencies know that marketing is just as essential to them as to the for-profit organizations.

Basic Marketing Issues

Four areas are involved in basic marketing issues for homecare organizations (Ingram and Hensel 1985):

1. Expectations of marketing.

2. Level of commitment to marketing by the homecare agency.

3. Market definition.

4. Implementation of marketing plans, strategies, and tactics.

Oram (1985) labels the three key components of marketing in a similar vein, as organizational commitment, research, and targets and strategies. Further, she identifies the fundamental tenets of marketing as the four Ps, in the following manner:

- *Product*   Services provided by the organization

- *Price*   Direct and indirect costs
  Reimbursement
  Demand for service

- *Place*   Geographic distribution
  Access to service

- *Promotion*   Advertising
  Direct mail
  Formal presentation

Obviously, thinking about professional services as a product may be difficult for some health care professionals. Nevertheless, the professional literature is replete with such ideology; some health care journals read more like the management/business publications. Each procedure may be a different product, such as IV antibiotic infusion, ventilator therapy, or meal preparation. In fact, each homecare agency has to differentiate its products from those of its competitors, as do all the appliance manufacturers. A *Home Health Care Handbook* is available from the National Association of Retail Druggists (1985) that "gives you the inside information and practical business tips you need to build a thriving home health care department . . . or even a separate home health care business."

Pricing out of specific services requires a cost accounting approach to enable homecare firms to market their variegated line of products while making a profit. Again, many health care firms are not accustomed to calculating fractions of personnel time, proportions of overhead, and support services to arrive at a bottom line cost for each product.

Place refers to how services are provided and distributed in the marketplace. Considerations include geographic boundaries, delivery sites, referral mechanisms, direct and indirect distribution alternatives, and the competitive advantages of each choice.

Promotion can include any method or technique to persuade, educate, and move potential consumers to take action regarding the available products (services). Brochures, bumper stickers, TV and radio ads, health fairs, a speakers bureau, seminars, newspaper ads, and any gimmick dreamed up by creative imagemakers can be used to promote homecare products.

In a case study of the VNA of Chester County in Wayne, Pennsylvania, Stewart (1985) reported that home visits rose 17.7 percent in one year. Her promotion activities included mass distribution of company brochures; a physician survey about the agency's services; quarterly patient question-naires; a mailing list for distribution of a newsletter; displays for store windows and at fairs and facilities; a slide/sound presentation for speaking engagements; and paid newspaper advertisements, along with press releases, feature stories, and letters to the editor.

Humboldt Senior Resource Center in Eureka, California, wanted to market homecare to physicians. Baginski (1985) reported on the creation of the Geriatric Humanitarian of the Year Award, honor presented at a dinner banquet.

A Marketing Plan

To achieve effective product management in homecare marketing, Wells (1985) lists three important concepts:

1. Know your products.
2. Marketing is not selling.
3. Your product's price should be determined by its value to your customers--not your costs.

Product identification is apparent and noted in other marketing elements. While marketing is more scientific, selling relies on interpersonal relations. Pricing involves variables that are not always within competitive market pressures, such as predetermined reimbursement values set by the government. However, Wells argues that "if a product is worth $1,000 to the client, then that is the price regardless of whether it costs you $1 or $950 to deliver."

Keeping the three concepts in mind, Wells' marketing plan has four action parts: segment your part or parts of the market; assess each part or parts of the market for needs, characteristics, and service profiles; evaluate the profitability of each segment; and choose the best distribution approaches. Strenski (1985) discusses marketplace perceptions and the homecare communications plan, while developing similar crucial marketing questions.

Taking an entrepreneur's approach, Trotter (1985) outlines nine elements of a business plan for home health agencies: prepare a written summary of the overall objectives and goals; examine the operational structure of the agency; specify the product(s) of the agency; assess the industry and the marketplace; analyze the marketing for your product(s) and your marketing strategy; make business operations efficient, economical, and effective; plan for research and new product development; plan to respond to emerging or rapidly changing situations; and develop financial projections.

Jay and Logsdon (1985) of the VNSA of Schenectady County, New York, faced an unanticipated change that could undermine their financial solvency. Two local hospitals expressed interest in forming their own home health agencies and the VNSA got 80 percent of their referrals from those hospitals. Considering five options, including doing nothing, fighting the hospitals, operating it alone, merging with one or both hospitals, or negotiating a plan with both hospitals, the VNSA chose the latter. With a representative group from the hospitals and the VNSA, a new broader-based governing board was developed for the VNSA that satisfied all the parties. VNSA staff increased from 145 to 208, and home visits rose 41 percent from 1983 to 1984--from 88,166 to 124,154.

Ten Marketing Rules

Considering the principles, concepts, issues, and planning guidelines, marketing seems to be the application of American business knowhow to a new area. Halamandaris (1985) agrees that the notion of marketing may be distasteful to homecare providers who have been taught to "associate health care promotion with hucksters and quacks." Given all of the above, he still comes up with his ten rules of marketing.

- Be the best.
- Be the nicest.
- Reach out to the poor/needy.
- Give, don't ask.
- Get involved politically.
- Say thank you.
- Identify the caring.
- Do unto others.
- Teach.
- Remember to love.

Marketing in the Future

Due to the unpredictable nature of a rapidly growing homecare industry, Ingram and Hensel (1985) anticipate complex marketing issues in the next decade. To make it in the future, home health agencies will need to have a deeply ingrained orientation and commitment to marketing to resolve problems effectively. These authors cite a quote from Dek Hagenburger, President of the Home Health Services Division of Beverly Enterprises, as strong support for marketing as a top home health agency priority.

> Home health will be the domain and those that will be preeminent in that arena will be the companies that have a solid background in understanding and creating a sensitivity to what is involved in delivering health care services.

Homecare Trade Associations

National homecare trade associations exist to foster the growth of the industry. These groups engage in a host of activities, such as legislative lobbying, inservice training, professional education, standards and quality of care, reimbursement, public education and awareness, and the promotion of the good and welfare of the homecare field. Although there is a good deal of cooperation, each organization does have its own goals. Homecare trade associations include: American Federation of Home Health Agencies, Inc. (AFHHA), Silver Spring, Maryland; American Hospital Association, Division of Ambulatory Care, Chicago, Illinois; Health Industry Manufacturers Association (HIMA), Washington, D.C.; Home Health Services and Staffing Association (HHSSA), Washington, D.C.; Hospice Association of America, Washington, D.C.; National Association for Home Care (NAHC), Washington, D.C.; National Association of Medical Equipment Suppliers (NAMES), Washington, D.C.; National HomeCaring Council (NHCC), New York, N.Y.; National Hospice Organization (NHO), Arlington, Virginia.

Recently, HHSSA entered into an arrangement with NAHC, wherein HHSSA received representation on NAHC's governing board but retained a separate corporate entity. It could be considered a sort of merger. However, if there are distinct issues, HHSSA is free to pursue those independently of NAHC. HHSSA includes about 20 investor-owned homecare firms with over 1,100 offices in 46 states that employ more than 175,000 persons: 60 percent home health aides and 15 to 20 percent in nursing.

"Differing opinions on whether home health agencies need a single or dual voice on Capital Hill appears to be the major obstacle to a proposed merger of all national home health trade associations" (Borfitz 1986). NAHC passed a standing resolution in favor of a merger with all groups in 1983 and reaffirmed it in 1986. Val Halamandaris, NAHC president, spoke in favor of mergers and noted conversations with the NHCC and the NHO (Borfitz 1986). However, AFHHA members unanimously approved a resolution against a merger May 7, 1986, at their annual meeting.

While there may be some merging, a total melding of all homecare trade associations is not likely.

Joint Ventures for Growth

Nobody would fail to guess that the growth of homecare follows the track of the money tree, governmental and otherwise. A quick perusal of the glossy advertisements in professional publications immediately calls your attention to the wizardry of expert consultants and computers, which can solve all your problems in homecare and related fields. One solution often suggested is a joint venture, which means exactly what the words suggest: a combined undertaking. In reporting on the eagerness of hospitals to capture a share of the home health care business, Louden (1984) advised them to be cautious and to "carefully evaluate the growing joint ventures that some product firms are offering." Similarly, Albertson (1984a) spoke about homecare involvements as a new horizon for hospitals and durable medical equipment suppliers. Riffer (1985a) noted that PPS was a major force driving hospitals to consider homecare activities as a springboard to diversification.

Facilities spurred to enter the homecare market have a number of options open to them other than establishing their own home health agency. Joint ventures could be undertaken with other facilities; there could be arrangements with established home health agencies through contract, purchase, or other mechanisms; similar deals could be made with health care products companies and/or manufacturers. Options in joint ventures appear to be limited only by the creativity of the people and organizations involved in putting the package together. *Medical Product Sales* (1984), the official journal of the Health Industry Distributors Association, even told its readers that, "Among the most important sales calls dealers make this year will be to hospitals testing the home health care waters."

Advantages and Disadvantages

Advantages and disadvantages of a joint venture have been identified by Sandrick (1986):

> *Risk is Reduced* -- Working with firms and people experienced in homecare management allows for possible augmentation of marketing power to gain a large enough share for financial stability and eventual profitability.

> *Patient Volume is Assured* -- Facilities by themselves may not have the patient volume for efficient and economical delivery of homecare ser-

vices, but affiliation with an established firm can integrate a steady patient referral flow in both directions.

High Technology is Accessed -- Relationships with firms constantly engaged in research and technology improvement as well as therapy upgrading enhances the status of the joint arrangement.

Management Expertise is Available -- Success in homecare ventures is abetted considerably because acute care is significantly different; specific homecare management expertise can go a long way toward making a successful program.

Disadvantages relate to the fact that facilities entering into joint ventures are financially and legally liable for the services provided. In addition, funding may or may not be required to set the arrangement into operation.

Not Lucrative?

Although some express rationales that homecare joint ventures will add to the coffers of institutions, Swoboda (1984) says, "For the most part, the 'lucrative return' does not exist." Traska (1986) quoted a hospital consultant expert as stating that most hospitals are seeing only 1 to 2 percent of their revenue from homecare, with small hospitals expecting 10 to 15 percent of their revenue from homecare. To that point, Gordon Clemons, president of Caremark, a for-profit home health services firm with a number of joint ventures with hospitals, comments: "Homecare is a thin piece of the health care world, in which margins are so low and competition is so high, that it often doesn't make sense for hospitals to get into it on their own" (Sandrick 1986).

Key Role of Physicians

Remarking on the key role of physicians in homecare programs, Lorenz (1985) notes that physicians can be financial investors in joint ventures with hospitals. In fact, he says that "some agencies (HHAs) even loan physicians the money to invest in their joint venture." He then proceeds to list 14 business operational points for HHAs to include in negotiations with hospitals in regard to joint ventures.

Caveat Emptor

At a conference on "Home Care . . . The Hospital's Business?," the attendees were told to approach homecare with caution and foresight. "As a business moves away from the services and products it is familiar with, the risk factor increases. The risk is not necessarily to be avoided, but to be understood and planned for" (Albertson 1984b). Eckel also urged caution before entering the tricky homecare industry at an annual meeting of hospital pharmacists (*IT News* 1985). In fact, he offered a quick test where two no-answers to any of the six following considerations/questions indicates that the homecare business is not for you or your organization:

1. Are you prepared to make a strong capital investment?

2. Do you have trained, competent people?

3. Do you have people oriented regarding consultation with and counseling of patients?

4. Can you cope with the ill-defined market and flux situation?

5. Can you acquire necessary technical knowledge?

6. Can you rely on third-party payments?

Typical Joint Ventures

Citing economic, social, and demographic forces, Pear (1986) gives examples of the linkages developing between hospitals and nursing homes. Beverly Hospital in Beverly, Massachusetts, entered into a joint venture with Hillhaven Corporation, a National Medical Enterprises subsidiary, that resulted in the building of a 122-bed nursing home on its grounds in December 1985; Sutter Health System in Sacramento, California, purchased a 162-bed nursing home in February 1986; Stamford Hospital in Stamford, Connecticut, is building a 120-bed nursing home on its grounds. These are examples of a joint venture, a takeover, and an independent venture, respectively.

Yale-New Haven Hospital in Connecticut offers patients "one-stop shopping for homecare products and services through its forprofit subsidiary, York Enterprises" (Riffer 1985b). In turn, York Enterprises created two subunits: Medical Center Pharmacy and Home Care Center, and Hospital Home Health Care of Connecticut; a consulting service was added later. Services provided include prescriptions, durable medical equipment, rehabilitation supplies, respiratory therapy services and oxygen, medical and surgical supply sales, parenteral and enteral nutrition, IV therapy and antibiotic services, and a variety of in-home professional services. Where needed, York Enterprises secures outside expertise. A link exists to a national durable medical equipment company to keep that component on the right track. David Tanner, a Yale-New Haven Hospital administrator, recognizes that, "We have to be realistic about where we have expertise" (Riffer 1985b).

Four major teaching hospitals and the University of Medicine and Dentistry of New Jersey entered into a joint venture creating a nonprofit corporation, University Health System of New Jersey, Inc. (Leebaw 1986). Through collective resources and new partnerships, the new corporation aims to develop new ventures; to reduce the stress on institutional care; to explore ambulatory and home health care opportunities; to establish new primary care networks; and to regionalize technology and tertiary care. This joint venture employs 14,250 people, receives $576 million in gross revenue, owns $532 million in physical assets, has more than 2,000 beds, and admits one of every 15 hospitalized patients in New Jersey.

Sandrick (1986) reported that Caremark had 10 joint ventures with hospitals and more on the way; Abbott Laboratories' Home Care Division had more than 100 partnerships with hospitals; and TravaCare Home Therapy Division of Baxter Travenol had joint ventures with several hundred hospitals and anticipated the ventures to grow at a rate of 30 percent.

While an Institute of Medicine study (*Home Health Journal* 1986) revealed no significant difference in the quality of care delivered by for-profit health care firms, the panel of experts did express concern over the surge of for-profits into the homecare field. Their list of big health care complexes in the industry included Abbott Laboratories, American Medical International, Baxter Travenol, Beverly Enterprises, Hospital Corporation of America, National Medical Enterprises, Personnel Pool of America, Quality Care, Inc., and Upjohn Health Care Service.

Legal Aspects of Joint Ventures

Legally, Pyles (1985) says that joint venture arrangements can be partnerships, corporations, or contract/arrangements. Pyles, an attorney, then proceeds to elaborate the advantages and disadvantages of each form of venture. His legal checklist covers areas such as revenue distribution, decision-making, resolving disputes, common ownership, third-party payers, flexibility of organizational structure, licensure, certification, certificate of need, tax status, conflicts of interest, liability, fraud and abuse violations, and seeking opinions from the HHS Inspector General on doubtful issues. Major attention has to be given to antitrust considerations and liability issues. Moomjian (1985) legally advises that "acquisitions of existing homecare offices are viewed as a cost effective and less risky method of entering the market."

Essentially, the antitrust issue deals with the curtailment of competition through joint actions taken with an anti-competitive purpose and to achieve an anti-competitive effect (Philip 1985). Of course, the legalities are not that simple, and both Pyles (1985) and Philip (1985) enumerate the court actions and the interpretations that are still being untangled in legal decisions. Joint ventures will be in trouble if they contrive to fix prices, to distribute sections of the market, to boycott other firms, to mandate tie-in purchases, to arrange exclusive deals, or if they try to monopolize the market. Referral arrangements between HHAs and hospitals are the most likely candidates for antitrust problems (Philip 1985). "Antitrust laws are now clearly applicable to the health care industry. Hospitals, nursing homes, and insurers have already become familiar with the threat of antitrust litigation, and home health agencies can expect to as well. This means that home health agencies should be aware of the basic antitrust concepts and must be attuned to what may be antitrust sensitive areas" (Philip 1985).

Greenberg (1986) and Mackowiak (1984) also cover antitrust issues and add cautions regarding civil liability. Professionals providing services in the joint venture must be aware of and meet appropriate standards of care to avoid liability for negligence. Issues of comparative and contributory negligence upon the part of homecare patients ministering to themselves is also discussed.

Legal issues in joint ventures are compounded by the fact that the parties involved become responsible for each others' actions. HHAs can be held accountable for what the hospital does and vice-versa. It is apparent that joint ventures have to be evaluated thoroughly before signing the agreement.

Hospital-based Homecare

With market research firms predicting large dollar volume homecare business, with the marketing of health care receiving emphasis, and with the movement to joint ventures, hospitals are entering or planning to enter the homecare field in increasing numbers.

Moore (1985a) reported that in a national survey of chief executive officers of hospitals, 75.6 percent planned to add or expand home health services. By the end of that same year, Moore (1985b) reported the same overall planned increase in homecare services, but the larger hospitals (over 400 beds) jumped to 82.3 percent of the anticipated expansion. A survey by the AHA (*Hospitals* 1986) confirmed that 64 percent of the hospitals planned to move into the homecare field. In addition, that survey showed hospitals planning to go into adult day care (28 percent), hospice centers (16 percent), and home birthing centers (16 percent). In a survey of 450 hospital administrators, Jensen and Jackson (1985) revealed geographic differences in the growth of hospital-based homecare, with the Midwest leading at 61 percent, followed by the Upper Midwest (57 percent), West (54 percent), Southwest (47 percent), Northeast (44 percent), and the Southeast (28 percent). The hospitals most likely to offer homecare are midsized (200 to 299 beds), independent nonprofit (55 percent), and religious sponsored (57 percent), as compared with the overall 47 percent offering homecare. Medicare certified hospital-based home health agencies exhibited the most growth of all--up 118 percent from 579 to 1,260 HHAs (Sandrick 1986), in the two years from December 1983 to December 1985.

Four reasons are cited for the interest of hospitals in homecare: a need to diversify; awareness of the public's preference for care at home; cost containment through PPS; and the efforts of insurers, employers, and employees to curtail costs through alternative forms of health care (Riffer 1984). Emphasizing that hospitals are the primary source for patient referrals, Louden (1984) noted the key factors for hospitals to consider in entering the homecare field: market factors; organizational auspices; internal factors such as case mix, liability, and physician acceptance; operations such as billing, coordination, and inventory control; and technology factors. Dan Lerman, program manager of the AHA's Division of Ambulatory Care, says that, "Hospitals must start to think big and creatively about their opportunities for providing homecare services" (Riffer 1985c). It was also noted that hospital-based HHAs receive about 13 percent more than freestanding HHAs in their cost reimbursement rates.

Christy and Frasca (1983) wrote about the benefits of hospital-sponsored homecare in a nursing journal. In letters to the editor, Flanders (1984) and Ziegler (1984) took contrary views. Flanders said hospitals are not the best source of home health care because they are task oriented, create inappropriate dependency of patient and family, and promote greater hospital utilization. Ziegler urged hospitals to use existing home health agencies in the community. "The last entity that most communities need is another home health agency." In response, Christy and Frasca (1983) cited the comprehensive resources of the hospital as a rationale and did not feel that "quality" homecare agencies were available in quantities to meet the need.

While it is obvious that the number of hospital-based homecare agencies is increasing, it is also apparent that there are bound to be battles about the add-on cost reimbursement to hospitals. Furthermore, it is likely that the mergers and takeovers will continue.

Proprietary Homecare Growth

Of all the Medicare certified HHAs as of December 1985, proprietary agencies constitute the largest number--1,927 (about 33 percent). Furthermore, between December 1983 and December 1985, the growth rate was 93 percent, second only to the hospital-based HHA growth rate (Sandrick 1986).

Even before PPS, homecare growth among for-profits was touted as a solid investment bet in *Barron's* (Donlan 1983). He mentioned a variety of players of all sizes and financial shapes, including Upjohn Home Care Services, Johnson & Johnson, Superior Care, Quality Care, National Medical Care, Baxter Travenol, Home Health Care of America, National Medical Enterprises, Health Extension Services, and the AFHHA. After PPS, Kuntz (1984) reported that investor-owned hospital chains were adding home health care to aid their bottom lines in the profit and loss columns. Borfitz (1985) reported that Humana, Inc. was testing the homecare waters by acquiring the Louisville, Kentucky, office of Medical Personnel Pool. Cautioning physicians that "you'd better learn to love homecare," Lavin (1985) summed up the for-profit impact: "Fueling the expansion is the entry of such big corporations as Humana, Inc., Beverly Enterprises, American Hospital Supply Corp., American Medical International, Upjohn Co., and others providing home services for inhalation therapy, kidney dialysis and--unimaginable just a few years ago--parenteral nutrition and cancer chemotherapy."

This growth in for-profit HHAs can be illustrated by looking at two of the largest proprietary HHAs in the field: Upjohn Health Care Services and Quality Care, Inc.

Upjohn started with 37 offices in 1969 and now has close to 300 homecare offices in almost every state in the U.S. Employing more than 60,000 people, Upjohn registers about 20 million patient care hours annually, producing more than $2 billion in annual revenue (*Caring* 1985; Edmonson 1985). At the moment, Upjohn concentrates on the service aspects of homecare and is not into ancillary products.

Quality Care had five offices in 1974 and generated about $3 million from services. Today, the firm maintains 165 offices in almost every state and in Canada. Employing about 1,000 full-time and more than 500 part-time employees, the firm provides approximately 12 million hours to about 120,000 patients per year. Total revenue is greater than $100 million, with a 600 percent increase in revenue since 1978. Quality care stresses complete homecare management and also is into durable medical equipment and supplying supplemental staff to institutions. On January 2, 1985, Quality Care was acquired for about $124 million and became a wholly-owned subsidiary of GrandMet USA, Inc., a diversified British company (Scheinman 1986; *Inside GrandMet* 1985; Grand Metropolitan Annual Report 1984; Edmonson 1985).

Voluntary Nonprofit Agency Growth

Founded in the late 1890s, Visiting Nurse Service of New York (VNSNY) is the largest nonprofit VNA in the U.S. In 1983, VNSNY underwent a corporate overhaul and became a parent company, VNSNY, and four subsidiaries: VNS Home Care, VNS Family Care Services, Partners in Care, and the National Education Center for Home Health (Rogatz 1985). Professional visits to patients in the boroughs of Manhattan, Queens, and the Bronx grew from 449,000 in 1980 to 766,000 in 1984. At the same time, aide hours went from 2,408,000 to 3,264,000. VNSNY employs over 500 full-time RNs and contracts for an additional 250 + RNs. In its wholly-owned for-profit subsidiary, Partners in Care, this unit started with 300 employees serving all five boroughs in October of 1983, and 14 months later had almost 1,800 employees (Visiting Nurse Service of New York 1985).

This nonprofit example illustrates that nonprofits are mixing up their corporate structures to include a combination of profitmaking and non-profit subdivisions. Eventually, it may become necessary to separate the wholly nonprofits from the mixed nonprofits.

Utilization as a Measure of Growth

When people were cared for in their homes, nobody compiled statistics. However, with the passage of federal legislation calling for reimbursement of homecare services, the numbers began to accumulate automatically and form the basis for an evaluation of the growth of the industry.

Early Growth

With the emergence of Medicare in 1965, there was quick growth in the number of homecare agencies and programs. In the early 1960s, there were more than 1,100 agencies offering nursing care to the sick. However, only about 250 could qualify to participate in the Medicare program by meeting the minimum requirement of providing nursing plus one other service (War-hola 1980, 6). From 1966 to 1976, there was a 71 percent increase in agencies participating in the Medicare program: from 1,275 to 2,165. Agency auspices also changed during that period, with the VNAs falling from 40 percent to less than 25 percent of all the home health agencies; the slack was taken up mainly by the private nonprofits, the hospitals, and the proprietaries. Only the combined government/voluntary agency declined dramatically.

Home Health Agencies from 1966 to 1985

Exhibit 10-1 compares the numbers and percentages of home health agencies participating in the Medicare program for selected years from 1966 to 1985. In 1966, official health agencies and VNAs combined to account for 85 percent of the providers. Even as early as 1972, the VNAs had already dropped to 24 percent, with hospital-based agencies gathering steam and the officials picking up 12 percentage points. By 1975, it was evident that the private nonprofits were moving into the market. Between 1975 and 1977, the private nonprofits almost tripled their share of the total, moving to 14 percent of all HHAs. Proprietary agencies did likewise, moving from a 2 percent share to 5 percent during the same two years. VNAs continued to decrease, while the officials remained fairly constant. By 1980, the VNAs were down to 17 percent, and most of the others were still claiming a higher percentage of the total number of agencies.

Between December 1983 and December 1985, hospital-based home health agencies experienced the greatest growth of all types of agencies: 118 percent, going from 579 to 1,260 HHAs. Remember that PPS/DRG went into effect on October 1, 1983, and a HCFA official attributes the growth of hospital-based HHAs to the new Medicare prospective payment system incentives for early discharge (*Home Health Journal* 1985). At the same time proprietary agencies grew at a 93 percent rate: from 997 to 1,927 (Sandrick 1986). An Institute of Medicine study (*Home Health Journal* 1986) commented on the "particularly striking" growth of for-profit HHAs from 1980 to 1982; a threefold increase attributed to the easing of HCFA requirements for proprietaries to have state licenses.

On examination, Exhibit 10-1 reveals that the VNAs, the official agencies, and the combined government/voluntary agencies remained almost static in absolute numbers of operating agencies from 1972 to 1985. Among the others, the numerical growth is dramatic: hospital-based went from 231 to 1,255 (a 500 percent increase); proprietary from 43 to 1,929 (up almost 5,000 percent); and private nonprofit from 72 to 833 (up almost 1,200 percent). As of December 1985, there were 5,962 Medicare certified HHAs with the proprietary and hospital-based accounting for 53 percent of the total. This trend appears likely to continue into the future.

Variability in Growth by State

If asked to guess which states have the largest number of home health agencies, most people would tend to name those with the largest populations. However, that would not always be the correct answer--there are some surprises. Texas is at the top with 516 HHAs, followed by California (368), Tennessee (353), Pennsylvania (280), Illinois (268), and Ohio (255). Surprisingly, Missouri (211) and Minnesota (185) both top New York (148) and

Exhibit 10-1 Medicare-Certified Participating Home Health Agencies, Selected Years 1966 - 1985

Year	Official Health Agency*		Visiting Nurse Associations		Combined Govt. and Voluntary Agency		Hospital Based	
	No.	Percent	No.	Percent	No.	Percent	No.	Percent
1966	579	45%	506	40%	83	7%	81	6%
1972	1,255	57	531	24	55	3	231	10
1975	1,228	55	525	23	46	2	287	13
1977	1,212	47	491	19	45	2	293	11
1980	1,253	41	506	17	59	2	401	13
1982	1,211	33	517	14	59	2	507	14
1983	1,230	29	520	12	58	1	579	14
1985	1,217	20	519	9	56	1	1,255	21

Year	Proprietary		Private Nonprofit		Other**		Total
	No.	Percent	No.	Percent	No.	Percent	
1966					26	2%	1,275
1972	43	2%	72	3%	97	4	2,284
1975	47	2	109	5	103	4	2,345
1977	129	5	359	14	69	2	2,589
1980	230	8	520	17	83	3	3,022
1982	628	17	632	17	85	2	3,639
1983	997	23	674	16	200	3	4,258
1985	1,929	32	833	14	153	3	5,962

*An agency administered by a state, county, or other local unit of government.
** Includes skilled nursing facility-based program, rehabilitation-based programs, and others.

Sources: Department of Health, Education and Welfare. Health Resources Administration. *Health Resources Statistics: Health Manpower and Health Facilities, 1976 -1977*, p. 394; Department of Health and Human Services. Health Care Financing Administration; *Medicare: Use of Home Health Services, 1977*. Pub. No. HCFA-03064. Jan. 1981, p. 12; *Home Health Line*. Vol. IX, Feb. 6, 1984; Reiss, K. *Federal Programs that Finance Home Health Care Services*. 1981. Congressional Research Service, Library of Congress, (1 March) p. 4; Department of Health and Human Services, Health Care Financing Administration, unpublished data, Dec. 17, 1985.

Massachusetts (152). States with large elderly populations are also not among the leaders: Florida (167) and Arizona (78). Massachusetts has the most VNAs, (76) followed by Connecticut's 58. Few have any combined government/voluntary HHAs, with the exception of Tennessee (13). Iowa (89) has the most official agencies followed by Mississippi (80) and Minnesota (71). Texas (143) far outdistances the other states in the number of hospital-based HHAs, followed by California (91), Illinois (61), and Pennsylvania (61). Again, Texas (257) has the highest number of proprietary agencies, while the others trail: Tennessee (192), California (176), Pennsylvania (110), and Louisiana (103). In private nonprofit agencies, Texas (75) likewise leads over Illinois (49), Florida (44), Pennsylvania (42), Tennessee (41), and Ohio (40). In three states--Texas, California, and Pennsylvania-- more than half the Medicare certified HHAs in each state are proprietary organizations; Tennessee approaches 50 percent proprietary. Exhibit 10-2 gives the complete frequency breakdown for each state by type of home health agency sponsorship.

Reasons for the variability among the states may relate to the legislation and regulations governing home health agencies, such as licensing and certificate of need requirements. HCFA reports a strong correlation between the existence of certificate of need laws and the establishment of new HHAs. Explosive growth in Texas and Tennessee occurred after both states abolished the certificate of need law. A HCFA official, Arthur J. Forest, commented: "A lot of the future growth among proprietary HHAs will depend on whether states retain or eliminate certificate of need provisions there" (*Home Health Journal* 1985). Additional growth was spurred after HCFA changed the regulations in 1980 eliminating the requirement that proprietary HHAs be licensed by their home states as a precondition for Medicare certification. Furthermore, the absolute number of agencies may not mean that the VNAs, for example, are serving fewer people. Therefore, it is appropriate to examine the growth in the number of home visits.

Growth of Home Visits

In the early years of the Medicare program, the total number of home visits declined by about two million a year between 1969 and 1971. Since 1972, home visits have climbed each year. Between 1975 and 1984, Exhibit 10-3 shows that the number of home visits almost quadrupled: from 10.8 million to 40.4 million. As cost containment activities took hold, the increase slowed down, but the total number of visits still rose. During that period, visits per person served increased slightly from 21.6 to 26.7, but the services per 1,000 Medicare enrollees rose more than 200 percent, accounting for the total visits surge. More people were using about the same amount of home visits per person. Findings from the National Medical Care Expenditure Survey (Berk and Bernstein 1985) also conclude that "it is apparently

Exhibit 10-2 Medicare: Participating Home Health Agencies by Locality, by Type of Agency, December 1985.

	Number of active, participating HHAs	Visiting nurse association	Combined government and voluntary agency	Official health agency*	Rehabilitation facility-based program	Hospital-based program	SNF-based program	Proprietary	Private Non-profit
All Locations	5,692	519	56	1,217	20	1,255	128	1,929	833
Alabama	124	2	0	64	0	6	1	24	27
Alaska	6	0	0	0	0	1	0	2	3
Arizona	78	2	0	12	0	18	2	36	8
Arkansas	159	1	0	69	1	30	3	23	32
California	368	46	3	9	1	91	14	176	28
Colorado	114	7	1	19	2	25	6	31	23
Connecticut	117	58	0	17	0	7	0	33	2
Delaware	27	2	0	6	2	6	0	6	5
D.C.	9	1	0	1	0	1	0	4	2
Florida	167	15	1	10	0	7	0	90	44
Georgia	71	1	1	6	0	7	0	20	36
Hawaii	12	0	0	2	0	6	1	3	0
Idaho	31	0	0	4	0	15	2	10	0
Illinois	268	23	0	42	1	61	2	90	49
Indiana	136	16	1	10	0	40	1	59	9
Iowa	155	13	3	89	1	26	0	17	6
Kansas	138	3	4	44	1	47	2	21	16

Exhibit 10-2 continued

	Number of active, partici-pating HHAs	Visiting nurse associa-tion	Combined government and voluntary agency	Official health agency[a]	Rehabili-tation facility-based program	Hospital-based program	SNF-based program	Proprietary	Private Non-profit
Kentucky	83	1	2	18	0	29	2	28	8
Louisiana	174	0	0	5	1	49	1	103	15
Maine	15	6	0	0	0	2	0	2	5
Maryland	99	2	0	17	0	24	10	34	12
Massachusetts	152	76	0	19	1	14	0	27	15
Michigan	188	12	1	49	0	12	2	74	38
Minnesota	185	1	2	71	1	43	9	39	19
Mississippi	135	0	3	80	1	17	0	10	24
Missouri	211	4	3	37	1	63	7	62	34
Montana	29	1	0	8	1	12	1	1	6
Nebraska	34	1	1	1	0	23	1	6	1
Nevada	16	2	0	2	0	3	1	8	0
New Hampshire	40	27	1	1	0	2	1	5	3
New Jersey	59	23	1	14	0	12	0	7	2
New Mexico	47	5	0	2	0	15	0	18	7
New York	148	18	3	58	0	44	18	0	7
North Carolina	111	2	1	57	0	10	2	16	23
North Dakota	32	0	1	7	0	16	1	6	1

Exhibit 10-2 continued

	Number of active, partici- pating HHAs	Visiting nurse associa- tion	Combined government and voluntary agency	Official health agency[a]	Rehabili- tation facility- based program	Hospital- based program	SNF- based program	Proprietary	Private Non- profit
Ohio	255	25	4	57	1	39	3	85	40
Oklahoma	165	1	1	56	0	44	0	46	17
Oregon	66	1	0	10	0	30	0	17	8
Pennsylvania	280	56	0	2	0	61	6	110	42
Rhode Island	13	10	0	0	0	2	0	0	1
South Carolina	42	0	0	16	1	6	0	10	9
South Dakota	24	2	1	2	1	13	1	1	3
Tennessee	353	2	13	65	0	39	1	192	41
Texas	516	9	0	12	3	143	16	257	75
Utah	25	1	0	4	0	12	2	5	1
Vermont	20	14	0	3	0	1	0	0	2
Virginia	138	4	1	37	0	32	3	55	6
Washington	54	4	0	8	0	16	1	9	16
West Virginia	47	3	0	18	0	8	0	5	13
Wisconsin	149	12	2	54	0	17	5	40	19
Wyoming	30	0	0	20	0	4	0	6	0
Puerto Rico	40	4	1	1	0	4	0	0	30

a. An agency administered by a state, county, or other local unit of government.

b. Guam and Virgin Islands excluded.

Source: Department of Health and Human Services. Health Care Financing Administration. Bureau of Health Standards and Quality. 1985. Unpublished data. (17 Dec.).

Exhibit 10-3 Medicare: Home Health Agency Services: Persons Served and Visits by Region Selected Years, 1975 - 1984

Region and Year	Persons Served		Visits	
	Number in Thousands	Per 1,000 Enrollees	Number in Thousands	Per Person Served
Total, All areas				
1975	499.6	20.2	10,805	21.6
1977	689.7	26.1	15,548	22.5
1982	1,171.9	39.7	30,787	26.3
1983	1,351.0	45.2	36,844	27.3
1984	1,516.0	49.8	40,357	26.7
Northeast				
1975	175.9	29.2	3,655	20.8
1977	229.7	36.5	5,106	22.2
1982	360.9	53.1	9,914	27.5
1983	398.0	57.8	11,333	28.5
1984	422.0	60.8	11,855	28.1
North Central				
1975	101.5	15.2	1,858	19.3
1977	142.2	20.4	3,029	21.3
1982	260.4	34.6	6,015	23.1
1983	297.0	38.8	7,002	23.6
1984	336.0	43.6	7,661	22.8
South				
1975	139.0	17.7	3,519	25.3
1977	199.3	23.7	4,870	24.4
1982	352.6	36.7	10,497	29.8
1983	429.0	43.7	13,366	31.2
1984	495.0	49.6	15,152	30.6
West				
1975	78.4	19.9	1,495	19.1
1977	108.3	25.5	2,188	20.2
1982	180.0	36.6	3,913	21.7
1983	207.0	41.0	4,593	22.2
1984	241.0	46.6	5,196	21.6

Source: Department of Health and Human Services. Health Care Financing Administration. *Medicare: Use of Home Health Services, 1977.* 1981. Pub. No. HCFA-03-64, (Jan.) p. 4.
_____.*Medicare Data: 1982 Home Health Agency Person File.* Table 2.
_____.Division of Program Studies. Office of Research. 1986. (Unpublished data)
(5 March.)

incorrect to perceive home health care as a service delivered exclusively to the elderly."

Geographic Variability of Home Visits. Residents in the Northeast section of the U.S. show the most absolute numerical growth in the number of persons served per 1,000 Medicare beneficiaries between 1975 and 1984 (Exhibit 10-3). Each of the four regions in the nation increased the number of persons served by more than 300 percent. North Central areas revealed the smallest number of persons served with home visits per 1,000 enrollees in each of the five years. Conversely, the Northeast exceeded the national average per 1,000 enrollees in each of the five years. In effect, the Northeast accounted for raising the national average since the other three regions were all below those figures per 1,000 enrollees served.

The number of home visits per person, however, shows a different picture. Here, the South is the leader, exceeding the national average for home visits per person served in each of the five years ranging from 25.3 in 1975 to 30.6 in 1984. In visits per person served, the South brought up the national average.

Exhibit 10-4 shows the average number of home visits per 100 Medicare eligible persons by state for selected years from 1975 to 1984. Note that in 1984, six states provided more than 200 visits per 100 Medicare beneficiaries: Missouri (375); Delaware (271); Tennessee (245); Rhode Island (226); Connecticut (219); and Michigan (209). On the other end of the scale, four states provided less than 50 home visits per 100 eligibles: Alaska (31); South Dakota (33); Mississippi (43); and Arizona (49).

Changes occurring in various states during the 1975 to 1984 time period can be observed. These trends may be due to legislation and regulations, as well as specific state initiatives.

Hospital executives surveyed plan to expand homecare activity greatly, by 52.5 percent, in the Great Plains states (Iowa, Kansas, Minnesota, Missouri, Nebraska, North Dakota, South Dakota) and by 51.8 percent in the West (Alaska, Arizona, California, Colorado, Idaho, Montana, Nevada, New Mexico, Oregon, Utah, Washington, Wyoming). Growth of new programs will be greatest, 40.6 percent, in the Northeast (Connecticut, District of Columbia, Maine, Massachusetts, New Hampshire, New Jersey, New York, Pennsylvania, Rhode Island, Vermont) and by 32.6 percent in the Southeast (Alabama, Delaware, Florida, Georgia, Maryland, Mississippi, North Carolina, South Carolina, Tennessee, Virginia West Virginia) (Traska 1986).

Home Visits by Type of Agency. Home visits for nursing care, home health aide services, physical therapy, and other services by the type of HHA are compared for selected years from 1975 to 1984 in Exhibit 10-5. In each of the five years, VNAs provided the largest number of the total home visits

Exhibit 10-4 Medicare: Home Health Agency Services: Visits by State
Selected Years 1975 - 1984

Number of Home Health Care Visits per 100 Medicare Eligibles

U.S.	1975	1977	1982	1983	1984
Alabama	50	70	134	143	164
Alaska	4	70	23	24	31
Arizona	37	51	27	42	49
Arkansas	12	16	85	90	89
California	39	63	84	99	111
Colorado	50	62	129	122	120
Connccticut	82	124	196	220	219
Delaware	76	96	153	204	271
District of Columbia	47	91	101	129	120
Florida	71	102	154	187	198
Georgia	21	34	89	103	110
Hawaii	51	55	50	52	58
Idaho	52	97	73	88	132
Illinois	28	67	91	103	120
Indiana	19	25	46	59	78
Iowa	19	24	70	71	64
Kansas	15	21	93	114	113
Kentucky	32	43	52	63	70
Lousiana	93	139	115	143	180
Maine	57	130	95	104	101
Maryland	57	130	95	104	101
Massachusetts	37	59	98	114	125
Michigan	73	103	224	254	209
Minnesota	21	41	72	95	111
Mississippi	25	30	43	44	43
Missouri	93	202	240	312	375
Montana	57	89	169	205	189
Nebraska	26	68	52	62	81
Nevada	23	32	58	65	68
New Hampshire	57	58	47	73	81
New Jersey	75	105	103	109	122
New Mexico	81	108	145	165	165
New York	88	86	93	99	101
North Carolina	45	62	103	111	119
North Dakota	40	60	60	80	91

Exhibit 10-4 continued

Number of Home Health Care Visits per 100 Medicare Eligibles

	1975	1977	1982	1983	1984
Ohio	9	17	71	51	57
Oklahoma	42	52	69	69	76
Oregon	10	14	61	70	72
Pennsylvania	45	50	74	77	92
Rhode Island	67	93	162	189	226
South Carolina	73	56	95	121	157
South Dakota	12	22	41	35	33
Tennessee	54	77	142	224	245
Texas	48	66	103	131	141
Utah	35	43	57	78	118
Vermont	124	195	150	159	167
Virgina	21	29	56	68	88
Washington	24	49	88	94	95
West Virginia	29	51	79	92	102
Wisconsin	43	51	71	83	97
Wyoming	31	67	115	122	151

Source: Department of Health and Human Services. Health Care Financing Administration. Medicare Data: 1982 Home Health Agency Person File, Table 2.
——————————— .Division of Program Studies. Office of Research. 1986 Unpublished data, (5 March)

for the specific services as well as the highest percentage. By 1984, the VNA provided a total of 12.1 million home visits, with the proprietaries closing in at 9.8 million and the private nonprofits at 7.2 million. In fact, the proprietaries showed an absolute increase from 1983 to 1984 of about 2.3 million home visits, while the VNAs were almost static with a slight drop.

For each type of home visit, the growth ratio of the proprietary HHAs exceeded each of the other agency types from 1975 to 1985 (Exhibit 10-5). For all types of visits combined, the proprietary's growth ratio was 16.3 compared to hospital-based (4.6), private nonprofit (4.4), VNA (2.7), government (2.1), and combined (1.1); the average for all agencies of 3.7. Interestingly, the proprietaries' growth ratio for physical therapy visits exceeded that of the hospital-based agencies by 18.4 to 4.3. One would think the hospital-based agencies would make greater use of the therapists on staff.

Nursing care constituted 48.2 percent of all home visits for all agencies in 1984, ranging from 45.1 percent for proprietaries to 52.5 percent for hospital-based. Home health aide visits averaged 34.6 percent, with ranges from 29.2 percent for hospital units to 38 percent for government agencies. Physical therapy visits averaged 12.2 percent of all visits, with 8.9 percent for government agencies and 13.5 for combined units. Home visits for other disciplines averaged 5 percent of the total home visits, ranging from 3.2 per-

Exhibit 10-5 Medicare Home Health Agency Services: Visits (in thousands) by Type of Agency and Type of Visit, Selected Years 1975–1984

Type of Visit	1975 No.	1975 %	1977 No.	1977 %	1982 No.	1982 %	1983 No.	1983 %	1984 No.	1984 %	Growth Ratio 1975–1984
Visiting Nurse Association											
Nursing Care	2,942	64.6	3,385	59.8	5,582	50.8	5,937	48.9	5,977	49.2	2.0
Home Health Aide	1,095	24.0	1,616	28.6	3,655	33.3	4,152	34.2	4,036	33.2	3.7
Physical Therapy	407	8.9	474	8.4	1,242	11.3	1,418	11.7	1,457	12.0	3.6
Other[1]	112	2.5	181	3.2	502	4.6	636	5.2	670	5.5	6.0
Total	4,555	100%	5,655	100%	10,981	100%	12,143	100%	12,139	100%	2.7
Combined Government and Voluntary											
Nursing Care	213	64.2	230	62.8	202	54.7	190	52.7	180	51.6	.8
Home Health Aide	74	22.3	93	25.4	105	28.4	106	29.3	107	30.8	1.4
Physical Therapy	30	9.0	28	7.7	48	13.0	49	13.6	47	13.5	1.6
Other[1]	5	1.5	15	4.1	14	3.7	16	4.4	14	4.1	2.8
Total	322	100%	366	100%	369	100%	361	100%	348	100%	1.1
Government											
Nursing Care	1,493	64.0	1,782	60.0	2,306	52.4	2,380	51.0	2,429	49.9	1.6
Home Health Aide	610	26.2	878	29.6	1,595	36.2	1,743	37.3	1,848	38.0	3.0
Physical Therapy	188	8.1	244	8.2	376	8.5	404	8.7	435	8.9	2.3
Other[1]	39	1.7	65	2.2	125	2.9	143	3.1	157	3.2	4.0
Total	2,331	100%	2,969	100%	4,402	100%	4,670	100%	4,869	100%	2.1
Hospital-Based											
Nursing Care	743	64.0	938	59.9	1,850	52.7	2,285	52.0	2,773	52.5	3.7
Home Health Aide	206	17.8	356	22.7	1,008	28.7	1,293	29.4	1,545	29.2	7.5
Physical Therapy	160	13.8	203	13.0	457	13.0	577	13.1	681	12.9	4.3
Other[1]	51	4.4	68	4.3	192	5.6	243	5.5	286	5.4	5.6
Total	1,159	100%	1,565	100%	3,507	100%	4,397	100%	5,285	100%	4.6

Exhibit 10-5 continued

Visiting Nurse Association

Type of Visit	1975 No.	%	1977 No.	%	1982 No.	%	1983 No.	%	1984 No.	%	Growth Ratio 1975–1984
Proprietary											
Nursing Care	262	43.4	398	39.9	1,674	44.0	3,362	44.5	4,436	45.1	16.9
Home Health Aide	256	42.4	325	43.5	1,416	37.3	2,830	37.4	3,651	37.1	14.3
Physical Therapy	70	11.6	95	12.7	538	14.2	1,016	13.4	1,286	13.1	18.4
Other[1]	16	2.6	29	3.9	171	4.5	354	4.7	474	4.8	29.6
Total	604	100%	847	100%	3,799	100%	7,562	100%	9,847	100%	16.3
Private Nonprofit											
Nursing Care	889	53.7	1,918	50.5	3,458	47.4	3,397	47.5	3,391	46.9	3.8
Home Health Aide	552	33.3	1,256	33.1	2,518	34.6	2,494	34.8	2,559	35.4	4.6
Physical Therapy	166	10.0	465	12.2	912	12.5	908	12.7	924	12.8	5.6
Other[1]	49	3.0	161	4.2	397	5.5	359	5.0	362	5.0	7.4
Total	1,656	100%	3,800	100%	7,285	100%	7,158	100%	7,236	100%	4.4
All Agencies											
Nursing Care	6,647	61.5	8,888	57.1	15,297	49.7	17,804	48.3	19,453	48.2	2.9
Home Health Aide	2,840	26.3	4,599	29.6	10,427	33.9	12,799	34.7	13,939	34.6	4.9
Physical Therapy	1,037	9.6	1,536	9.9	3,637	11.8	4,459	12.1	4,936	12.2	4.8
Other[1]	281	2.6	527	3.4	1,426	4.6	1,735	4.8	2,009	5.0	7.1
Total	10,805	100%	15,550	100%	30,787	100%	36,847	100%	40,337	100%	3.7

1. Includes speech or occupational therapy, medical social services, and other health disciplines.
Sources: Department of Health and Human Services. Health Care Financing Administration. 1981. *Medicare: Use of Home Health Services, 1977.* HCFA Pub. No. 03064, (Jan.) p. 14.
—— *Medicare Data: 1982 Home Health Agency Person File, Table 7.*
—— Division of Program Studies. Office of Research. 1986. Unpublished data, (5 March).

cent for government units to 5.5 percent for VNAs. Home visits for nursing care dominates the volume of services, but home health aide care is not that far behind.

Exhibit 10-6 looks at home health aide utilization by type of HHA for 1984, percent of persons receiving such visits, percent of an HHAs' total visits, and the average number of visits per person served. Only the proprietary agencies (52.2 percent) and the private nonprofits (44.4 percent) exceed the average of 41.6 percent of persons served who receive home health aide visits. In percent of total visits for home health aide care, three types of HHA do better than the average of 34.6 percent: government (38 percent); proprietary (37.1 percent); and private nonprofit (35.4 percent). Although the same three HHA types also exceed the average number of home health aide visits per person served, the range is small, 18.1 to 24.0 percent. From 1975 to 1984, the percent of home health aide visits increased from 26.3 to 34.6 percent of all home visits by all types of agencies.

Persons served, number of home visits, and average visits per beneficiary by type of HHA is shown in Exhibit 10-7 for 1984. VNAs still lead, as they serve 31 percent of the beneficiaries with 30 percent of the home visits. Proprietaries follow at 20 and 24 percent, respectively, but they exceed the VNA in visits per beneficiary by 31.9 to 25.8. Private nonprofits also deliver more visits per beneficiary than the VNAs, 30.0 to 25.8, despite the fact that the private nonprofits serve about half the beneficiaries the VNAs do.

Analysis of Exhibit 4-6 reveals another type of growth pattern in home visits. Note that 38 percent of the beneficiaries accounted for only 6.7 of all the visits, with an average of 4.7 visits per person. Conversely, 14.6 percent, the total of the two highest user groups, accounted for 52.6 percent of the total visits, and about 122,000 persons in this grouping received an average of 109.7 visits each.

Utilization Impact

Despite the rapid expansion of HHAs and the homecare utilization growth shown in the exhibits, homecare still remains only a small portion of the total expenditures of the Medicare and Medicaid programs--in the 1 to 3 percent range. In comparison to the dollars spent for nursing home care, the expenditures for homecare are the proverbial drop in the bucket. With the cost containment mentality taking hold and the probability of prospective payment for homecare services, future utilization may slow down even though need will most likely increase. Nevertheless, it is clear that there is still plenty of room for expansion of the utilization of homecare services. In fact, a survey of changes in company health plan provisions (Business Roundtable Task Force on Health 1985) showed that since January 1982 about 32 percent of the firms added home health care benefits for salaried

Exhibit 10-6 Medicare: Home Health Aide Utilization by Type of Agency, 1984

Measure of aide utilization	All Agencies[1]	Visiting nursing association	Combined government and voluntary	Government	Hospital-based	Proprietary	Private non-profit
Percent of persons receiving visits	41.6	39.3	32.2	35.9	35.4	52.2	44.4
Percent of total visits	34.6	33.2	30.8	38.0	29.2	37.1	35.4
Average number of visits per person served	22.1	21.8	19.6	24.0	18.1	22.7	23.9

1. Includes rehabilitation agency and skilled nursing facility-based agencies.
2. Usually jointly administered by a state or local health department and a VNA.

Source: Department of Health and Human Services. Division of Program Studies. Office of Research. 1986. Unpublished data, 5 March.

Exhibit 10-7 Medicare: Persons Served, Number of Home Visits, and Average Visits per Beneficiary by Type of Agency, 1984

Type of agency	Benificiaries Served (thousands)	%	Visits Per Number (thousands)	%	Visits Per Beneficiary Served
Visiting nurse associations	470	31	12,139	30	25.8
Proprietary	308	20	9,846	24	31.9
Hospital-based	242	16	5,286	13	21.9
Private nonprofit	241	16	7,236	18	30.0
Government	215	14	4,869	12	22.6
Other**	22	1	612	2	27.8
Combined government and voluntary*	17	1	348	1	20.5
All agencies	1,516***		40,337		26.6

*Usually jointly administered by a state or local health department and a VNA.
** Includes rehabilitation and skilled nursing facility-based agencies.
*** Does not add exactly because of rounding.

Source: Department of Health and Human Services. Health Care Financing Administration. Division of Program Studies. Office of Research. 1986. Unpublished data 5 March.

employees, and 21 percent added them for hourly employees; 41 percent added hospice benefits for salaried workers and 26 percent for hourly workers. About 80 percent of companies cover home health care, and 75 percent of the Fortune 500 companies do likewise.

Barriers to Homecare Growth

Weller (1978) devised a 13-point list of barriers to the growth of homecare:

- Therapeutic orientation of the American health care system emphasizes episodic and crisis care.
- Skepticism, indifference, and lack of knowledge exist on the part of physicians and the public.

- An inadequate number of personnel are trained to deal with the diverse needs of homecare patients.

- Physicians and consumers are unaware of the availability and use of homecare in their communities.

- Geographic barriers exist that restrict or prohibit access to patients' homes as in rural areas.

- Funding is limited in the high cost of providing a comprehensive array of homecare services.

- Deficiencies exist in program planning, development, management, and coordination.

- Strict and inconsistent interpretation of Medicare guidelines by fiscal intermediaries and statutory restrictions on covered services inhibits growth.

- Bureaucratic red tape abounds in the myriad requirements of local, state, and federal government agencies and programs.

- There is a lack of mechanisms for assessing patients' needs and matching them with available services.

- Standards for the quality of homecare are not universally accepted.

- Inadequate utilization review procedures exist to prevent overutilization and the resulting cost increases.

Interestingly, Weller's list was published before the onset of PPS/DRG reimbursement but yet manages to cover all the barriers that are so often mentioned after that dramatic change in the funding of health care in the U.S.

Dunlop (1980) countered the rush to expand homecare services by asking if the expansion was a solution or a pipedream? He asked how we know that families really want more homecare services and if there is a true demand. How much expansion of homecare is warranted? Dunlop explains that he is not opposed to the concept but feels that an objective investigation is appropriate before allocating resources.

Governmental reports that cite unnecessary home visits also put a dampening chill on efforts to expand homecare. A GAO (1981, 25) investigation found 5,070 of 18,586 home visits to be improper or of questionable need. In addition to administrative gaps, the GAO also found physicians not actively participating in the homecare program, incomplete documentation, poor intermediary supervision, and uninformed intermediary decisions.

Suggestions to lower the barriers to homecare growth include a liberalization of the Medicare Conditions of Participation, elimination of a certificate of need for HHAs, revision of regulations to encourage homecare services in underserved areas, use of tax incentives to families providing care at home to their relatives, raising of reimbursement rates to reflect economic reality, and the use of senior citizens for personnel in underserved areas.

These barriers are often noted by a variety of individuals and organizations, but they relate to the generic health and social services delivery system in America, rather than solely to the homecare industry.

Physicians and Homecare Growth

In a cover story about home health care's growing pains in *Medical World News*, Turbo (1986) states, "Physicians are often uncertain middlemen in an industry trying to work out the kinks while in the grip of a financial vise." While the physician should not be made to be the heavy standing in the path of homecare growth, the literature often cites the doctor's unawareness of the homecare alternative. Turbo adds that physicians resent not receiving case management fees for overseeing and coordinating homecare. In fact, poor Medicare reimbursement is cited as a reason for rare housecalls by physicians. "When a doctor implements homecare, it's usually because of good marketing by the agency," says Dr. Frank Randolph, a family physician in California. As Dr. Randolph points out: "I'm for homecare, and most doctors seem to be for it. But I sense a lot of concern about when it's indicated, the lack of outcome studies, and the fact that private business is becoming so heavily involved that it's sometime hard to tell whether it's the patient or the homecare agency who's benefiting" (Turbo 1986).

Writing in *Medical Economics*, Carlova (1986) advises physicians to make the most of the homecare boom. He quotes Dr. John Berger, former president of the San Diego County Medical Society: "Organized homecare has made tremendous advances, and it has benefits for attending physicians as well as for patients. Given the economics of medicine today, I'd say homecare is a big wave of the future. Doctors would be wise to learn how to ride that wave, not be swamped by it."

With the explosive growth in HMOs and preferred provider arrangements, physicians are being recruited to join those groups providing services. These prepaid health care arrangements also are expanding their use of homecare services (Firshein 1986). In practice, the Bay Pacific Health Plan, an IPA covering much of northern California, stimulates their physicians: "We pay the attending a $100 administrative fee up front for each homecare case he has, which goes toward the time he spends managing the patient" (Carlova 1986).

Since the physician is considered the sun around which the rest of the homecare services revolve, it is obvious that he/she can be a major impetus to the growth of homecare. In a GAO report (1981,25), it was noted that "the intent of the authorizing legislation was that physicians would play an active role in the home health care program. In practice, however, this does not seem to be the case." That situation reiterated an earlier GAO (1979) report citing the lack of physician involvement.

Based on the literature, the position statements of professional organizations, and the legislation, there seems to be no doubt that physicians should be involved in homecare. Now, with stimulation from the PPS/DRG plan, from the prepaid group health care plans, from Blue Cross/Blue Shield plans (Crenson 1985) and for-profits, it remains to be seen if physicians can enhance or hinder homecare growth.

Referrals--The Touchstone of Homecare Growth

For homecare services to grow, people have to be referred for care. Usually, the physician makes the referral and prepares the required written treatment plan. Some critics raise doubts about who actually makes the referral in practice, but the responsibility remains with the attending physician. A 1984 survey of the Lackawanna County Medical Society, with responses projected to the entire membership, revealed that 85 percent of the doctors expected to increase referrals to home health care. Furthermore, 71 percent anticipated that their patients would need higher levels of care. Primary referral diagnoses were given as cerebrovascular accident (64 percent), orthopedic problems (56 percent), and congestive heart failure (53 percent) (Frayne 1985).

Louden (1985) asked who controls homecare referrals? She described the historical changes moving from providers to hospitals to current and future movement to physician groups and third-party payers.

Considering legal aspects of homecare referrals, Philip (1985) talked about "captive patient" referrals, "steering," monopoly, tying arrangements, and the withholding of information to affect referrals. Captive referrals arrange, formally or informally, for a hospital to direct their patients to a specific HHA. Steering takes place typically when a discharge planner recommends a particular HHA. Monopoly is exactly what the term means in the business world. Tying deals occur when a hospital touts its own homecare services to the detriment of all others. Withholding information could take place when the hospital allows a specific HHA to participate in its discharge planning and effectively limits information about competing services. Philip points out the possibilities of antitrust litigation in these variations of referral techniques.

Referrals cannot stand in isolation from other factors involved in the growth of homecare services. A homecare referral is merely the mechanical procedure that starts the ball rolling. Observers continually call for increased professional education about the ins and outs of homecare and for integration into the curriculums of the educational institutions. In the interim, homecare referrals will initiate more growth in the field. However, that increase in referrals may occur because of economic pressure. Hopefully, professional education will achieve proper motivation and understanding as time goes on.

Homecare--Growing! Growing! Growing!

Based on the available data, homecare is still growing rapidly. New agencies continue to appear, home visits keep going up, and total expenditures are still rising. On the other side, the percentage of funds spent by the Medicare and Medicaid programs remains minute, although a minute portion of a multibillion dollar budget still means substantial dollars. Despite apparently discharging people sicker and quicker because of PPS/DRG, legislators, budget analysts, and governmental bureaucrats are heeding to a hard cost containment line.

A three-volume study looked at alternate site providers managing during a period of transition (Health Industry Manufacturers Association 1985,16). Dividing the alternates into life cycles of introduction, growth, maturity, and decline, the study placed homecare in the growth cycle. "The homecare market is difficult to analyze. The diversity of services and products, the rapidly changing market structure, and the lack of a standard definition complicate market analyses." This study then went on to identify the market for manufacturers, distributors, and professionals, and consumers. Statistics in the study drove the growth point home: "Overall, U.S. expenditures for home healthcare have risen from less than $4 billion in 1980 to an estimated $10 billion in 1985 to a projected $15 to $20 billion in 1990. The annual percentage growth from 1983 to 1990 is projected to be 13 to 20 percent" (Health Industry Manufacturers Association, 17).

Despite difficulties with a lack of knowledge on the part of professionals and a bias toward institutionalization, homecare services are still growing. While homecare experts seek to alleviate the difficulties and the barriers, homecare services continue to expand unabated.

References

Albertson, D. 1984a. Home care involvements. A new horizon for buyers. *Hospital Purchasing News* 8(3):1,10,49.

Albertson, D. 1984b. Hospitals review options for home care involvement. *Medical Product Sales* 15(11):86-87.

Arthur Andersen & Co. 1984. *Health care in the 1990's: trends and strategies.* Dallas, TX.

Baginski, Y. 1985. Marketing home care to the doctors. *Caring* 4(9):34-40.

Berk, M. L., and A. Bernstein. 1985. Use of home health services: some findings from the National Medical

Care Expenditure Survey. *Home Health Care Services Quarterly* 6(1):12-23.

Borfitz, D. 1985. Humana tests homecare service 'water.' Medical Personnel Pool has contract - sort of. *Home Health Journal* 6(3):3.

Borfitz, D. 1986. AFHHA/NAHC merger proposal defeated again. *Home Health Journal* 7(7):1,11.

Business Roundtable Task Force on Health. 1985. Corporate health care cost management and private sector initiatives. Indianapolis (May).

Caring. 1985. Upjohn Healthcare Services: responsive leadership, quality services and an eye on the future. 4(6):44-51.

Carlova, J. 1986. Make the most of the homecare boom. *Medical Economics*:129-141.

Christy, M. W., and C. Frasca. 1983. The benefits of hospital sponsored home care programs. *Journal of Nursing Administration* 13(12):7-10.

Cohen, L. Z. 1986. Personal communication. Springhouse Corporation, Springhouse, PA (20 Feb.).

Crenson, C. 1985. Blue Cross and Blue Shield Association survey shows growth in home health care programs. Washington, DC (23 July).

Curtiss, F. R. 1986. Recent developments in federal reimbursement for home health care. *American Journal of Hospital Pharmacy* 43(1):132-139.

DeCosta, T. 1984. Home healthcare. It's red hot and right now. *Nursing Life* 4(2):54-60.

Donlan, T. G. 1983. No place like home. That's increasingly true these days for health care. *Barron's* (21 March).

Douglas, A. S. 1984. Look before leaping into homecare. *Modern Healthcare* 14(5):132.

Dunlop, B. D. 1980. Expanded home-based care for the impaired elderly: solution or pipe dream? *American Journal of Public Health* 70:514-519.

Edmonson, B. 1985. The home health care market. *American Demographics* 7(4):28-33.

Firshein, J. 1986. Prepaid use of home health services booming. *Hospitals* 60(8):66-67.

Flanders, D. M. 1984. Hospitals not best source of home health care. *Journal of Nursing Administration* 14(3):6.

Frasca, C., and M. W. Christy. 1984. The authors respond. *Journal of Nursing Administration* 14(3):6-8.

Frayne, L. J. 1985. DRGs - the impact on physician home health referrals. *Caring* 4(3):60-63.

Freudenheim, M. 1985. Profit squeeze in home care. *New York Times* (13 Aug.).

Frost & Sullivan. 1986. Home/self healthcare--an industry in constant flux. *Home/self healthcare '86.* New York, NY.

Garland, S. B. 1984. Rising costs, population spur home health care. *Star-Ledger,* Newark, NJ, (14 Oct.).

General Accounting Office. 1974. *Home health care benefits under Medicare and Medicaid.* Washington, DC: Government Printing Office (9 July).

General Accounting Office. 1981. *Medicare home health services: a difficult program to control.* Washington, DC: Government Printing Office. Pub. No. HRD 81-155 (25 Sept.).

Grand Metropolitan. 1984. Annual report. London, England.

Greenberg, R. B. 1986. Legal implications of home health care by nonprofit hospitals. *American Journal of Hospital Pharmacy* 43(2):386-390.

Halamandaris, V. J. 1985. Caring thoughts. *Caring* 4(9):48.

Harris, P. 1983. House calls with a hard sell. *Sales and Marketing Management* 131(4):49-51.

Health Industry Manufacturers Association. 1985. *Alternate site providers - managing during a period of transition. Executive summary.* Washington, DC (Dec.).

Health Industry Manufacturers Association. 1985. *Vol. I. Alternate site providers - an encyclopedia; Vol. II. Their role in a changing health care system; Vol. III. Challenges for product distribution.* Washington, DC (Dec.).

Home Health Agency Gazette. 1985. AFHHA continues public awareness program on home care. 5(1):4.

Home Health Journal. 1985. Certified agencies' growth dramatic. 6(1):11.

Home Health Journal. 1986. For-profit health care cost more, quality high, including home care. 7(7):1,5.

Hospitals. 1984a. Study: product market $5.43 billion in '87. 58(5):40.

Hospitals. 1984b. Rapid growth pattern tracked. 58(5):33.

Hospitals. 1985a. Demystification of home health care spurs growth for self-test products. 59(13):57.

Hospitals. 1985b. High tech home care market has greatest growth. 59(7):45.

Hospitals. 1986. AHA survey. 60(4):75.

Ingram, T. N., and P. J. Hensel. 1985. Marketing in home health organizations: issues in implementation. *Family & Community Health* 8(2):22-32.

Inside GrandNet. 1985. Quality Care joins GrandNet. 14(1):3.

IT News. 1985. Former president of ASHP urges caution before entering tricky homecare industry. 12(8):1,22.

Jay, T., and J. Logsdon. 1985. The marketing impact of a joint venture. *Caring* 4(9):42-45.

Jensen, J., and B. Jackson. 1985. Half of hospitals offer home care; one-quarter plan to start programs. *Modern Healthcare* 15(21):76, 80.

Kuntz, E. F. 1984. For-profits adding home healthcare to aid bottom lines. *Modern Healthcare* 14(7):168,170.

Lavin, J. H. 1985. You'd better learn to love home care. *Medical Economics* (29 April).

Laxton, C. E. 1985. Editorial intro. *Caring* 4(9):2-3.

Leebaw, J. 1986. UMDNJ and 4 major N.J. teaching hospitals incorporate to develop new health care delivery systems. *Healthwire* (June).

Lenz, E. A. 1985. Testimony before House Select Committee on Aging. Washington, DC: Home Health Services and Staffing Association (30 Sept.).

Lorenz, B. R. 1985. Prospective reimbursement: planning for the future. *Caring* 4(10):47-54.

Louden, T. L. 1984. Hospitals eager for a larger share of growing home health care market. *Modern Healthcare* 14(2):66,68.

Louden, T. L. 1985. Who controls homecare referrals? *Caring* 4(10):17-19.

Mackowiak, J. 1984. Legal issues in hospital based home health care. *Topics in Hospital Pharmacy Management* 4(3):16-25.

McCormick, B. 1986. High-tech home care becomes new growth area. *Hospitals* 60(13):86.

Medical Marketing & Media. 1986. The new magazine that meets a new need. 21(1):52.

Medical Product Sales. 1984. Hospitals eye potential for DME dealer alliances. 15(2):1,16,18.

Moomjian, G. T. 1985. The legal aspects of homecare company acquisitions. *Home Health Journal* 6(3):16.

Moore, W. B. 1985a. CEOs plan to expand home health, outpatient services. *Hospitals* 59(1):74-77.

Moore, W. B. 1985b. CEOs plan resource shift for 1986. *Hospitals* 59(24):60-70,72.

National Association of Retail Druggists. 1985. *Home health care handbook.* Alexandria, VA.

Newald, J. 1986. Home health care for the elderly: a real comer. *Hospitals* 60(6):63.

New York State Association of Health Care Providers, Inc. 1986. Licensed home care agency development seminar. Massapequa, NY (Feb.-March).

Oram, D. 1985. The challenge of marketing professional services. *Caring* 4(9):11-15.

Pear, R. 1986. Change in Medicare prompts hospital-nursing home ties. *New York Times* (16 April).

Philip, M. S. 1985. Antitrust and home health agencies. Presentation at annual meeting of the National Association for Home Care. Las Vegas, NV (16 Oct.).

Philip, M. S. 1985. Home health referrals: some legal guidelines. *Hospitals* 59(23):72-75.

Pyles, J. C. 1985. Legal issues raised by home care joint ventures and corporate reorganizations. Presentation at annual meeting of the National Association for Home Care, Las Vegas, NV (15 Oct.).

Rich, S. 1985. Home care regulations are termed too tough. *Washington Post* (28 May).

Riffer, J. 1984. PPS prompts home care rise; few hospice benefit takers. *Hospitals* 58(24):54.

Riffer, J. 1985a. PPS, diversification push home care rise. *Hospitals* 59(24):52,54.

Riffer, J. 1985b. One-stop shopping protects market share. *Hospitals* 59(10):72.

Riffer, J. 1985c. Home care agencies up 25 percent since '84. *Hospitals* 59(10):64,68.

Rogatz, P. 1985. Visiting Nurse Service of New York. Outline of major programs. *Manhattan Medicine* 4(6):25-27.

Rx Home Care. 1985. Report predicts healthy market. 7(4):13.

Sandrick, K. 1986. Home care: cutting health care's safety net. *Hospitals* 60(10):48-52.

Scheinman, D. A. 1986. Personal communication. Quality Care, Inc. Rockville Centre, NY (8 Jan.).

Smythe, S. 1984. Marketing home health care. *Texas Hospitals* 40(3):22-24.

Stewart, N. 1985. Marketing tools & methods for small home health agencies. *Caring* 4(9):30-33.

Strenski, J. B. 1985. Marketplace perceptions and the homecare communications plan. *Caring* 4(9):18-19.

Swoboda, R. J. 1984. Home health care: bane or boon for hospitals? *American Journal of Hospital Pharmacy* 41(1):149-151.

Taylor, I. 1984. Big growth likely for home health care. *Star-Ledger,* Newark, NJ, (8 April).

Traska, M. R. 1986. Home health care: hospital activities vary by region across the nation. *Hospitals* 60(3):54,56.

Trotter, J. 1985. The entrepreneur's approach. Business planning for home health agencies. *Caring* 4(9):20-24,25.

Turbo, R. 1986. Home health care encounters growing pains. *Medical World News* 27(3):76-88.

Visiting Nurse Service of New York. 1985. *A report to the community. 1984 annual report.* New York, NY.

Warhola, C. F. R. 1980. *Planning for home health services: a resource handbook.* Washington, DC: Government Printing Office. Pub. No. HRA 80-14017 (Aug.).

Washington Report on Medicine & Health. 1985. HHS targets home health costs. Washington, DC (5 Aug.).

Weller, C. 1978. Home health care. *New York State Journal of Medicine* 78(12):1957-1961.

Wells, J. B. 1985. Homecare marketing and product management. *Caring* 4(9):5-9.

Ziegler, K. 1984. Utilize existing home health agencies. *Journal of Nursing Administration* 14(3):7.

Chapter 11

Homecare Evaluation

Evaluation depends upon your viewpoint--some see a glass half full of water and others see a glass half empty. Additionally, there are gradations of evaluation ranging from simple to sophisticated and related to investigative goals and methodology. Regardless of the type of evaluation or the level of application, evaluation is an integral part of any operating program. Formally or informally, evaluation is undertaken to assist in determinations about the value of activities and to make adjustments as required.

Homecare Evaluation Questions

More than 30 years ago, Dr. E.M. Bluestone (1954), the originator of the Montefiore homecare program, listed almost 40 questions that should be considered in evaluating the practice of homecare. Questions covered administration, choice of patients, unique homecare characteristics, relations to other groups, finances, and a comparison of hospital and homecare. Typical questions follow:

- Has full advantage been taken of the services of other health, social, and charitable agencies in the community for the benefit of the homecare patient?

- Does the homecare program take full advantage of the principles of group medicine?

- Does medical continuity keep pace with social continuity as between intramural and extramural care?

- Does the homecare program share all of the highly specialized equipment of the hospital?

- Is chronicity in itself, or "incurability," a fair reason for homecare?

- Does the homecare program help to break down the outmoded distinctions that still prevail between "acute" and "chronic" hospitals?

- Does the roster of diagnoses indicate that patients have been properly classified and assigned?

- What opportunities does the homecare program offer to the teacher and the student of medicine, social service, nursing, and the like?

- Are medical and other facilities available in the home around the clock?

- What is the length of stay in the extramural service as compared to the intramural service?

- Is homecare expensive or inexpensive in relation to the total effort?

- Are the medical records, financial records, social statistics, and vital statistics of homecare adequate and immediately available?

- Have the medical and financial possibilities of homecare been considered to the full in connection with a prepaid voluntary health insurance plan?

- Has the homecare program been popularized and publicized to the point of maximum response?

- What is the relative success of homecare?

Only 15 of Dr. Bluestone's questions have been listed, and the viewpoint of a hospital-based homecare service is apparent. Nevertheless, with minor modifications, that evaluative question list is as current today as when it first appeared in print. In fact, many of the queries have already been addressed in this book and come as no surprise. Thus, early in the homecare movement, evaluation of a comprehensive nature was part and parcel of its fundamental principles and practices.

Specific Areas for Homecare Evaluations

Areas for evaluation are limited only by the creativity of the mind. A large body of existing medical literature can supply endless ideas for investigation and guidelines for research. Investigative topics should be selected according to their usefulness to patients, to homecare agencies, and to the community. Exhibit 11-1 lists 24 possible evaluative topics from an evaluation handbook for home health agencies (Kleffel and Wilson 1975). Note that many of the topics can be used as starting points for more diversified studies.

Exhibit 11-1 Possible Subjects for Homecare Evaluation Studies

1. Adequacy of admission information.
2. Necessity of admission to agency.
3. Comprehensiveness of patient care plan.
4. Most common diagnosis(es) and the type and number of visits by staff.
5. Quality and adequacy of teaching and supervision of diabetic regime (or congestive heart failure patients, etc.).
6. Teaching and supervision of patients with colostomies.
7. Whether patients actually follow therapeutic diets.
8. Frequency of urinary tract infections in patients with indwelling catheters.
9. Effectiveness of bowel and bladder training.
10. Care of decubiti.
11. Differences in characteristics of patients receiving physical therapy from those receiving restorative nursing.
12. Need for social work services (nutritional services, home health aide, etc.).
13. Drug study (amounts, interactions, adverse effects).
14. Appropriate use of consultants.
15. Adequacy of weekend services.
16. Indicators of change in level of care needed by patient.
17. Assessment of psychosocial problems of patients; intervention, if any.
18. Effectiveness of physical therapy services, social work services, etc.
19. Outcomes of patient care as related to objectives of care.
20. Patient satisfaction with care.
21. Number of cases not admitted, with reasons.
22. Care of dying patients.
23. Frequency and reason for readmission.
24. Effectiveness of discharge planning.

Source: Kleffel, D. and E. Wilson. 1975. *Evaluation handbook for home health agencies.* Washington, D.C.: Government Printing Office. Pub. No. HSA 76-3003.

Cost Containment and Evaluation

In a climate of cost containment, evaluations tend to stress the money aspects, proving that services are cost-effective. Federal grants are awarded to develop cost-saving techniques and methods of delivering health care. Policymakers await each new evaluation that can bolster their cost-cutting decisions. Critics of PPS/DRG also claim that the methodology was untested before the government implemented the program primarily as a cost curtailment device, without regard for the quality of care and the patient's wellbeing. At a Senate committee hearing on a piece of homecare legislation, Dr. Philip W. Brickner (1981,9), a physician prominent in the homecare movement, put the evaluation emphasis on cost containment and dollar expenses into perspective: "I think it would be an error to concentrate solely on dollars here. Dollars obviously are very important, but the issue of what human beings are entitled to in their lives--a choice--I think equally important. We should never ignore that in the concern about dollars." In a similar fashion, Dr. Peter Rogatz (1985), who reported on the impact of homecare programs on hospital services in 1958 (Rogatz and Crocetti), said that viewing homecare as primarily an economy measure would be a mistake. "I believed then that this was unwise; I believe it is equally unwise today."

What is the Best Evaluation Method?

In many instances, the choice of evaluation methods and techniques can become a political battle. Ultimately, evaluation calls for a judgment as to what is and what is not worthwhile. Evaluation experts, in classic publications, comment that there is no single best way to evaluate. Weckwerth (1969,1) said that "the crucial element in evaluation is simply who has the power, the influence, and the authority to decide." That statement contrasts with the popular attitude that evaluation is objective, scientific, and without bias or political influence.

In discussing the evaluation design, Suchman (1967,91) reiterates that there is no single best evaluative method:

- It seems to us futile to argue whether a certain design is "scientific." The design is the plan of study, and as such, is present in all studies. It is not a case of scientific or not scientific, but rather one of good or less good design.

- The proof of hypotheses is never definitive. The best one can hope to do is to make more or less plausible a series of alternative hypotheses.

- There is no such thing as a single "correct" design. Hypotheses can be studied by different methods using different designs.

- All research design represents a compromise dictated by the many practical considerations that go into social research.

- A research design is not a highly specific plan to be followed without deviation, but a series of guideposts to keep one headed in the right direction.

Home health agencies should use the evaluation style that fits their individual needs while achieving effectiveness with easy implementation. In talking about community nursing care evaluation, Davidson (1978) added relevant points: "Evaluation is a continuous integrative process, and . . . program evaluation and clinical record review that are mandated by Medicare law are only a beginning to the type of evaluation that should be performed in a home healthcare agency."

Evaluation Defined

Definitions of evaluation usually deal with determinations of value, an examination, or a judging. Commonly, explanations talk about whether or not a program achieves its goals and how well it does so with specific measurements. Impacts of key program variables and comparisons with external variables are often included. In an analysis of the effects of federal government evaluation policies on public programs, Wholey, Scanlon, Duffy, et al. (1970,23) put the various parts together in an expanded definition of evaluation: "Evaluation (1) studies the effectiveness of an ongoing program in achieving its objectives; (2) relies on the principles of research design to distinguish a program's effects from those of other forces working in a situation; and (3) aims at program improvement through a modification of current operations."

Generally, all evaluation definitions detail measures such as mortality, morbidity, functional status, or cost savings and attempt to pinpoint the relevant factors that are part of the cause and effect.

Homecare Evaluation Study Characteristics

Homecare evaluation studies, similar to the medical evaluation studies required by the Medicare Conditions of Participation, are mainly concerned with quality of care. Usually, the homecare evaluation is a multidisciplinary effort resulting in recommendations to benefit the patient, agency, and/or the community. Kleffel and Wilson (1975,67) identified the following general characteristics of homecare evaluation studies:

- Specifically designed in-depth studies focusing on particular potential problem areas.
- Usually of short duration.

- May be prompted by statistical reports which show significant deviation patterns. May also focus on subjectively perceived problems.

- Usually focus on the care provided a group of patients by a group of practitioners, rather than on care provided to individual patients by individual practitioners.

- Results of homecare evaluation studies can be utilized for developing appropriate inservice and continuing education programs.

- Results of homecare evaluation studies often identify needed changes in the organization and delivery of care.

Similarly, Davidson (1978) lists critical evaluation generics as objective criteria, full documentation, flexibility, and resulting logical actions.

Skeptics may contend that this type of evaluation is a continuous part of their agency's activities. However, it is vital to examine the differences between informal and formal research (Michnich, Shortell, and Richardson 1981).

Characteristics of evaluation studies are more alike than not, and the steps involved usually proceed in a scientific methodology: define the problem; appraise the data; formulate hypotheses; test the hypotheses; and analyze the results. Regardless of the variations in the evaluation steps, there are specific evaluation "dos and don'ts." Exhibit 11-2 lists the guidelines. Although they were compiled some time ago and appear simplistic, the test of experience and application has proven their durability and value.

Exhibit 11-2 Evaluation Dos and Don'ts

- Do bring in the evaluator early. Allow the evaluator to become fully involved. Waiting until the end of the project to employ an evaluator indicates lack of value attached to the evaluation.

- Do pre-evaluative investigation. It is worthwhile to secure a grass roots feeling for what is happening.

- Do engage in systematic study and exploration. This is an evaluation prerequisite. There is no need to reinvent the wheel; history is well known for repeating itself with regularity.

- Do include other disciplines in the evaluation effort. Statisticians, sociologists, social workers, nurses, and others can add to the evaluation with their diversity.

- Do coordinate efforts. This saves time, effort, and wear and tear on staff members.

- Don't use sophisticated evaluative techniques if other alternatives serve as well. Seek the simple approach first.

Exhibit 11-2 continued

- Don't use existing case records as your only source of data for evaluation. An obvious bias occurs in this method; the reservations must be stated.

- Don't undertake evaluation unless adequate resources are available. Efforts will be wasted on gerrymandered evaluations.

- Don't undertake lopsided evaluations. It is not necessary to use a high-powered rifle to kill an ant.

- Don't underestimate unpretentious evaluation techniques. Sometimes, a simple yes or no questionnaire is powerful. Merely asking patients "why" can be most revealing.

- Don't believe in the fantasy of a neat, precise, utterly objective science in evaluation. Reliability and validity can be questionable on numerous occasions, as well as other variables.

- Don't overvalue loosely used terms in evaluation activities. Jargon can cloud a study and its results.

Source: Herzog, E. 1966. *Some guidelines for evaluative research.* Washington, DC: Government Printing Office. Pub. No. Children's Bureau 375-1959.

Political and Other Evaluation Pitfalls

Frequently, decision-makers may use evaluation to solidify political ends. However, Day (1984) observes, "Neither system objectives, nor that criteria for measuring progress toward objectives, are addressed sufficiently in public policy debate and analytic literature on the several types of services which compose what is known as long term care." Both evaluators and administrators should be aware of the possibility of political ends in considering the following listing of pitfalls that can cause evaluation difficulties (Kleffel and Wilson 1975,12):

- Agency policy and practice are assumed to be compatible.

- The quality of a total program is judged on the basis of an assessment of one segment.

- Evaluation is seen as an isolated activity rather than as a continuous integrated process.

- Positive evaluation reinforces agency objectives which have been met, but objectives can remain inappropriately static.

- Evaluation outcomes are not shared with persons to whom the evaluation is most pertinent.

- Evaluation recommendations are not implemented by administrators.

- Personality conflicts contaminate the objectivity of the evaluators.

- New programs are implemented without making provisions for evaluating them.

- Statistical data aren't used or, even worse, are used improperly.

- Objectives/outcomes aren't stated in measurable terms and thereby lead to subjective evaluations.

- There is no feedback to evaluators to maintain their interest in the process and to monitor their recommendations.

Additional pitfalls occur in homecare evaluations that involve interviews or surveys with clients, professionals, or community members. Bias and inconsistency could take place, resulting from respondent motivation, fatigue, or mood; weather, location, or time; ambiguous or poorly worded questionnaires; mechanical and/or coding errors in data processing (Suchman 1967,118). Identification of control subjects for comparison evaluations is cited as another problem by Lurie, Chan, Kasch, et al. (1985) with regard to the long lead time required for data collection, the nature of the subjects, the possibility of shifting goals/objectives, and the possible lack of generalization from the study. Of course, reliability and validity considerations also affect potential problems. Evaluators should also be aware that it is quite common for clients/patients to try to please the interviewers by saying what they think the investigators want to hear.

Homecare raises unique problems in evaluation through the fact of the environment in which care is rendered, the organizational development of the diverse agencies involved, and the broad ranging diseases/conditions being treated. Branch and Stuart (1984) raise an underlying ethical issue relating to withholding care in the interests of upholding the scientific integrity of the evaluation. "Admittedly the random clinical trial (RCT) is the experimental method of choice. . . Ethical and other considerations suggest that a definitive RCT is not soon forthcoming."

Furthermore, homecare evaluation is affected by Medicare regulations, PROs, consumers, and professional associations. By law, the Medicare Conditions of Participation mandate evaluations of policy and administration as well as clinical record reviews. Where they exist, Health Systems Agencies (HSAs), certificate-of-need requirements, and licensure programs also influence evaluations. There are efforts to have Peer Review Organizations (PROs) monitor the quality of care provided by home health agencies (*Home Health Journal* 1986). Consumers are provided with a variety of checklists and guides to evaluate and compare home health agencies for quality services and standards (American Association of Retired Persons 1984,22; Nassif 1985,386). Professional organizations have long maintained an interest in evaluation and use instruments such as the Homemaker-

Home Health Aide Evaluation Questionnaire (H/HHA-PEQ) to measure the quality and adequacy of services rendered (Fashimpar 1985).

When evaluators sidestep or avoid the input from influential sources, difficulty is assured. Evaluators should attempt to involve all those who will be affected by the outcomes of the study to ensure fairness.

Data Collection

Homecare data collection exhibits problems common to all evaluation and research efforts. Philosophic program distinctions contribute to inconsistencies in definitions, in the timing of data collections, and in establishing a uniform set of statistics that mean the same thing to all parties. States may gather Medicaid information that does not concur with federal Medicare data. Individual home health agencies may still have a unique one-of-a-kind statistical accounting system, although Miller (1986) may be coming to the rescue. She has prepared a comprehensive guide to homecare record documentation and management that includes field tested forms, a recommended uniform minimum data set, Medicare reimbursement documentation guides, ICD-9-CM coding instructions, quality assurance guides, and management aid.

Uniform Basic Data Set

An expert consultant panel on health statistics (Department of Health and Human Services 1979,4) explains the importance of a uniform basic data set: "In a country like the U.S. with its exceedingly complex health care system, these data sets are an essential means of communication. They permit variety and flexibility in health information systems without loss of the essential ability to make basic comparisons. In addition, through arrangements like the Cooperative Health Statistics System, they make it possible to share data and to keep to a minimum the demands made on health providers by external agencies and associations." Furthermore, the panel said that a uniform basic data set "defines the central core of data about a given dimension of health and health services needed on a routine basis by the majority of users and established standard measurements, definitions, and classifications of this core."

A uniform basic data set could gather information about demographic variables (sex, age, birthdate, race/ethnicity, marital status, living arrangements, court-ordered constraints, and personal identification); health status items (vision, hearing, communication, and ADL--bathing, dressing, toileting, continence, eating, walking, mobility, behavior problems, etc.); service factors (provider identification, admission date, direct services, source of payment, charges, discharge data, and discharge status); and procedural data on the date and type of report (Department of Health and Human Services 1976,12-34).

While most of the homecare associations support a uniform data collection system, the range of sophistication and expertise among the almost 6,000 Medicare-certified home health agencies would mandate a system that is relatively easy and inexpensive to implement and maintain.

Deterrents to Data Collection and Use

Evaluative use of data requires essential patient information and the use of cost accounting methods as well. Day (1984) referred to a CBO study which contended that the dearth of adequate data on nonfacility-based health care utilization is a serious methodological obstacle to cost-effectiveness analysis. With the emphasis upon cost containment, this lack of data could be disastrous. To fill at least part of that information gap, the NAHC cooperated in a Congressional survey of Medicare-certified home health agencies (House Subcommittee on Health and Long Term Care 1985). Information garnered from a statistically significant sample of HHAs detailed agency profiles, agency budgets, agency operations, client populations, agency programs/case flow, cost per visit, and cost per hour.

In using instruments with statistical applications, Liang, Partridge, Larson, et al. (1984) caution that the measurement error of instruments used may exceed the anticipated numerical differences, particularly in functioning abilities, and especially among elderly homecare patients where limited progress may be the norm. Combs-Orme, Reis, and Ward (1985) also warn about evaluations of maternal and child health homecare programs where the statistical power of the data is so low as to not find significant differences even when they do in fact exist. Small samples and high attrition in field trials often undermine the ability to use meaningful statistical applications.

A special problem occurs when evaluation seeks to measure attitudes and behaviors. Spiegel and Backhaut (1980) review a good deal of the literature on the problematical variables involved in areas such as patient and provider satisfactions, nonobservational ascertainment of behavior of patients and providers and expressed attitudinal stances of patients and providers. Development and testing of satisfaction and preference scales to measure attitudes toward the medical care of chronically and terminally ill patients and their families was reported by McCusker (1984). Her home care study sought satisfaction dimensions in the following areas: (1) general satisfaction; (2) availability of care; (3) continuity of care; (4) physician availability; (5) physician competence; (6) personal qualities of the physician; and (7) communication with the physician. Preference dimensions included: (8) place of care; and (9) patient and family involvement in treatment decisions. Her terminal care study included all of the above dimensions except for 3 and 4, and added satisfaction measures on freedom from pain and pain control. In developing the instruments, five methodological issues were addressed: ability to differentiate the multidimensionality of attitudes; scaling methods using a continuum of response; use of direct and indirect questioning approaches; balancing positive and negative items to minimize acquiescent response set where respondents tend to agree regardless of the question content; and the selection of pretested attitudinal questions. Versions of the measurement scales were developed for patients, and for caretakers. There was also a postbereavement version.

Based on discriminant validity, convergent validity, and internal consistency, the tests of general satisfaction, physician availability, freedom from pain, preference for homecare, pooled physician communication, and physician personal qualities performed well. Availability of care, involvement of patient and family in treatment decisions, and pain control did not. The others show promise but need further development.

Obviously, the collection of valid and reliable data on attitudes is quite complex and certainly requires considerable time and effort, as well as money, to do well. In addition, generalities are often tempered by the variables that are beyond the evaluator's ability to control and by the particular characteristics of the respondents.

Warhola (1980,32) summed up the deterrents: diversity of HHA sponsorship; variable agency size; type of staff and staff sophistication; the complexity and diversity of homecare services; the difficulty of describing patients in functional terms along with medical diagnosis and treatment; and the difficulty of measuring quality of care relative to goal achievement.

Evaluation Using Five Ds

Among the most common evaluative measurements are the five Ds: death, disease, disability, discomfort, and dissatisfaction (Blum 1974; Elinson 1972). Details of each measure follow:

Death--Statistics are usually readily available and broken down by various variables. However, the population base may be uncertain, there may be incomplete records, and there may be a time lag in securing up-to-date information.

Disease--Data are usually collected and available from a number of sources on acute, chronic, self-terminating, and incurable conditions. There are indications of the severity and survival predictions but little on disability or discomfort. Problems with the data relate to clinical determinations and other variables involved in causation.

Disability--Measures note the inability to carry out customary roles and to perform customary duties related to school, work, or leisure. Acute and chronic disability is counted along with the degree of impairment and the number of disability days. Relation of the disability to the individual's social role raises questions, as does the judgment distinction between handicapped or disabled. Again, the population base for data may overlook many individuals who are not reported with disability.

Discomfort--In both acute and chronic forms, measurements note the degree of discomfort as well as the number of days involved. These measures include scientific and subjective information. Since discomfort is usually self-reported, other variables of a sociocultural nature influence the data.

Dissatisfaction--Measurements can cover a broad spectrum of variables relating to physical, intellectual, emotional, and social factors, such as the physician's attitude, the cost of care, and the mood of the patient. Both degree and intensity of dissatisfaction should be documented. Yet, these data will be subjective for the most part and seriously tainted by other variables.

Typical Homecare Evaluations

For the most part, up to this point the abstract nature of evaluation has been discussed. It is important for people in homecare to understand that the methods and techniques of evaluation apply equally well to the entire health care delivery system. Fortunately, a huge body of literature exists that can be tapped for suggestions, ideas, and even resolutions to perplexing problems.

Grouping typical homecare evaluations into classifications can be troublesome and as varied as the methods themselves: surveying; opinion polling; program descriptions; comparisons; data analysis; participant observation; and position papers. Furthermore, each study could use more than a single type of evaluation tool. Therefore, the examples will be grouped, but there may be overlapping of methods and techniques.

Each method can make use of existing records, annual reports, vital statistics, questionnaires, interviews, discussions, expert opinions, and other data sources. Some evaluations make generalizations based on their outcomes, while others limit their conclusions to the group(s) being investigated. Some seek statistical significance using appropriate mathematical tests, while others report trends. In essence, each form of evaluation is variegated. Readers need to approach the written material with a wary eye and an inquisitive mind while the methods, analyses, and conclusions are weighed.

Reviews of Evaluations in the Literature

Community-based Long-term Care Evaluations. Reflecting a major evaluation difficulty, Hughes (1985) reviews evaluations of community-based long-term care and calls attention to the inappropriate comparisons of apples and oranges. A total of 13 studies are grouped into three models: four look at the effect of "traditional" skilled nursing services following acute care hospitalizations; five examine the impact of "expanded" homecare programs providing both medical and social services, and four examine how well "case managed" community care works. All evaluations were reviewed as to internal validity: study design; sample size; instrumentation; length of observation; and method of analysis. In addition, Hughes examined construct validity: explicit statement of theory and rationale; sample appropriateness and congruence with at-risk population; presence of treatment utilization data indicating operationalization; and appropriateness of outcome measures for the sample and the treatment.

Traditional studies dealt with stroke patients, with five surgical procedures, and with veterans discharged to homecare, to hospital-based nursing homes, or to community-based nursing homes. Despite the differences in methodology, a trend of consistently beneficial treatment was observed. Hughes (1985) states that "the similarity of findings across this group of studies is therefore interpreted to suggest that when a population is well matched with an intervention appropriate to its needs, and outcomes are plausible, consistent findings across studies are likely."

Expanded care studies provided services to the mentally impaired, to patients with chronic disease, a majority of patients with circulatory disease, and in two studies to geriatric patients needing rehabilitation. All five studies were randomized experiments with similar methodologies (Hughes 1985). Despite that, "findings vary widely across these studies, ranging from no effect, to both positive and negative effects." That variation may be due to the imprecise definitions of what services constitute "expanded care" and the selection of inappropriate target populations: "confused conceptualization." "Although the demonstrations were intended to substitute for institutional long-term care, in fact, they served disparate, heterogeneous populations which in some cases exhibited risk characteristics of long-term care users and in some cases did not." This attribute seriously weakens the usefulness of these findings in shaping long-term care policy. These five "expanded care" evaluations stress the need to have multiple independent investigators test new interventions. In addition, these studies point out the need to be cautious before generalizing the results of a single study or grouping generalizations across studies.

Case management studies included four of the federally funded "channeling" demonstrations: Triage, Inc. (Hicks, Raisz, Segal, et al. 1981); Monroe County Long Term Care ACCESS (Eggert, Bowlyow, and Nichols

1980); Wisconsin Community Care Organization (CCO) (Applebaum, Seidl, and Austin 1980); and the Georgia Alternative Health Service (AHS) (Skellie and Coan 1980; Skellie, Mobley, and Coan 1982). The homecare service was a major component of the case management demonstrations, with the agency providing a single entry system and acting as the broker to arrange for comprehensive care.

Relating the findings of the four case management studies is difficult because of the differing study methodologies. Additionally, the heterogeneity of the study populations confounds generalizations: some were mainly Medicare beneficiaries; some Medicaid groups; ages varied considerably; and minimally impaired, acutely ill, and chronically ill adults were eligible for the project services. Hughes (1985) concludes that "it is likely that this lack of agreement on risk characteristics of target populations account for a substantial degree of the variation in study findings." On top of all these disparities, the services tested also varied widely.

Importantly, three of the four case management studies suggest that overall health cost expenditures are not reduced. Other services are substituted at about the same cost or a somewhat higher overall cost.

In a summary of the 13 community-based long-term care evaluations, Hughes (1985) identifies conditions to facilitate unambiguous evaluations: random assignment of subjects to experimental and control groups; use of multiple design strategies; awareness of rival hypotheses; capture the content and context of treatment to enhance replicability and theory development; and include measurement of treatment implementation in the design. She notes that it may be difficult to meet all those conditions in a single study. For the "expanded and case management" experiments that seek to deter institutionalization, Hughes suggests attention to better assessment of at risk populations, gearing services to the chronically ill, matching treatment outcomes to the specific characteristics of the people served, and using multivariate analysis to test for effectiveness.

In all fairness to the evaluators, the determinants of nursing home admissions are not clear, nor are the characteristics of services that truly substitute for institutional care, and the appropriateness of services for people not at risk of institutionalization. Hughes concludes that "although the issues which require further research in this area are numerous and pressing, they do not appear to be insurmountable if approached in a systematic way. . . When one considers the fact that field research on community-based long-term care is barely a decade old, there is room for considerable optimism."

Homecare Effectiveness and Cost Evaluations. Hedrick and Inui (1986) review 12 studies aimed at chronically ill populations that used experimental or quasiexperimental designs. Six basic review criteria were used, dealing with randomization, comparisons of study groups, patient outcome status, and patient follow-up. Each of the 12 investigations was compared in reference to mortality, physical function, nursing home placement, hospitalization, outpatient visits, and cost. Results showed that homecare programs do not appear to affect mortality rates (9 of 11 studies support that contention); no impact on physical function (5 of 8 studies); a majority of the experimental studies (4 of 8) suggest that homecare has no effect on nursing home placements, no effect on inpatient hospitalization (7 of 10 studies) or actual increase in bed days (2 experimental studies); homecare may actually increase ambulatory outpatient visits by approximately 40 percent (4 studies); costs would be unaffected (3 studies) or increased (2 experimental studies), "with the suggestion that costs would be increased by approximately 15 percent for the homecare group."

These literature evaluation analyses are tempered by the fact that the number of studies may be insufficient--only 12 could be located; that the studies may differ substantially from one another--particularly in the nature of the homecare services provided; that important information may not be in the reports; and that there may be substantial problems with the study methodology. Hedrick and Inui (1986) list some methodology problems, such as subject selection, attrition, and assessment; reporting of methods, analyses, and results; and lack of data for statistical power calculations.

"Surely the safest conclusion from this summary analysis would be to contend that, while the preponderance of evidence does not support the expectation that homecare programs of the type studied have a positive impact on the outcome assessed here, the existence of some contradictory findings and methodological problems in these studies supports the need for additional methodologically rigorous research to assess the effectiveness of homecare." Based on their review, Hendrick and Inui come up with the following suggestions for future evaluations: give greater attention to the choice and description of subjects and setting; improve the targeting of high risk populations and the evaluation of services delivered to the group; give careful attention to the sample sizes and the expected power of statistical observations; minimize subject attrition; note and assess subject crossovers; for dependent variables take into account patient intake characteristics known to affect treatment, such as age, living arrangement, recent facility stay, and clinical status; and observe strict, complete standards for reporting research results. In addition, Hendrick and Inui recommend that "outcome measures include the technical and interpersonal quality of homecare, patient satisfaction with home versus other modalities of extended care, and the impact of homecare on other measures of physical health status, psychosocial status (mental status, contentment, life satisfaction, behavior problems, social role), adherence to medical regimens, unmet need for services, family burden and family finances."

Maternal and Child Health Home Visits Evaluations. Combs-Orme, Reis, and Ward (1985) review eight evaluations that study the effectiveness of home visits by public health nurses to women and children. Home visits were for assessment, teaching, counseling or support, referral, and clinical service. Two major problems were noted in the eight studies: there were theoretical gaps detailing the link between the needs of the population served and the services provided, as well as between the outcomes measured and the nursing services being assessed; and limited statistical power due to the small samples and the high attrition. "In conclusion, while the public health nursing literature does not provide convincing evidence of the effectiveness of PHN, neither does it indicate that PHN is not effective."

Descriptive Evaluations

Retrospectively reviewing the records of all 23 patients discharged from a hospital to an intravenous (IV) antibiotic therapy regimen at home, Harris, Buckle, and Coffey (1986) described the unit's experience. Clinical features and antimicrobial therapy are listed along with age (range from 7 to 68 years; average 44) and duration of treatment (7 to 35 days with a mean of 22 days). Results of treatment showed that 78 percent were cured; 21 percent suffered side effects; and 30 percent were able to resume work while on IV antibiotic home therapy. Financial analysis indicated a cost saving of $115,783.34 for third-party payers. Investigators concluded that their study confirmed that IV antibiotic therapy can be given at home safely and effectively and at substantially less cost.

A Geropsychiatric Outreach Team of the Illinois State Psychiatric Institute evaluates and treats physically impaired elderly over the age of 60 who reside in Chicago. Wasson, Ripeckyj, Lazarus, et al. (1984) detail the experiences of the team relative to 66 of the 83 patients treated in the first 11 months of operation, using initial diagnostic reports and the three-month follow-up interviews. Diagnoses, age, socioeconomic status, sex, race, living arrangements, ethnicity, and family ties are given along with the process of intervention. At the three-month evaluation, the 66 patients are grouped into three improvement categories: improved (34/52 percent); stabilized (14/21 percent); and unimproved (18/27 percent). "Even though most patients had a considerable number of physical, social and psychiatric problems, 86 percent of the 66 patients assessed at the 3 month follow-up were still at home . . . From the results of this study, we believe that home evaluation and treatment of psychiatrically impaired elderly can be instrumental in alleviating suffering and in providing a viable alternative to hospitalization and long term institutionalization."

Holman (1986) explored the feasibility and costs of providing hospice care to patients without caregivers at home. In an eight-month study at Montgomery Hospice Society, Maryland, 20 patients were admitted to the program. A chart gives the age, sex, diagnosis, length of stay, referral source, location at death, and number of visits by the nurse and social worker. Comparison data from other studies were used in the evaluation, along with historical logs on each patient, and measurements from two quantitative tools: one observed activities of daily living, and the other tracked who provided what type of care to the patient. Based on the study, Holman urges that the federal government continue its policy of not requiring Medicare hospice beneficiaries to have caregivers. Under certain conditions, safe and comfortable hospice homecare can be provided even if the individual does not have live-in caregivers.

Researchers at Toronto General Hospital in Canada undertook an economic evaluation of 73 patients on a home parenteral nutrition program measuring the incremental costs and health outcomes (Detsky et al. 1986). Descriptions are given of the setting, the population, the program, the patients, and the evaluation methodology. Costs and health outcomes were measured against the costs and outcomes for patients treated with alternative strategies. "In summary, our best guess is that home parenteral nutrition results in decreased expenditures"--a net savings in health care costs of $19,232 per patient. Additionally, there was an increase in survival of 3.3 years, adjusted for quality of life.

Descriptive evaluations often rely on looking at program characteristics and answer the who, what, where, when, why, and how type of questions. At times, descriptive evaluations can extend over a long period. Investigators examine an activity and use a variety of mechanisms to determine the value of the operation. Data could be compared to studies in the literature, measurement tools could be applied to the statistics, survey and interviews could add additional information for analysis, and statistical significance tests could be applied. Existing data sources, such as annual reports, service statistics, patient records, billings, management reports, and other official documents are used. Yet, the baseline data may still be experiences from a single program, and generalizations may be difficult to make and support. Conclusions may be value judgments rather than scientific fact. Generally, descriptive evaluations do not have true research designs, and the uncontrolled variables could significantly influence any outcomes.

Survey/Polling Evaluations

"There has been no systematic examination of the extent to which the absence of primary caregivers inhibits provision of hospice service," according to Kieffer and Wakefield (1986). To rectify the situation, they used a mail survey and collected information from 31 of the 35 hospices in Iowa (88.6 percent response rate). Questionnaires contained 23 questions; 16 dealt with organizational characteristics and seven related to the unavailability of primary caregivers. Results indicated that the majority of hospices used paid care providers (13/68 percent) to overcome the absence of a suitable primary caregiver. Females appear to be lacking caregivers more frequently, and few hospice programs had formal training for primary caregivers. "Our data document that the absence of a suitable primary caregiver for some patients seeking care in the home is a potential barrier to hospice care." Furthermore, the investigators note that the problem may be underestimated in their data. Kieffer and Wakefield also call for further research including specifically controlled trails.

Scharlach and Frenzel (1986) evaluated institutional respite care provided by the Veterans Administration Hospital in Menlo Park, California. They looked at the "degree to which the availability of expended respite care affects the physical and mental well-being of impaired adult males and their caregivers, the caregivers' ability to continue to provide care over a prolonged period of time, and the reported likelihood that the care recipient would require permanent institutional placement within the next 12 months." A survey questionnaire was mailed to 150 principal caregivers with open-ended and fixed-choice questions on their use of respite services, effect on their own health, relationship with the patient, the patient's health, and their ability to continue to keep the patient at home. Questionnaires were returned by 99 people, a 66 percent response rate. "According to the reports of the program's participants, the availability of respite care has resulted in better physical and mental health and more rest for the caregivers, better health for their patients, and an improvement in caregiver/patient relationships."

Based on the results of their mail survey, Scharlach and Frenzel suggest areas for further investigation: testing the objective validity of the caregivers' self-reports; determining whether decreased burden actually translates into improved care and delayed institutionalization; the replicability of the findings in other settings and types of respite care; benefit determinations related to caregiver/patient characteristics, cost, and effectiveness; and the development of instruments to evaluate the quality of homecare. Interestingly, the authors stated that they knew of no previous attempt to examine their hypothesis.

Generally, surveys ask: what is happening and where do we stand? Evaluations are descriptive in nature and usually aid in planning and development. This common technique gathers data on knowledge, attitudes, and behavior via questionnaires that are administered, self-administered, or mailed although other methods such as small discussion groups can also elicit similar data. In any event, this evaluation technique always raises the question about the honesty of the respondents. Because of this doubt, surveys and polling are risky, even when researchers plan and test for the accuracy of responses. Furthermore, respondents are often self-selected, perhaps creating a bias. How can we be sure that the sample is representative? Can we be sure that questions are understood? Can we control the influence of the staff and others on the responses? Despite these nagging queries, surveys and polls can still serve a useful purpose indicating trends or suggesting areas for further exploration.

Evaluations Using Personal Interviews

A literature review produced few studies that looked at the post-hospital needs of patients; Wolock, Schlesinger, Dinerman, et al. (1985) were eager to initiate one. Using a semistructured interview schedule, 13 master's level social work students interviewed 69 patients, in person or by telephone, 6 to 11 months after discharge from 12 area hospitals. Questions centered on the services needed and received; the services needed but not received; barriers to receipt of service; informal patterns of help and support; and the physical, economic, social, and psychological impact of the illness on the patient and his/her family. Results echoed other studies showing the overwhelming burden falling on family members. While data on community resources were positive, the scope seemed minimal because of the extensive needs documented. However, the respondents did not agree that services were minimal and the authors attribute the disagreement to the high level of family support, low expectations re: community services, and limited knowledge of available services. "Although this was a small scale exploratory study, the findings are of sufficient importance to suggest the need for a larger more rigorously designed study."

Branch and Stuart (1984) reported on a statewide stratified area probability sample of noninstitutionalized persons involved in the Massachusetts Home Care Corporation program to provide home support services to elders in need. Data came from personal interviews with 1,317 of the original first wave sample of 1,625, and from third wave interviews with 825 members at year six of the study. Thus, the interviews presented information on a five-year history of targeting homecare services to prevent institutionalization. Fourteen characteristics were analyzed, including age, gender, marital status, household composition, income, education, perceived health, reality orientation, Title XX eligibility, morale, instrumental tasks of daily living, ADL dependence, functional dependence, and the use of ambulatory aids. Results strongly supported the contentions that homecare services can be targeted to vulnerable groups and that the services can be maintained over a five-year period. Findings moderately supported the theory that the program did in fact target services to those who would later be classified in the high risk group. "These data lend support to the underlying issue that home based support services can in fact be an *alternative* to institutional services because they can consistently serve individuals with the same risk factors" (author's emphasis).

Personal interviewing as an evaluation technique exhibits problems similar to surveys and polls. Bias on the part of the interviewer; honesty of respondent replies; questionnaire reliability and validity; coding errors; representativeness of the sample; respondent and interviewer fatigue; influence of time, weather, and mood on responses are only a few of the difficulties. In addition, personal interviews are an expensive evaluation technique relative to staff time. Still, the personal interview does assure a definitive response.

Evaluations Using Data Analysis

These types of evaluation usually use data collected by other sources to test hypotheses retrospectively or to analyze the statistics to discover what happened and why. Investigators seek to gather accurate data representative of the study population. If the data are reliable, conclusions can be drawn with assurance and used in complex computer statistical packages to look for statistically significant findings.

Meiners and Coffey (1985) used 1980 data on all short-term, nonfederal Maryland hospital Medicare patients discharged to nursing homes, home health care, or self-care: 103,635 people. In addition, data on 478 patients from 18 randomly chosen for-profit, skilled nursing home facilities in San Diego, California were added. Their study looked at hospital DRGs and the need for long-term vs. short-term services. Characteristics of patients most likely to be considered for earlier discharge to nursing home and home health care programs are identified. Cautioning that the results should be considered exploratory because the data were limited to Maryland and San Diego, Meiners and Coffey found differences in the most common DRGs of patients discharged to nursing homes, home health care, and self-care. Nursing homes received people requiring skilled rehabilitation services, reflecting mental or behavioral problems linked to the frailty of old age. Homecare got patients needing long-term care but not necessarily having debilitating conditions. Self-care patients tended to have shorter-term care expectations. In all three discharge groups, the top 10 DRGs account for a significant percentage of cases: 40.2 percent for nursing homes; 36.5 percent for homecare; and 28.5 for self-care. "These results suggest that the Medicare PPS gives hospitals a strong incentive for earlier discharge of patients needing long term care services."

Using 3,200 clinical charts from four private hospitals selected 18 months before and 18 months after initiation of the DRG system, Coe, Wilkinson, and Patterson (1986) examined the impact of DRGs on the patient's level of dependency at the time of discharge. Six scales were used to measure dependency: activity and mobility; bathing and hygiene; number of medications; procedures; signs and symptoms; and age. Three medical and two surgical DRGs with the highest post-hospital placement rates were selected for study: DRG 14 (specific cerebrovascular disorder [stroke], except transient ischemic attacks; DRG 89 (simple pneumonia/pleurisy) DRG

127 (heart failure and shock); DRG 209 (major joint replacement); and DRG 210 (hip-femur pin procedure). This study indicates that patients do leave the hospital with higher dependency levels as a result of a shortened length of stay, prompted by the PPS/DRG incentive toward earlier discharge.

Benjamin (1986) used data provided by Medicare fiscal intermediaries to HCFA, tabulated by service for Part A and Part B and by user category, and then summed for total home health users by state. Taking this 1982 program data, Benjamin sought the determinants of state variations in home health utilization and expenditures under Medicare. A chart lists total users, total expenditures, users per 1,000 enrollees, and expenditures per user for each of the 50 states and the District of Columbia. Variables in the analysis included demographic need based on age, bed disability, and poverty level; home health agency supply; service substitutes such as Title XX allocations, SSI payments, and nursing home beds; referral sources; costs of service inputs; state resources; and geographic region. Data on state social and economic conditions came from a variety of sources and from other research. Sophisticated statistical techniques were applied to the data to find significant differences. Findings revealed that supply factors strongly and consistently explained both utilization and expenditure variations among the states. Significant correlates of home health utilization included population need, presence of service alternatives and referral sources, in addition to HHA supply. Expenditures are most influenced by case-mix severity, input costs, available alternatives, and HHA supply. Nearly 75 percent of utilization variability is explained by seven state characteristics, while 60 percent of expenditure differences can be explained by six state factors. "Results suggest the need to give more analytic attention to the impact of the market share of proprietary HHAs in explaining expenditure variations and the effects of total supply on utilization and spending" (Benjamin 1986).

Data analysis evaluations depend upon the reliability and validity of the external sources for their value. An assumption is made that the supplier of the data has accurately compiled the statistics over the time period in question. If that assumption is true, then evaluations using large bodies of collected information can be a very powerful technique for all types of investigations. There is an advantage of being able to work with a universe allowing for matching samples and for representative groups, and for even using a total population of patients, providers, or payers. Evaluations of this type can be invaluable for determining policies and procedures. However, the amassed data may lag behind several years, and the environment may have changed by the time the material is analyzed. For example, Meiners and Coffey used 1980 data (DRGs were implemented in 1983) to test questions related to DRGs and discharge. Despite that drawback, the pool of collected data available for this type of evaluation is huge and worth investigating.

Comparison Evaluations

Probably the most common evaluation forms are those that compare services or care choices using two or more experimental and control groups. Designs vary from simple to complex, from crude to sophisticated; the conclusions reflect the diversity of evaluative skills being applied in the study. Usually, some variation of a scientific method involves hypotheses, data collection, testing of theories, statistical analyses for significance, and conclusions and recommendations.

Diseases/Conditions Comparisons. Wade, Skilbeck, Langston-Hewer, et al. (1985) reported on a controlled trial of a homecare service for acute stroke patients in England. After their strokes, 440 patients received the new service and 417 patients were in the control group for a comparative period of six months. A care team based at Frenchay Hospital treated patients only in their own homes and did not treat those in the hospital. Results indicated that the trial group used more hospital bed days, had a slightly higher admission rate, and did not show better emotional adjustment to stroke than did the control group. There was no difference between the two groups in stress on relatives. Functional recovery was equal. "Our failure to show any advantage for the homecare service may have been because patients were not randomized at entry. . . The service may not have been sufficiently different from those already available. . . One cannot conclude that homecare is ineffective, but only that a small increase in the services already available locally did not have any effect."

Comprehensive rehabilitation services for elderly homebound patients with arthritis and orthopedic disability were evaluated by Liang, Partridge, Larson, et al. (1984). Patients were randomized into a treatment group of 29 and a usual treatment control group of 28. Patients in the experimental group received an additional eight-week rehabilitation program. Evaluations were made at the beginning, at two, four, and six months after the study. Two months into the study the experimental and control groups switched so that each group actually experienced the special rehabilitation intervention. Findings compared program activities, outcome variables, quality of life, hospitalization, falls, and functional status. "In this study, stepped-up outreach and physical and occupational therapy services did not reverse functional decline in the group as a whole." Rationales included the fact that the patients in this study were considerably sicker than in other studies, and their overall condition limited anticipated potential improvement. Indications were that 25 percent of the homebound population could benefit from such services but that few patients would avail themselves of the service, even if free. It is suggested that community nurses and home health aides be taught to identify and manage reversible deficits in their patients with arthritis disability.

An eight-session, two-hour-weekly group support program was designed for 22 family members and relatives caring at home for patients with Alzheimer's Disease. That experimental group was compared with 18 others on the waiting list for the group support program. Kahan, Kemp, Staples, et al. (1985) measured family burden, levels of depression, and knowledge of dementia among the two groups using pre- and post-questionnaires on family burden, a self-rating depression scale, and a dementia quiz. "In conclusion, this study indicated that a relatively short but intensive training experience that offers practical knowledge about dementia (its effects on the patient as well as on the family) and the opportunity to discuss individual problems can have a positive effect in reducing perception of burden and levels of depression in caregivers."

Pai, Channabasavanna, Nagarajaiah, et al. (1985) engaged in a comparative study of homecare by a trained nurse vs. hospital outpatient supervision in the management of chronic psychiatric patients in Bangalore, India. Matched groups of 25 each, with a mean duration of illness of nine years, were in each group, with clinical and social functioning assessments at intake and again after two years. "It is evident from the data presented here that a homecare service does seem to offer a viable alternative mode of follow-up care for the chronically mentally ill population . . . it may be possible to prevent repeated hospitalization . . . and offer them a better chance of long term community adjustment." Researchers cautioned on the ethnic factors as well as a number of questions to be investigated further.

A randomized study of the impact of home health aides on diabetic control and utilization patterns involved a comparison of a group receiving routine care (113 people), a group offered home health aides (114 people), and the subgroup of those offered who accepted aides (44 people). Hopper, Miller, Birge, et al. (1984) used outcome measures of fasting blood sugar as an index of diabetic control, number of eye clinic visits as an index of positive utilization of service, and an index of negative utilization that consisted of the total number of emergency room visits and the number of missed appointments to either the diabetes or eye clinic. Results showed that the group offered aides had fasting blood sugar declines, fewer missed appointments, and decreased emergency room use compared with the control group. Those in the group of 44 who accepted aides showed a significant increase in eye appointments as well as the greatest blood sugar decline. "While this intervention produced modest changes . . . the outcomes suggest the usefulness of aide interventions with low-income patients." Importantly, an editorial by Haug (1985) in the same issue of the journal carrying this study pointed out the contribution of the "unsung family caregivers" and the question of who really benefits from homecare services.

Long-term Care Comparisons. A homecare team approach to providing care to chronically or terminally ill elderly was the subject of a randomized controlled study by Zimmer, Groth-Juncker, and McCusker (1985). Randomization yielded a homecare group of 82 and a control group of 76. Hypotheses related to health care system utilization, patient health status, and satisfaction with health care. Trained interviewers collected data using an initial baseline questionnaire, a sickness impact profile, a morale scale, and a patient and caretaker satisfaction questionnaire. Additionally, a health service utilization diary was maintained by the patient or family caretaker. "This study failed to demonstrate any effect of the intervention upon patient functional status (physical or psychosocial) or morale . . . the strongest statistical results favoring the team were observed in caretaker satisfaction with health care. . . Trends in patient satisfaction were also strong, especially at six months."

Hughes, Cordray, and Spiker (1984) used an experimental group of 122 clients and a control group of 123 to evaluate the model long-term comprehensive coordinated homecare program of the Five Hospital Homebound Elderly Program in Chicago. Pre- and post-outcome measurements looked at mortality, comprehensive functional status, rate of hospitalization, and rate of institutionalization over the 31-month data collection period. Major findings include a significant reduction in nursing home admissions and nursing home days for the experimental group. Clients in the experimental group also increased their sense of well-being and decreased their previously unmet needs for community services. "Somewhat paradoxically, the experimental group also demonstrated a decrease in physical activities of daily living function." Mortality and hospitalization rates were about equal. Despite nursing home days savings, costs for the experimental group were 19 percent higher but that additional cost increased the quality of life for those clients. "A moderate and consistent use of expanded homecare services over an extended period of time was demonstrated to be associated with beneficial service effects."

Twelve community-based long-term care projects providing alternates to institutionalization were compared and evaluated by the Health Systems Agency of New York City (1985). Programs included those funded by the state's long-term home health care program such as Elderplan, Inc., ACCESS, and the VNS of NY, and eight of the programs target clients residing in the community. Comparisons were based upon project reported data or data supplied by the project upon request. Investigators noted that there was a limited capacity to retrieve data and that there was a good deal of inadequate data and, in a few cases, comprehensive data. The most striking similarity among the 12 programs was the adoption of overall goals related to client benefit and cost reduction along with the use of case management to coordinate and deliver long-term care. Other findings show that hospitals made 50 percent or more of the referrals; client follow-up was the most common case management activity, with 7 to 120 contacts per year, whereas client reassessment and updating of the care plan involved 3 to 9 contacts yearly; contact by telephone was most common; less than one-third of program costs related to coordination, assessment, and case management functions; direct care costs, particularly in-home services of personal care, accounted for about 70 percent of program costs; and reimbursement methods included variations of prospective, retrospective, social/HMO, and waiver projects. In conclusion, it was recommended that in-home and community-based services should include ongoing case management.

Gaumer, Birnbaum, Pratter, et al. (1986) evaluated the performance of the first nine LTHHCPs (Long Term Home Health Care Program) in New York over the first two years of operation. Comparisons are made of 724 clients enrolled in the LTHHCP and 649 persons eligible, but not yet clients. "Across all sites there is clear evidence that the program has been extremely successful in reducing levels of nursing home utilization." Upstate communities saved considerable money while improving patient survival. New York City sites also had favorable client outcomes, but at a higher cost than non-LTHHCP services. Targeting of eligible patient groups is suggested to improve cost-effectiveness.

Facilities vs. Homecare Comparisons. Greer, Mor, Morris, et al. (1986) compared care for terminally ill patients receiving care in homecare hospices (HC), hospital-based hospices (HB), and conventional hospital care (CC). A total of 1,754 patients from more than 50 facilities were in the follow-up group: 833 HC, 624 HB, and 297 CC. Data were gathered from personal interviews with patients and family members at different points, from a log of services used, and from clinical records. Comparisons included patient outcomes, pain control, satisfaction with care, family outcomes, costs, Medicare costs, and service utilization. Results confirmed that hospice care is different from conventional care and suggest that the hospice philosophy influences institutional behavior positively: hospice patients are less likely to receive diagnostic tests, X-rays, and aggressive antitumor therapy in the terminal period. With the exception of pain and symptom control, where hospice care may do better, the patient's quality of life was similar in all three settings. Satisfaction with care also was shown in all settings, with hospice patients likely to die at home. No consistent superiority of family outcome was associated with the hospice approach. Cost of HB hospice and CC care is roughly equivalent, while HC hospice costs are lower.

This National Hospice Study "appears to confirm that hospice is a viable alternative for the care of some terminal patients. . . Incentives might well be structured to encourage utilization of HC hospices since these seem less costly and more likely to keep patients in their home environments."

Community care for the mentally handicapped adult in a hostel, a home, and a hospital was evaluated by Locker, Rao, and Weddell (1984). Matched groups were chosen for the hostel (17 patients), home (12), and hospital (8). Using progress assessment instruments, individuals were evaluated on entrance, at 3, 6, and 12 months during the one-year study. Attention was given to changes in self-help, communication, socialization, and occupation. Hostel residents showed significant improvements in all four areas, while those living at home showed no such improvement, and the hospital group exhibited a less certain and less dramatic gain. "While the limited data presented here would support the case for additional provision of residential accommodation in the community, further evaluations of these forms using larger populations and controlling for more factors are necessary."

Home health care vs. nursing home care for the elderly is typified by an evaluation by Powers and Burger (1985). Patients were selected from the practice of a single physician and matched to provide 10 people in each group. Retrospective analysis of variables compared included ADL, laboratory tests, medications, physician visits, hospitalization, and costs. There were no significant differences in the two groups after six months of treatment. "Our data support the position, so far as financial considerations are concerned, home health care can be advocated perhaps only when disability is not severe and there is a desire to prevent or delay unnecessary institutionalization."

Kramer, Shaughnessy, and Pettigrew (1985) compared nursing home and home health case-mix relative to cost-effectiveness implications. Differences were sought between 653 home health patients and 650 nursing home patients, and between 455 Medicare home health patients and 447 Medicare nursing home patients. Random samples from 20 home health agencies and 46 nursing homes in 12 states in 1982 and 1983 provided the study population. Data came from the RNs and LPNs, randomly selected, who provided care at the sites, from the clinical records, and from ADL assessment tools.

Results suggest "that the general home health population differs considerably from the traditional nursing home population . . . home health care, to date at least, is oriented more toward the 'subacute' patient than the chronic, long-term care patient . . . homecare patients were younger, had shorter lengths of stay and were less functionally disabled than nursing home patients." In comparing Medicare patients only, nursing home patients were more likely to be dependent in ADL, although their long-term care problems and medical problems were similar. Hospital-based nursing homes also seem to have more functionally disabled patients than do freestanding nursing homes. "From the standpoint of cost effectiveness, it appears that home health care may provide a substitute for acute care at the end of a hospital stay and may prevent exacerbations of medical problems resulting in hospitalization for certain patients."

A comparative analysis of patient type and service mix of hospital-based and community-based home health care agencies was undertaken by

Balinsky and Rehman (1984). Data came from 30 patient records selected from each of the 19 participating agencies for a total of 570 cases: about two-thirds community and one-third hospital-based. Using a detailed questionnaire, information was taken from the records on age, living arrangements, primary payment source, primary diagnosis, ADL, admission expectations, referral source, preadmission site, utilization of services, certified services, and intensity of care. Hospital-based patients were significantly different from community-based patients. "Hospital-based home care patients were older, more limited in their functional ability, received a higher intensity of care and utilized a greater proportion of therapeutic services . . . a higher percentage were in an acute care facility prior to homecare, had cancer and circulatory disorders as their primary diagnosis and had Medicare as the primary payment source." Suggestions are made for taking case-mix into account when planning for reimbursement in the provision of homecare services.

Participant Observation

In an unusual evaluation study, Bregman (1980) lived with each of six different families for four days and four nights. Each family was caring for a child with progressive neuromuscular disease at home. In her observations of the family, Bregman kept a daily log supplemented with copious notes and interview material. Analysis involved the constant comparative method requiring the simultaneous coding and analysis of data. From this anecdotal information, the evaluator was able to identify five different family coping patterns, along with the specific strategies used by each family.

Participation evaluation is most often used in sociological and anthropological studies with the evaluators actually blending into the group being observed. Critics claim that the intimate relationship may color the observations, introducing a bias. Conclusions are highlighted by verbatim quotes and the reports may read more like a novel than a scientific paper.

Evaluation Constants

Considering the generic abstract foundation about homecare evaluation along with the concrete examples of evaluative techniques using descriptions, interviews, data analysis, and a variety of comparative studies, the importance of the guidelines can be readily seen. Simple dos and don'ts now become truisms to be followed in evaluations. Particularly important is the admonition to make sure to compare and measure the same items. Cost comparisons often evidence, however, that the cost of comparable factors are missing or ill stated; for example, the value of services provided by family members in the home and the value of their time lost from jobs or other activities.

The homecare industry has yet to develop accurate and reliable techniques to evaluate programs and to arrive at sound conclusions. Deterrents to homecare evaluations have to be addressed and removed prior to proceeding to valuable investigations. A sampling of reports by the investigative arm of the U.S. Congress, the General Accounting Office, illustrates the evaluation difficulties:

- Home Health-The Need for a National Policy to Better Provide for the Elderly. HRD-78-19, Dec. 30, 1977.

- Home Health Services-Tighter Fiscal Controls Needed. HRD-79-17, May 15, 1979.

- Evaluation of HCFA's Proposed Home Health Care Reimbursement Limits. HRD-80-84, May 8, 1980.

- Response to a Senate Permanent Subcommittee on Investigations' Queries on Abuses in the Home Health Care Industry. April 24, 1981.

- VA's Home Care Program is a Cost Beneficial Alternative to Institutional Care and Should be Expanded, But Program Management Needs Improvement. April 27, 1981.

- Medicare Home Health Services: A Difficult Program to Control. HRD-81-155, Sept. 25, 1981.

- Improved Knowledge Base Would Be Helpful in Reaching Policy Decisions on Providing Long Term In-Home Services for the Elderly. HRD-82-4, Oct. 26, 1981.

- Assessment of the Use of Tax Credits for Families Who Provide Health Care to Disabled Elderly Relatives. GAO/IPE-82-7, Aug. 27, 1982.

- The Elderly Should Benefit from Expanded Home Health Care, But Increasing These Services Will Not Insure Cost Reductions. GAO/IPE-83-1, Dec. 7, 1982.

- Medicaid and Nursing Home Care: Cost Increases and the Need for Services are Creating Problems for the States and the Elderly. GAO/IPE-84-1, Oct. 21, 1983.

- Simulations of a Medicare Prospective Payment System for Home Health Care. GAO/HRD-85-110, Sept. 30, 1985.

- Changes Needed in Medicare Payments to Physicians Under the End Stage Renal Disease Program. GAO/HRD-85-14, Feb. 1, 1985.

- Information Requirements for Evaluating the Impacts of Medicare Prospective Payment on Post-Hospital Long-Term Care Services: Preliminary Report. GAO/PEMD-85-8, Feb. 21, 1985.

While evaluation is an obvious necessity for homecare, the requirements should not be any different from those mandated for other health and social areas. All the evaluation literature exhibits the same difficulties in arriving at conclusions that are based upon accurate, reliable, and valid data from which generalizations can be made with confidence. Most evaluation studies have problems relating the process of care to outcomes. Furthermore, all evaluation suffers from the constant change taking place in the health care service delivery system. In a discussion of the social imperatives of medical research, Eisenberg (1977) poignantly stated that "what appears to be true in the light of today's evidence proves false by tomorrow's."

References

American Association of Retired Persons. 1984. *A handbook about care in the home*. Washington, DC.

Applebaum, R., F. Seidl, and C. Austin. 1980. The Wisconsin Community Care Organization: preliminary findings from the Milwaukee experiment. *The Gerontologist* 20(3):350-355.

Balinsky, W., and S. Rehman. 1984. Home health care: a comparative analysis of hospital based and community based agency patients. *Home Health Care Services Quarterly* 5(1):45-60.

Benjamin, A.E. 1986. Determinants of state variations in home health utilization and expenditures under Medicare. *Medical Care* 24:535-547.

Bluestone, E.M. 1954. The principles and practice of homecare. *Journal of the American Medical Association* 155:1379-1382.

Blum, H.L. 1974. Evaluating health care. *Medical Care* 12(12):999-1011.

Branch, L.G., and N.E. Stuart. 1984. A five year history of targeting home care services to prevent institutionalization. *The Gerontologist* 24(4):387-391.

Bregman, A. 1980. Living with progressive childhood illness: parental management of neuromuscular disease. *Social Work in Health Care* 5(4):387-408.

Brickner, P.W. 1981. Testimony on S.234 before Senate Committee on Labor and Human Resources. Washington, DC (4 March).

Coe, M.F., A. Wilkinson, and P. Patterson. 1986. *Depending at discharge: impact of DRGs final report*. Beaverton, OR: Northwest Oregon Health Systems (May).

Combs-Orme, J. Reis, and L.D. Ward. 1985. Effectiveness of home visits by public health nurses in maternal and child health: an empirical review. *Public Health Reports* 100(5):490-499.

Davidson, S.V. 1978. Community nursing care evaluation. *Family and Community Health* 1(1):37-55.

Day, S.R. 1984. Measuring utilization and impact of home care services: a systems model approach for cost effectiveness. *Home Health Care Services Quarterly* 5(2):5-24.

Department of Health and Human Services. National Center for Health Statistics. 1979. *Long term care minimum data set*. Report of the Technical Consultant Panel to the National Committee on Vital and Health Statistics. Washington, DC: Government Printing Office.

Detsky, A.S., J.R. McLaughlin, H.B. Abrams et al. 1986. A cost-utility analysis of the home parenteral nutrition program at Toronto General Hospital: 1970-1982. *Journal of Parenteral and Enteral Nutrition* 10(1):49-57.

Eggert, G.M., J.E. Bowlyow, and C.W. Nichols. 1980. Gaining control of the long-term care system: first returns from the ACCESS experiment. *The Gerontologist* 20(3):356-363.

Eisenberg, L. 1977. The social imperative of medical research. *Science* 198:1105-1110.

Elinson, J. 1972. Methods of sociomedical research in *Handbook of medical sociology*, edited by H.E. Frieman, S. Levine, and L.G. Reeder. Englewood Cliffs, NJ: Prentice Hall.

Fashimpar, G.A. 1985. A manual for the administration, scoring, and interpretation of the Homemaker-Home Health Aide Program Evaluation Questionnaire. *Home Health Care Services Quarterly* 6(1):65-84.

Gaumer, G.L., H. Birnbaum, F. Pratter, et al. 1986. Impact of the New York Long-Term Home Health Care Program. *Medical Care* 24:641-653.

Greer, D.S., V. Mor, J.N. Morris, et al. 1986. An alternative in terminal care: results of the National Hospice Study. *Journal of Chronic Disease* 39(1):9-26.

Harris, L.F., T.F. Buckle, and F.L. Coffey, Jr. 1986. Intravenous antibiotics at home. *Southern Medical Journal* 79(2):193-196.

Haug, M.R. 1985. Home care for the ill elderly--who benefits *American Journal of Public Health* 75:127-128.

Health Systems Agency of New York City. 1985. *Study of community based long-term care*. New York (June).

Hedrick, S.C. and T.S. Inui. 1986. The effectiveness and cost of home care: An information synthesis. *Health Services Research* 20(6):851-880 (Part 2).

Hicks, B., H. Raisz, J. Segal, et al. 1981. The Triage experiment in coordinated care for the elderly. *American Journal of Public Health* 71:991-1003.

Holman, M. 1986. Hospice patients without caregivers. *American Journal of Hospice Care* 3(3):19-26.

Home Health Journal. 1986. Quality Assurance Act could "watch" HHAs. 7(3):4,8.

Hopper, S.V., J.P. Miller, C. Birge, et al. 1984. A randomized study of the impact of home health aides on diabetic control and utilization patterns. *American Journal of Public Health* 74:600-602.

House Subcommittee on Health and Long Term Care. 1985. *Building a long term care policy: home care data and implications*. Washington, DC: Government Printing Office. Comm. Pub. No. 98-484.

Hughes, S.L. 1985. Apples and oranges? A review of community based long term care. *Health Services Research* 20(4):461-488.

Hughes, S.L., D.S. Cordray, and V.A. Spiker. 1984. Evaluation of a long term home care program. *Medical Care* 22:460-475.

Kahan, J., B. Kemp, F.R. Staples, et al. 1985. Decreasing the burden in families caring for a relative with a dementing illness. *Journal of the American Geriatrics Society* 33(10):664-670.

Kieffer, S.E., and D.S. Wakefield. 1986. The availability of primary caregivers: an emerging problem. *American Journal of Hospice Care* 3(3):14-18.

Kleffel, D., and E. Wilson. 1975. *Evaluation handbook for home health agencies*. Washington, DC: Government Printing Office. Pub. No. HSA 76-3003.

Kramer, A.M., P.W. Shaughnessy, and M.L. Pettigrew. 1985. Cost effectiveness implications based on a comparison of nursing home and home health case mix. *Health Services Research* 20(4):387-405.

Liang, M.H., A.J. Partridge, M.G. Larson, et al. 1984. Evaluation of comprehensive rehabilitation services for elderly homebound patients with arthritis and orthopedic disability. *Arthritis and Rheumatism* 27(3):258-266.

Locker, D., B. Rao, and J.M. Weddell. 1984. Evaluating community care for the mentally handicapped adult: a comparison of hostel, home and hospital care. *Journal of Mental Deficiency Research* 28(9):189-198.

Lurie, E., M.T. Chan, K. Kasch, et al. 1985. Identifying control subjects through referral. Presentation at a meeting of the Gerontological Society of America, New Orleans, LA (23 Nov.).

McCusker, J. 1984. Development of scales to measure satisfaction and preferences regarding long-term and terminal care. *Medical Care* 22(5):476-493.

Meiners, M.R., and R.M. Coffey. 1985. Hospital DRGs and the need for long term care services: an empirical analysis. *Health Services Research* 20(3):359-384.

Michnich, M.E., S.M. Shortell, and W.C. Richardson. 1981. Program evaluation: resource for decision making. *Health Care Management Review* 6(3):25-35.

Miller, S.C. 1986. *Documentation for home health care: a record management handbook.* Chicago: American Medical Record Association.

Nassif, J.Z. 1985. *The home health care solution.* New York: Harper and Row Publications.

Pai, S., S.M. Channabasavanna, Nagarajaiah, et al. 1985. Home care for chronic mental illness in Bangalore: an experiment in the presentation of repeated hospitalization. *British Journal of Psychiatry* 147(8):175-179.

Powers, J.S., and C. Burger. 1985. Home health care vs.nursing home care for the elderly. *Journal of the Tennessee Medical Association* 78(4):227-230.

Rogatz, P. 1985. Home health care: some social and economic considerations. *Home Healthcare Nurse* 3(1):38-43.

Rogatz, P., and G. Crocetti. 1958. Home care programs--their impact on the hospital's role in medical care. *American Journal of Public Health* 48:1125-1133.

Scharlach, A., and C. Frenzel. 1986. An evaluation of institution based respite care. *The Gerontologist* 26(1):77-82.

Skellie, F.A., and R.E. Coan. 1980. Community-based long-term care mortality:

preliminary findings of Georgia's Alternative Health Services project. *The Gerontologist* 20(3):372-379.

Skellie, F.A., G.M. Mobley, and R.E. Coan. 1982. Cost-effectiveness of community based long term care: current findings of Georgia's Alternative Health Services project. *American Journal of Public Health* 72:353-358.

Spiegel, A.D., and B. Backhaut. 1980. *Curing and caring.* Jamaica, NY: SP Publications.

Suchman, E.A. 1967. *Evaluation research. Principles and practice in public service and social action programs.* New York: Russell Sage Foundation.

Wade, D.T., C.E. Skilbeck, R. Langston-Hewer, et al. 1985. Controlled trial of a home care service for acute stroke patients. *The Lancet* 1(8424):323-326.

Warhola, C.F.R. Aug. 1980. *Planning for home health services. A resource handbook.* Washington, DC: Government Printing Office. Pub. No. 80-14017.

Wasson, W., A. Ripeckyj, L.W. Lazarus, et al. 1984. Home evaluation of psychiatrically impaired elderly: process and outcome. *The Gerontologist* 24(3):238-242.

Weckwerth, V.E. 1969. On evaluation: a tool or a tyranny. Minneapolis: Systems Development Project, University of Minnesota.

Wholey, J.S., J.W. Scanlon, H.G. Duffy, et al. 1970. *Federal evaluation policy. Analyzing the effects of public programs.* Washington, DC: The Urban Institute.

Wolock, I., E. Schlesinger, M. Dinerman, et al. 1985. The posthospital needs of patients: a follow-up study. Presentation at annual meeting of the American Public Health Association, Washington, DC (20 Nov.).

Zimmer, J.G., A. Groth-Juncker, and J. McCusker. 1985. A randomized controlled study of a home health care team. *American Journal of Public Health* 75:134-141.

Chapter 12

The Future of Homecare
Trends, Issues and Dilemmas

While considering trends, issues and dilemmas, the philosophical concepts associated with homecare should be kept in mind. Homecare services place emphasis upon the dignity and independence of the individual and homecare is recognized as an effective and economical alternative to unnecessary institutionalization. Programs have existed in the U.S. since the last quarter of the eighteenth century aiming to prevent, postpone and limit the need for institutionalization while enabling patients to remain independent at home.

Trends

Early and Developing Homecare Patterns

When the Boston Dispensary set up its homecare program in 1796, the policy was to "keep them out of the hospital" (Ryder 1967,1). Welfare or charity for the poor was the rationale. Much later, with the establishment of the Montefiore Hospital extramural homecare program in 1947, the pattern was to "get them out of the hospital." A rationale emphasized moving those inappropriately admitted to the hospital into homecare. About 1966, as Medicare was implemented, the policy became "give the patient the kind of care he needs." Reasoning related to the social insurance aspects of the Medicare program.

Today, all the policies and rationales blend together into a pattern to keep people out of the hospital in the first place, to seek early discharge to alternative care modes, and to provide health and social/personal care needs at home.

Current Patterns

Utilization and Expenditures. Using 1976 data on 7.5 million hospitalrelated episodes of illness, the General Accounting Office (GAO 1986) found that hospital care followed by homecare accounted for 5.2 percent of the episodes, with an average hospital stay of 22.9 days, and an average charge per episode of $4,610. Of course, today with the PPS/DRG payment plan, the length of stay will be shorter and the cost higher.

Medicare reimbursements for homecare services rose sharply from 1968 to 1980 with an average annual compound rate of 21.4 percent. Between 1982 and 1983 benefit payment grew by 31.4 percent and by 22.8 percent from 1983 to 1984. About $1.9 billion was spent in 1984 for Medicare homecare services (GAO 1986). A National Association for Home Care press release (NAHC 1986a) approximated total home health care 1985 expenditures at $10 billion, with growth to $25 billion by 1995.

Increased utilization and expenditures may also be related to the trend toward a more sophisticated technical level of care being rendered to patients in their own homes. Intravenous infusions for nutritional and/or chemotherapy treatment, respiratory therapy, and the rental and/or purchase of durable medical equipment are now common homecare services.

Growth of Home Health Agencies. From December 1983 to December 1985, the total number of Medicare certified home health agencies (HHAs) jumped from 4,258 to 5,964--an increase of 40 percent in the two years (Sandrick 1986). Hospital-based HHAs showed the greatest growth going from 579 to 1,260--up 118 percent. Sandrick also reported that more than 90 percent of the nation's Blue Cross/Blue Shield plans offer homecare; that of companies with 25 to 499 employees that had health insurance policies written between 1979 and 1984, 67,000 of the 99,000 employees were covered for homecare services; and that a survey of health maintenance organizations (HMOs) revealed that 17 percent already own HHAs, and that 60 percent are considering establishing homecare units.

Managed Care and Homecare. Prepaid health care plans currently expend 1 to 3 percent on homecare services with an anticipated increase to 5 to 10 percent in the next five years (Firshein 1986). Additionally, these organizations are considering establishing their own HHAs to serve their enrollees. Ernst & Whinney (1986) use the term "managed care" to include HMOs, PPOs (Preferred Provider Organizations), EPOs (Employer and/or Employee Provider Organizations), and Utilization Managed Insurance Products (similar to traditional insurance products).

These managed care entities seek provider arrangements with cost effective hospitals, home health agencies and physicians while taking advantage of the marketplace dynamics.

A Trend to Corporatization. In a review of the increasing opportunity in outside-of-hospital services, Stoesz (1986) listed 45 U.S. corporations in the health care industry with $10 million+ revenues in 1983/1984. Five companies specializing in homecare had income ranging from $13.8 million to $1.7 billion, with growth ranging from 14.6 to 121 percent. However,

Stoesz did note that the business approach could result in homecare providers "dumping" or "transferring" patients unable to pay for the services into publicly funded units.

Schutzer (1985) discussed the impact of DRGs and asked: "Will the Hospital Cost Squeeze Produce an Investor's Bonanza?" He answered in the affirmative and cited examples of home health care stocks for the 1990s adding a prediction that "homecare exotics could flourish."

In a cautionary vein, Pyles and Philip (1985) and Flanagan (1985) reviewed legal aspects of corporate joint ventures. Antitrust violations received particular emphasis.

Future Patterns

Joseph A. Califano, Jr. (1986), Health, Education and Welfare Secretary from 1977 to 1979, addressed the future of health care in this nation. "The revolution in the American way of health will be as profound and turbulent as any economic and social upheaval our nation has experienced. At stake are not only billions of dollars but who lives, who dies--and who decides." Califano pointed out "millions of dollars can be saved, and pointless anguish avoided by using home health and hospice care and by promoting healthier life styles . . . Medical technology makes it possible to provide at home . . . diagnosis and treatment that once could be delivered only in a hospital."

In discussing technological advances, Shaw (1985) gazed into the crystal ball of homecare high technology envisioning homecare for people who received artificial organs; mobile and home surgeries; telecommunications and video for homecare use; monitoring of vital signs and body chemicals with results transmitted to central bases; documentation of homecare therapy via video cameras in the home; and home robotics being used for medication reminders, delivery methods, compliance monitoring, IV adjustments, automated massage, and environmental control.

Other factors contributing to homecare growth include demographic trends producing an older population, cost-effectiveness activities and increased public demand for homecare services. Halamandaris (1985a) predicted that "homecare will grow at a meteoric rate through the end of this century" and develop "a cafeteria-style" system geared to ability to pay.

Medical Growing Pains. Turbo's (1986) cover story in *Medical World News* discussed the growing pains encountered by home health care from a medical standpoint. Problems related to the lack of physician awareness about homecare services, case management and coordination difficulties, the inroads of proprietary firms aggressively marketing durable medical equipment and services, and the pressures of the PPS/DRG plan to discharge earlier. "Despite these problems, home health care appears to be here to stay, and some observers believe physicians will increasingly rely on it as they become more familiar with available services."

Future Need for Homecare. In a current report on Americans needing homecare, Fellner (1986) reported on the types of help required by people with chronic health problems who live outside of institutions. Children, young adults, adults and the elderly were included in the calculations with the following resultant rates per 1,000 for those needing help: 6-17 years, 2.6; 18-44 years, 4.7; 45-64 years, 40.0; 65-74 years, 89.0; 75-84 years, 189.0; and 85+ years, 419.0. These rates take on greater importance when consideration is given to the Census Bureau projection that by 2050 the elderly will comprise 16 to 30 percent of the U.S. population. Furthermore, the 85+ group is expected to continue to show rapid growth surges. Fellner (1986,4) concluded that "Homecare is now considered as an alternative or supplement to institutionalization."

Cost Containment Peril. Despite the forecasts of current and future growth trends, the emphasis upon cost containment is also imperiling the homecare industry. Proposed cuts in Medicare are called "devastating," causing homecare to be in "jeopardy" (*Medical World News* 1985). In testimony before the House Select Committee on Aging, Florida's Governor Robert Graham said that "budget cuts to community and home-based services will drive the elderly back into hospitals and nursing homes at even higher medical costs." At the same hearing, Committee Chairman Congressman Edward R. Roybal stated that he was also concerned about sound fiscal policies but "I draw the line when it comes to hurting people -- particularly the vulnerable elderly" (*Medical World News* 1985).

Impact of Trends

Data leads to the assumption that the homecare industry will continue to show increased utilization and expenditures with a proliferation of home health agencies and managed care organizations. At the same time, the need for homecare services will keep track with the expansion. However, a "Catch 22" evolves as the current PPS/DRG reimbursement plan dramatically stimulates the need for homecare, while reimbursement to HHAs is being cut by at least five percent according to homecare industry analysts (*Medical World News* 1985). Obviously, multifaceted issues arise in this situation.

Issues

Homecare is affected just as is every other segment of the health care delivery system by the impact of the PPS/DRG payment plan. Spiegel and Kavaler (1986) present a comprehensive picture of issues generated by cost containment initiatives including those directly related to homecare services. Reductions in length of stay at facilities, lower occupancy rates and fewer admissions have combined to create pressing issues for the homecare industry.

Quicker and Sicker

A major issue is the proposition that elderly hospital patients are being discharged "quicker and sicker" to homecare services or other alternatives. Marosy (1985) told a House Select Committee on Aging about federal government cost containment policies pushing frail older people into a "No Care Zone." Since the Medicare program tends to restrict reimbursement to medical related services, the patient who needs social and/or personal care may be unable to secure that care. In fact, Azzarto (1986) noted the "medicalization" of the problems of the elderly. Health care providers, particularly physicians, are creatively turning social/personal needs into medical needs in order to provide care where the individual would not otherwise receive help. According to Azzarto, "One need only look at Medicare, which will pay for skilled nursing but not custodial care, to realize that concerns about illness overshadow those related to the quality of life in the eyes of policymakers."

Saving Money or Lives

A newspaper editorial (*Star-Ledger* 1986a) gave an overdue welcome to the "New Age of Cost-Effective Medicine" and praised the healthy competition and the projected better medical treatment at lower cost. In contrast, the local medical society lamented the eclipse of the Golden Age of Medicine into the economic realities of cost containment actions by the government, by third-party payers, by employers, and by consumers; all clamoring for a better return on their health care dollars.

Reasoning of this nature raises the basic issue of when saving dollars takes precedence over the health care an individual may need. Does the physician not order certain diagnostic tests because they are too costly? Does an individual with a poor prognosis receive fewer therapeutic interventions because there is less hope for recovery? Do people get discharged "quicker and sicker" because the hospital loses money if they overstay the guidelines? Does the physician become a "product line manager" instead of a "healer"? Smith (1986) discussed ethical, economic, and professional issues in home health care relating to hospital pharmacy services. He concluded that the resolution of these issues should consider how best the needs of the patient can be met, since that is the societal purpose of the professional. That resolution may not be universally accepted and the ethical, economic, and professional issues are not idle puzzlements within the health care cost containment environment. There are many ways to look at the problems.

Vantage Viewpoints

Homecare is much more than a business and the viewpoints of the self-interests of various groups raises pertinent homecare policy issues. Families can be concerned with training and emotional support to assist a loved one's recovery. Physicians may see homecare as a way to keep their professional commitment to provide a continuum of care. To administrators, homecare fills a community need and accomplishes the institution's mission in the face of the realities of reimbursement. Patients in need of care may see homecare as their safety net. Within these disparate vantage points, the issues are manifold and deal with areas such as professional ethics, community need assessment, business management, family support and hands-on therapy. However, almost all of the issues are in turn linked to the federal government's activities, and particularly those of the Health Care Financing Administration (HCFA), in cost containment.

Government Actions Initiating Issues

Passage of the Balanced Budget and Emergency Deficit Reduction Act (PL 99-177), also known as the Gramm-Rudman-Hollings Act, resulted in HCFA applying automatic across-the-board spending cuts of 1 percent with increases to 2 percent each subsequent year to home health care expenditures. Savings of $300 million were projected for 1986 with an additional $74.5 million savings in Medicare administrative expenses (Livengood 1986). Even though the U.S. Supreme Court declared the Gramm-Rudman-Hollings Act unconstitutional in a July 7, 1986 decision, members of Congress indicated their intentions to rectify the constitutional shortcomings to achieve a balanced federal budget.

Dismantling of Homecare Benefits. In a report prepared for the House Select Committee on Aging by the NAHC, it was charged that the Reagan administration "has set about the step-by-step dismantling" of the Medicare program's home health benefit (McIlrath 1986). Another article on the NAHC report (*Home Health Journal* 1986a) commented: "The administrative restrictions placed on homecare providers are punitive. They are designed to restrict the statutory Medicare benefit, to force providers out of business or to force them to subsidize Medicare with revenue raised from private contributions of Medicare patients."

Initiatives by HCFA raise issues of legality and governmental authority. At a hearing convened by Senator Bill Bradley (*Star-Ledger* 1986b), he heard about actions by HCFA intending to restrict eligibility for homecare benefits under Medicare. Senator Bradley said that HCFA has been circumventing home health care requirements. HCFA was accused of "rewriting" of the Medicare laws at a meeting of the Home Health Agency Assembly of New Jersey (Whitlow 1985). Representing the American Federation of Home Health Agencies (AFHHA), Thietten (1986) wrote to the Congressional appropriations committee members about the "onslaught of precipitous regulatory HCFA changes" resulting in increased denials of coverage and reductions in reimbursements.

A Senate Special Committee on Aging staff report (1985; *Star-Ledger* 1986c) highlighted a "growing number of inappropriate and perhaps even illegal denials of coverage by Medicare." Medicare denials of homecare claims soared from 18,121 at the end of 1983 to 47,855 in the first quarter of 1986. Reasons for the denials by the Medicare fiscal intermediaries usually had to do with discrepancies in the interpretation of what constitutes skilled care and the requirements for homebound status.

To add further insult to injury, the HHAs experienced considerable delay in actually collecting their money from the fiscal intermediaries. In a joint statement at the Senate oversight hearing on the Prompt Payment Act (PL 97-177), the National Association of Medical Equipment Suppliers (NAMES) and the AFHHA (Antone and Thietten 1986) complained strongly about the significant reimbursement delays in excess of 120 days and the resultant confusion for beneficiaries, carriers, and suppliers alike. They noted that Blue Cross/Blue Shield owed $4.9 billion to Medicare Part A and Part B providers, an 88 percent increase over 1985's backlog. Furthermore, the ensuing retroactive denials are causing HHAs to lose their eligibility for Periodic Interim Payments (PIP) which gave them regularly scheduled reimbursements and a steady cash flow. It was also noted that HCFA takes the position that the Prompt Payment Act does not apply to Medicare. NAMES and AFHHA are petitioning Congress for clarification and asking that HCFA not be allowed to violate the law.

Basically, HCFA has been accused of not meeting the intent of the Congress in the Medicare legislation and specifically as the law applies to homecare services.

Constancy of Homecare Issues

At a series of national regional hearings on homecare (Department of Health, Education and Welfare 1976), 514 individuals testified in person, and 725 written statements and exhibits were submitted. Analysis showed remarkable consensus on most issues at that time:

Issue	Yes	No
Need broader range of services	415	0
Expand delivery capacity	206	6
Broaden the eligibility	273	1
Provide a health/social service mix	290	0
Increase/improve quality assurance/standards	229	5
Unified national policy and definitions needed	154	0
Frustration with federal programs complexity	152	0
Proprietary agency participation in federal programs	72	0

Although the testimony achieved remarkable consensus on the issues, there was little agreement on the solutions. Interestingly, most of the issues are still unresolved. Note that the listing of issues was compiled before the tremendous impact of cost containment and the aftermath of the PPS/DRG reimbursement system.

Is A National Homecare Policy Missing?

A report of the House Subcommittee on Health and Long-term Care (1985,iii) by the Chairman, Congressman Claude Pepper, remarked that this was the fifth report in 10 years that had recommended the establishment of a national policy with respect to homecare. In a policy perspective on in-home health care services, Ramage (1985) stated the situation clearly:

> Lack of a current national policy on home health care with appropriate and adequate funding patterns impacts on the delivery of comprehensive care at home ... The fragmented irrational mix of funding mechanisms and regulations promotes disorder, lack of coordination, and further fragmentation. A proposal to expand inhome health care services that are comprehensive, coordinated, beneficial, accessible, and effective in costs is worthy of the time required of the public and private sectors to effect legislation and implementation.

Suggested Resolutions

Although Trager (1984,63) testified at a House Subcommittee on Health and Long-term Care Committee hearing on the need for a national long-term care policy, she addressed herself to homecare reform. Nine directions for action on care based in the community were enumerated:

1. A rational rearrangement of the present confusion in state and federal funding sources and eligibility requirements.

2. Planned development of homecare services to achieve equity of access and service range.

3. Realistic changes in home health services certification and eligibility requirements to better match needs and clients.

4. Requirement that all home health services provide paraprofessional care with activities of daily living and environmental maintenance.

5. Redefinition of the part-time intermittent care concept to allow for variation in the intensity of need.

6. An aggressive approach in preventive care in high-risk groups including outreach, health supervision, and health education.

7. Emphasis on hospital discharge planning with special attention to care in the community.

8. Implementation of the concept of the community network using adult day care, meal service, special needs transportation, and electronic security and monitoring devices.

9. Attention to the range of innovative housing arrangements to increase the feasibility of homecare planning.

In a comprehensive 32-page report, NAHC (1985) detailed its position on a host of issues aimed toward the development of a national homecare policy. Organized into six sections, the report begins with a series of facts about the homecare situation in America within the health care delivery system.

Section two contains 12 policy recommendations relating to areas such as gaps in care, using homecare as a cost containment strategy, and elucidating the advantages of alternative (prospective) forms of reimbursement.

Section three provides six recommendations to increase the availability of homecare services through the private sector.

Eighteen recommendations for legislative changes for consideration by Congress are included in the fourth section.

Descriptions of 22 administrative and regulatory impediments limiting the delivery of appropriate and cost-effective homecare services are enumerated in the fifth section. A list is given of a series of administrative changes made in the form of new guidelines to intermediary insurance companies which administer the Medicare program on behalf of the government. Taken together, these seemingly innocuous clarifications constitute a major diminution of the already narrow Medicare home health benefit.

In the last section of the report, six judicial interventions are described. These are issues that have not been resolved in negotiations with either intermediaries or HHS. As a last resort on matters of crucial concern, litigation has been brought to protect the vital interests of Medicare beneficiaries.

For each of the problems, NAHC presents the issue(s), follows with their position, and ends with the rationale for taking that stand. If HHS/HCFA or other governmental agencies are not responsive to the recommendations, NAHC is prepared to seek redress through regulatory clarification, Congressional support, legislative action, litigation, or other appropriate means.

Exhibit 12-1 illustrates NAHC's position on a sampling of the more than 60 issues addressed in this blueprint for action on a national homecare policy.

Dilemmas

Homecare trends continue to exhibit rapid growth and utilization patterns and that growth is projected into the future. However, at the same time the emphasis on cost containment will also remain as a constant trend. The conflict between use and expenditures has created numerous issues, mainly linked to the aftermath of the implementation of the Medicare PPS/DRG reimbursement scheme. In fact, the PPS/DRG plan may be at the crux of the emerging dilemmas.

Dilemmas Linked to PPS/DRG

In response to a Congressional recommendation that HHS funds be withheld until the PPS/DRG impact report is delivered to Congress, the GAO (1986) declared that efforts to evaluate Medicare PPS effects are insufficient. That GAO investigation concluded that, "HHS has not demonstrated--and does not plan to produce information that can validly demonstrate--whether the changes it does measure are due to the prospective payment system, and what effects, if any, the system had on Medicare beneficiaries and/or posthospital services" (GAO, 1986,48).

Five questions were identified in relation to PPS/DRGs: patient condition at discharge; use of post-hospital subacute services; expenditures for

Exhibit 12-1 Examples of NAHC's Position on Various Homecare Issues

HHS/HCFA Circumvention of the Regulatory Process -- HHS/HCFA must not be allowed to use written or verbal policy directives and manual issuances to accomplish substantive changes in the Medicare program. HHS/HCFA must not be allowed to promulgate regulations which do not include the projected impact on small business. HHS/HCFA must not be allowed to change rules/guidelines at will and apply them retroactively.

NAHC will seek appropriate changes in the Federal Administrative Procedures Act and urge Congress to use prospective implementation dates in any legislation affecting home health.

Application of the "Intermittent Care" Requirement -- NAHC supports the reintroduction of legislation like that proposed in the last Congressional session defining "intermittent care."

Application of the "Homebound" Requirement -- NAHC will monitor the administration of the homebound requirement by HCFA and its intermediaries to ensure consistent and nonrestrictive application of the current HIM-11 guideline, and will seek regulatory or legislative clarifications of this requirement, if necessary.

Application of the "Skilled Nursing" Requirement -- NAHC believes intermediaries should apply the skilled nursing requirement in a consistent manner and in keeping with accepted clinical standards. NAHC believes that there should be coordination between State Nurse Practice Acts and the HCFA guidelines defining skilled nursing. NAHC will review these Acts and other national models in more detail and make recommendations to HCFA and Congress, as appropriate.

Lack of Specificity in Denial Notices -- The regulation should be changed to (a) require that either the denial notice and/or appropriate accompanying papers from the fiscal intermediary must specify each visit denied and the specific reason for each visit denial; (b) require that denial notice be sent to HHAs and patients in a timely manner, and in understandable language; and (c) require that HHAs get notification of denials prior to or, at a minimum, simultaneous with notification to patients.

Technical Denials -- The "technical denial" should be abolished.

[A technical denial is a denial of a visit based on the FI's determination that the visit failed to meet a statutory or regulatory requirement, other than medical necessity.]

Appellate Rights of Provider -- HHAs should be given the right to appeal directly any claim denial, regardless of the basis of the denial.

Ability of Beneficiaries to Designate HHA Employees as Representatives in the Claims Appeal Process -- The Section 257-A [prohibiting HHA employee representation] issuance is illegal on a constitutional basis, in terms of lack of promulgation through the Federal Administrative Procedure Act process, and in terms of existing regulation allowing beneficiaries to designate representatives. On March 26, 1984, NAHC filed a lawsuit to contest the issuance (NAHC, et al. v. Heckler, Civil Action No. 84-0957, U.S.D.C., District of Columbia).

Exhibit 12-1 continued

Removal of Waiver of Liability Provision -- NAHC opposes the elimination of the waiver presumption and believes that HCFA should retract this proposal. NAHC opposes this proposed change but supports the removal of presumptive status for new HHAs. NAHC believes the permissible rate of error should be changed back to 5 percent from 2.5 percent. [This waiver allows HHAs to be reimbursed for Medicare services provided in good faith to individuals later determined to be ineligible.]

Design and Implementation of a System of Ten or Fewer Intermediaries for Home Health Agencies -- NAHC supports the acceleration of the implementation of a system of ten or fewer fiscal intermediaries by HCFA.

Alternative Forms of Reimbursement for Home Health Agencies -- Demonstration projects should be conducted and evaluated before any prospective payment system is put into place for HHAs. Any PPS should be scientifically valid; independently evaluated by experts; based on final data, not preliminary results; consider any valid and reliable results of the impact of the Medicare hospital DRG system, which won't be fully phased in until 1987; and should maintain at least the current levels of quality of care.

Cost Caps -- The sum allowable should be in the aggregate and not applied independently [HCFA regulations limit cost per discipline rather than in the aggregate.]

Medical Coinsurance for Durable Medical Equipment -- NAHC opposed this proposal and continues to oppose any other form of coinsurance which would force Medicare beneficiaries to pay more out-of-pocket costs for their health care. NAHC will urge Congress to mandate a GAO study of the newly enacted 20 percent coinsurance provision; a cost comparison of providing DME under Part A vs. Part B; and with a potential sunset requirement for Section 2321 based on the results of the study. [Copayments for Medicare/Medicaid patients are also opposed.]

Approval of Technologies for Homecare Coverage -- NAHC believes that as long as a technology has the necessary approval from the Food and Drug Administration (or PHS, as appropriate) and is prescribed for use at home pursuant to a physician's order, the skilled and/or supportive services necessary to administer (or train others to administer) the technology should be Medicare Part A reimburseable, and the necessary supplies and equipment should be Medicare reimburseable.

Proper Interpretation of the Anti-fraud and Abuse Sections of the Social Security Act -- NAHC will meet with the HHS Inspector General's staff to discuss joint ventures and other contractual arrangements among health care entities and suppliers of medical supplies and equipment and the trend toward exclusive and semiexclusive referral arrangements. The very broad language of the criminal provisions of the statute as applied to the Medicare program are of concern to the IG's staff as well as to the healthcare industry, since there are no clear guidelines for behavior nor clearcut bases for successful prosecutions.

Intermediate Sanctions for Home Health Agencies Prior to Termination from Medicare Program -- NAHC will work with HCFA to establish an appropriate mechanism to provide interim sanctions for HHAs found not to be in compliance to avoid abrupt prehearing terminations. If necessary, NAHC will seek a legislative resolution to this problem.

Exhibit 12-1 continued

Lack of Medicare Certification Requirement for HMOs -- NAHC believes the regulations should require any HMO providing homecare from in-house sources to be required to meet the Medicare HHA conditions of participation as part of the HMO's certification process (not that the HMO's HHA would have to be a separately certified HHA). If the regulations are not so amended, corrective legislation should be pursued.

Qualifications of Home Health Agency Administrators -- Expanded and specific minimum mandatory standards should be developed by NAHC for discussion with HCFA. The goal of the standards should be to ensure that the person administering the HHA has the skills and experience necessary to run the agency and maintains these skills on an ongoing basis. This should include exploration of the feasibility of a licensure program for administration and a certification program.

State Licensure and Regulation of Home Care -- NAHC will analyze existing state laws, work with state homecare associations to develop model laws, and prepare a strategy for advocating state adoption of the model laws. This model law will provide guidance to the states re HHA licensure, regulations and enforcement of the law to ensure the quality of homecare services.

Need for Supervision and Training Requirements for Homemaker-Home Health Aides -- Both the Social Services Block Grant program (Title XX) and the Older Americans Act (Title III-B) should have at least the same federal minimum mandatory training and supervision requirements for H-HHAs and personal care givers.

Individuals as Providers: Case Management and Brokering of Home Care Services -- NAHC opposes subcontracting by either federal or state governments with individuals for the direct provision of homecare services. NAHC also objects to the practice of individuals rendering H-HHA care on their own, through independent solicitation or employment agencies, where there are inadequate training, supervision and liability safeguards. NAHC will work to amend the SSBG (Title XX), OAA (Title III-B), and state laws to rectify this problem.

NAHC favors and supports the following:

- Greater homecare coverage in major medical plans.

- Development and marketing of long term care insurance.

- Expanding the concept of IRAs to long term care.

- Tax incentives for families who provide long term care.

- Greater coverage of homecare in collective bargaining contracts between labor and management.

- Use of home equity conversion to fund homecare.

- Expansion of programs to provide homecare coverage for mothers and children.

- Expansion of homecare in the Veterans Administration services.

- Funding of home health agencies to provide care to American Indians and Alaskan natives.

Exhibit 12-1 continued

- Creation of a nutritional services homecare benefit.
- Expansion of the basic Medicaid minimum coverage for homecare.
- Physician involvement in homecare services.

Source: National Association for Home Care. 1985. *Toward a national homecare policy. Blueprint for action.* Washington, DC (Jan.).

those services; access to those services; and the quality of care delivered in those services (GAO, 1986,2). Relevance of those PPS/DRG questions for homecare services are apparent and have been raised constantly as dilemmas by representatives of the industry.

Medicare Dilemmas and Reforms

With the questions raised about Medicare's reimbursement plan and the lengthy list of complaints engendered, it naturally follows that there should be talk about reforming Medicare to resolve the dilemmas. Dr. William Roper, the new HCFA administrator, "cited problems with the home health benefit as an example of the need for fundamental changes in the Medicare program" (*Home Health Journal* 1986b). Specifically, Dr. Roper mentioned the disputes over the definition of intermittent care by Medicare fiscal intermediaries as a strong argument for reform. Acknowledging homecare industry concerns about HCFA's efforts to dismantle home health benefits and to limit the availability of homecare services, Dr. Roper also cited the sharp cost increases in the Medicare home health benefits. Dr. Roper said he would push strongly for a fixed price capitation system for Medicare acceptable to both providers and beneficiaries.

In a sweeping study of Medicare by Harvard University researchers (Blumenthal, Schlesinger, Drumheller, et al. 1986; Pear 1986), 40 proposals were made for changes over the next 10 to 15 years. Recommendations affected the existing dilemmas and the future of the Medicare program.

Reforms directly affecting beneficiaries included decreased copayments and increased premiums; premiums adjusted to the ability to pay; and expansion of coverage for long-term care and chronic illness, "especially of home health care and mental health services"; improvement of primary care; and administrative simplification.

Reforms in payment of physicians included paying doctors according to a relative value scale (RVS); setting a target budget for total expenditures for physicians' services; requiring physicians to accept Medicare's fee as full payment; and encouraging physicians to participate in prepaid health care organizations.

Reforms in payment of hospitals included prospectively set target budgets for hospitals; requiring all payers to use the same method for paying for care; setting up systems to cover uninsured patients; and providing access to hospital care for uninsured patients.

Reforms related to prepaid health care included allowing HMOs to recruit up to 75 percent of their members from the Medicare population; providing beneficiaries with easily understandable information about the benefit packages and costs of participating HMOs; and monitoring of HMO performance by Medicare.

These Medicare reform researchers declared that "the financial impact of our proposals on Medicare expenditures in the year 2000 could range from a net savings to a net cost of approximately $3 billion (1985 dollars) depending on the assumptions used" (Blumenthal, Schlesinger, Drumheller, et al. 1986).

Long-term Care Dilemmas

Usually, discussions of long-term care include mention of homecare as a modality to be considered in the scope of treatment and/or care regimens. A GAO (1986,172) report defined long-term care as follows: "Health care or related personal care services provided on a sustained basis to individuals whose functional capacities are chronically impaired. The range of services cover a continuum of care provided in home or institutional settings including personal care assistance, adult day care and foster care, and skilled nursing care provided by home health agencies and in nursing homes."

Using that definition, it is obvious that homecare has strong direct links to long-term care activities. Part of the dilemma can be noted by the fact that family members and friends provide at least 80 percent of the needed long-term care at home and those caregivers consider that practice normative behavior (Brody 1985).

Raising an obvious dilemma when he called cost control the key to Medicare's future, HHS Secretary Bowen (1986) commented that Medicare was not established to cover long-term care needs. Therefore, Secretary Bowen expressed concern for the solvency and survivability of Medicare if coverage for long-term care was included. He did note that skilled nursing care and home health care were used in the Medicare program to bridge the gap between acute care and long-term care.

In an examination of the financing and delivery of long-term care services, O'Shaughnessy, Price, and Griffith (1985,59) pointed out three dilemmas that plague policymakers: how to strike a balance between institutional and community-based care; how to offer more consistent and adequate protection for long-term care expenses; and whether or not community-based care is more cost-effective than institutional care. A number of issues were raised pertaining to the dilemmas, including the appropriate roles for the private and public sectors, how to respond to the needs of diverse populations, the uncertainty of the costs of community-based care, the most desirable options, the contributions of family members, the controls for coverage, and long-term care in a managed care setting.

While Shaughnessy (1985) noted similar public policy dilemmas, he said, "Some optimism may be found in the opportunity to change and adapt our long-term care system through reimbursement due to the high proportion of public financing."

Mollica (1986) identified the goals of a long-term care program, again asserting the obvious relation to homecare services. He posited that the program aims to maintain and improve independence; to facilitate hospital discharges; to avoid or delay nursing home placement; to broaden in-home service funding; to cover middle income groups; to supplement family care and to do all this without increasing costs. Within those goals, long-term care dilemmas must address the issues of administration of programs, financing, delivery of services, benefits and eligibility.

Administration of Programs. What is readily apparent in the administration dilemma is that same situation that applied when only homecare was an issue--the lack of a national policy. Obviously, programs will flounder awash in administrative red tape and confusion if there is no unifying national policy. At a hearing before the House Subcommittee on Health and Long-Term Care (1984,4) on the need for a national long-term care policy, Congressman Claude Pepper commented:

> Long-term care for *all* Americans stands as the most troubled, and
> troublesome, component of our entire health care system . . . Our
> health care systems virtually rule out financial assistance for care that
> may prevent or postpone costly and premature institutionalization, such
> as immunizations, pediatric and adult homecare and other supportive
> services . . . The purpose of our hearing will be to explore what the
> federal role might be in structuring a comprehensive continuum of care
> -- a long-term care policy -- capable of addressing the preventive,
> acute, and chronic care needs of our nation's citizens.

In a policy analysis examination of health care, the Heritage Foundation (1984,14) reinforced the connection between long-term care and homecare in a conclusion that, "The keystone of a long-term health care policy should be a comprehensive program fostering home service."

Financing. In talking about long-term care and the alternatives to institutionalization, Rice (1985,62) points out that "the initial policy issue is not whether home health services are less costly, but how these services should be organized and financed for maximum efficiency and effectiveness." That approach could apply to all the services before consideration of the sources of funding. It appears that national policymakers feel that the long-term care dilemma is being adequately handled through individual family arrangements for care at home and that there is no need to interfere at this time. Should that attitude prevail, the dilemma of financing will not be adequately resolved. Funding will remain a muddle of interconnected agencies reimbursing for a tangle of unitary services.

Long-term care insurance, including homecare benefits, is attracting attention as a resolution to the financing dilemma (Scheier 1986). Employees put aside money during their working years to pay premiums for "cafeteria-style" benefits including nursing home care, acute medical care, homecare, disability benefits, and life insurance with adjustments as the needs of the insured change. Northwestern National Life Insurance Company in Minnesota calls the coverage LifeScope, and has put $2 million into an advertising campaign to increase awareness and to stimulate a demand for such coverage. A typical print advertisement uses the headline, "In America, the fear of dying early has been replaced by the fear of living too long." That ad features a drab home environment with an elderly woman sitting in a rocking chair (Scheier 1986).

In addition to lack of awareness and the subsequent lack of a demand, Knickman and McCall (1986) find three other reasons for a disinterest in long-term care insurance: state regulations stifle innovation; fears by insurance companies that the coverage would be uncontrollable; and the public's conception that Medicaid is always the insurance of last resort when they run out of money. They also said that including long-term care in prepaid or managed care plans, such as a Social/Health Maintenance Organization (S/HMO), was a good idea.

Financing alternatives have also delved into the use of reverse equity mortgages and life care communities as possible resolutions of the dilemma. However, the resolution of the funding dilemma is not so easily solved.

Delivery of Services. With the difficulties in establishing a national long-term care policy and then funding those decisions, dilemmas in the delivery of services will be constant for some time. It is likely that a large portion of the services will be delivered in institutions. Many observers have commented on the apparent bias towards institutionalization in the American health care delivery system. Trager (1984,62) sums it up neatly: "Public policy in long-term care has not only favored the institution, it has made any other choice almost impossible." Add to that the statistics that nursing home care costs an average of $35,000 per year; that the U.S. spent about $32 billion in 1984, up 11.1 percent over 1983, for nursing home care; and that custodial homecare services cost about $10 per hour (Knickman and McCall 1986).

Major suppliers of homecare services are now proprietary and hospital-based home health agencies. Obviously, the delivery of services must be influenced by the commercial overtones of the management of the sponsoring agencies.

Benefits. A constant dilemma regarding benefits concerns the division made between medical/health related services and the personal/social care services. Frequently, the health benefits are the only services that individuals can receive under either governmental programs or private insurance coverage. Benefits also tend to have restrictions relative to the number of visits, the length of time and the total expenditures allowable. In addition, the dilemma of benefits is compounded by the fact that whatever does exist is often poorly coordinated for the individual receiving the care.

Again, with the other dilemmas unresolved, it is unlikely that there will be substantial progress on clearing up the benefits maze.

Eligibility. Under the Medicare program, eligibility dilemmas relate to determinations of homebound status, skilled nursing care and whether or not the care is intermittent. Those eligibility problems have caused considerable distress among providers of home health care. On the other hand, if individuals have the funds to pay for services, the eligibility dilemma is a mute question.

Consideration of when an individual qualifies for long-term care services, including homecare, is often also intermingled with the family's ability to render care at home. How much care should family members be required to provide at home? Is there a legal and/or moral obligation to do so? What is society's obligation? These are all facets of the eligibility dilemma awaiting resolution.

It is easy to realize that these five long-term care dilemmas will require considerable effort by all concerned parties to arrive at solutions.

Homecare/Long-term Care Reforms

In a report of the House Subcommittee on Health and Long-Term Care (1985,65) on "Building a Long-Term Care Policy: Homecare Data and Implications," nine recommendations were made for Congress to consider to meet the "massive unmet need for homecare services" as part of a national long-term care policy. Congress was urged to examine a comprehensive homecare benefit to address the long-term care needs of Medicare and

Medicaid populations; to consider a general extension of the home health benefit targeted to those individuals most likely to be placed in a nursing home because they lacked assistance at home; to move toward establishing a prospective payment system for all homecare providers; to encourage homecare contributions by family members through an appropriate tax reduction; to stimulate the development of long-term care insurance; to require a certification before nursing home placement that homecare is either unavailable or inappropriate for the patient; to initiate a national long-term care policy founded on the principle of treatment in the least restrictive environment and based on prospective payment; to alter HCFA's home health agency classifications to reflect hospital-based, -sponsored or -owned agencies; and to have HCFA, in cooperation with the NAHC, develop a common set of key definitions to compute an unduplicated clients count, to indicate primary and secondary diagnoses, and to develop a methodology for computing average lengths of stay per visit.

In a discussion of innovative approaches to community-based long-term care by the states, Benjamin (1985) raised five policy dilemmas regarding long-term care reforms:

1. Who gets into the long-term care system and, more importantly, where in that system do they enter?

2. How can traditional modes of community care, including self-care and family care, be reinforced and supported?

3. How can present payment methods be altered to reduce the costs of community care?

4. How can the fragmentation be reduced among the various public funding streams that support long-term care services?

5. How can the level of resources available for community long-term care services be increased?

While the questions relate to federal long-term care reforms as well, Benjamin (1985) divided political support in the states into three types. There are states where commitment and funding are available (e.g., Massachusetts); states where some commitment is present but funding is not (e.g., Connecticut); and states where next steps are being discussed (e.g., most of the others).

Specific reforms that could be evaluated for each of the dilemmas include preadmission screening programs prior to institutional placement with increased hospital discharge planning; family support programs such as respite care; use of reverse equity home mortgages; private health insurance coverage; movement from retrospective to prospective reimbursement methods; use of assessment and screening procedures for need determinations; use of case managers; the setting up of single administrative mechanisms; and the seeking out of new resources. But Benjamin (1985) commented that the increases from new resources, "however real, remain much too small--relative to the needs of the elderly, disabled, and others--to stir much excitement yet."

Legislation to Resolve Dilemmas

In American society, reforms are often tested in the public arenas of legislative bodies and in courtrooms. Bills passed and decisions rendered determine the directions that homecare will follow in the future. Actions of the legislative assemblies and the courts engender considerable concern among the professionals and the public alike. Currently, national legislative solutions appear to focus upon the provision of acute medical care. Harnett (1986) commented that "if we are to avoid a political and social failure of major proportions . . . a national long-term care policy must become a legislative priority."

Picking up on the acute medical care aspect, Collier (1986) stated that "it has become clear to me that long-term care policy is not best served by being centered around medical care . . . What seems clear to me is that long-term care policy over the next several years, and even for a generation or two, should be centered around housing and social support efforts." He cited three reasons why it will take a long time to effect changes in policies: the enormous deficit in the federal budget resulting in legislative attitudes on savings and budget cutting; the 20-year evolution of Medicare and Medicaid policies creating an inertia of not easily reversed events; and the need for time to develop models and then carefully consider, modify, and establish new policies.

From his perspective as Director of the Health and Human Resources Staff of the Senate Labor and Human Resources Committee, Sundwall (1986) discussed federal legislation and initiatives. Pointing out that critics of the Reagan administration's health care policies label the actions as "retrenchment, withdrawal and disengagement," he also notes that others feel those policies are the only hope for resolving the problems of escalating expenditures, overwhelming regulations, and access to services. Despite an almost unanimous agreement on the need for change, the priority of budgetary issues towers over all else. Vladeck (1985,115) also noted that the consensus of policymakers is greater than it has been in many years; the body of knowledge is also greater about long-term care clients, services, and funding than in prior years. Yet, Vladeck feels that there exists a constant federal administration aversion to systematic policy reform and even to small-scale experimentation. In explanation, Vladeck says: "At one level the current stasis in long-term care reflects primarily the inability of policymakers to address fiscal conflict between federal and state government . . . Which level of government will get stuck with the bills? . . . Other principles are at stake . . . The current policy stalemate may arise from conflicts about the appropriate role of government, families, and individual responsibility so profound that only creative and aggressive policy leadership, of a kind now nowhere to be found, can end it."

Sundwall (1986) closed by saying, "There are not, however, any measures for major long-term care reform . . . I am concerned that the Secretary-designate of Health and Human Services, Dr. Otis Bowen, has no specific plans or recommendations for long-term care reform."

Homecare Legislative Priorities. Six key issues were identified by NAHC (1986b) as the top legislative priorities:

1. Relief from the HCFA regulations establishing cost limits by discipline for HHAs; legislative extension of the waiver of liability; and extension of the hospice benefit along with an increase in the reimbursement rates.

2. Opposition to the 5 percent copayment proposed for Medicare users of the home health benefit.

3. Seek exemption from the Gramm-Rudman-Hollings budget cuts for Medicare home health benefits.

4. Legislative action requiring HHS/HCFA to abide by the Federal Administrative Procedures Act requiring appropriate notice and opportunity for public comment before proposed changes in federal programs.

5. Legislation to clarify the term "intermittent care" in Medicare statutes including the fact that daily care up to 90 days is within the definition.

6. Legislation authorizing reimbursement for pediatric homecare to be specifically included in the statutes.

Halamandaris (1985b) enumerated 14 legislative goals which elaborate on the six priorities noted above. Combined, these homecare legislative priorities and goals comprise an ambitious undertaking.

Federal Bills. Proposed bills in Congress indicate a great deal of concern about homecare. A number of members of Congress have been quite active introducing legislation year after year in relation to home- and community-based care. A sampling of recent federal proposals follow:

• Medicare and Medicaid Patient and Program Protection Act

- Medicare Solvency and Health Care Financing Reform Act
- Medicare Home- and Community-Based Services Improvement Act
- Allow Medicare Coverage for Home Health Services on a Daily Basis
- Extend Hospice Benefits Under Medicare for Three Years
- Prohibit the Secretary of Health and Human Services from Changing Reimbursement Levels or Methodologies for Home Health Services under the Medicare Program prior to October 1, 1986 or during a Freeze Period to Eliminate the Sunset Hospice Benefits under the Medicare Program
- Medicare and Medicaid Budget Reconciliation Amendments
- Older Americans Alternative Care Act
- Home- and Community-Based Services for the Elderly
- Long-term Care Insurance Promotion and Protection Act
- Health Care Data Systems Clearinghouse Act
- National Home Health Clearinghouse
- Home Respiratory Care Act
- Alternatives to Hospitalization for Medical Technology Dependent Children's Act
- Increase the Amount of the Credit for Dependent Care Expenses, to Make Such Credit Refundable, and to Provide that Certain Respite Care Expenses are Eligible for Such Credit
- Add-Ons to the Reimbursement Limits for Home Health Agencies May No Longer be Made for Hospital-Based Agencies
- Quality Assurance Reform Act
- Deficit Reduction Amendments

This rather impressive list of federally-sponsored bills concern a wide variety of dilemmas in the homecare industry. It also attests to the ability of the homecare trade associations to get their messages across and to prompt action.

While the intent of federal legislation may be commendable, governmental employees do not always prepare rules and regulations consistent with the legislative goal. In that event, lawyers jump into the fray to represent their clients' reactions to what is considered ill-determined policy. Of course, there may also be legal reaction to the original legislation.

Quality: The Bottom Line Dilemma

All of the dilemmas related to long-term care and to homecare ultimately lead to the question: Is the quality of care better or worse? Quality of care is difficult to measure because of the long-term nature of the patient's illness/ condition and the subsequent equally long-term treatment modalities, including homecare.

A GAO (1986) report made comprehensive proposals for studies to evaluate quality of care as affected by PPS/DRGs. A report prepared for the House Select Committee on Aging by the American Bar Association (ABA) (*American Medical News* 1986) cited the fact that the service location at home puts the monitoring of homecare beyond the easy reach of public or professional scrutiny. They found that existing monitoring was mostly a paper exercise and compared the position of homecare with that of nursing homes 20 years ago. A state survey found 40 percent deficiencies in coordination and a 70 percent deficiency in conforming with the orders of physicians. Other quality care dilemmas included a failure to require H-HHA training, a failure to routinely interview clients about quality, no regulation of H-HHAs, and a lack of investigations of complaints.

In relation to the ABA study results, Congressman Edward Roybal introduced legislation to require PROs to do quality assurance, to require states to monitor homecare, to require HHS to be involved in training, and to require states to develop certification for H-HHAs and personal care workers. At a House hearing on a prior Medicare quality protection bill, the AFHHA (1986) strongly supported the actions to improve the quality of care.

Quality of care is a major concern of the American Association for Continuity of Care (1986). These professionals seek to upgrade homecare via sound discharge planning and the case management approach to supplying coordinated services to people in need. Their 1986 annual meeting had sessions on cost-effective discharge planning, performance standards for discharge planning, the team approach, clinical and ethical decisions, and management of the AIDS patient in the community. Gallivan (1986) reported on the impact of PPS on discharge planning in the Medicare Conditions of Participation.

Malpractice. Directly connected to the quality of care dilemma is the problem of malpractice. Most articles deal with medical malpractice, but Connaway (1986) specifically discusses whether or not a home health nurse should carry her own professional liability insurance. Among the reasons cited in favor of personal policies for nurses are the following: the nature of homecare; the increase in lawsuits against health professionals; the trend in lawsuits to name nurses as defendants; the inclusion of subrogation or restitution clauses in malpractice policies; and that exclusions in an employer's policy may affect a nurse's coverage. A final argument by Connaway may be the most telling--in 1986, it cost about $60 for $1 million per occurrence and $2 million aggregate malpractice coverage for nurses.

Impact of Trends, Issues and Dilemmas

Taking simple dictionary meanings, a trend signifies a general direction; an issue is a topic for discussion; and a dilemma is a predicament of choice between alternatives. There is a clear cut trend toward increased use of homecare with a motivating force of saving dollars. Issues cover the gamut and include the use of high technology, the rental or purchase of durable medical equipment, eligibility definitions, reimbursement caps, eligibility determinations, claims denials, ethical and moral overtones, and a host of day-to-day operational components. Finally, the predicament arises in choosing between meeting the steadily increasing need for homecare services or using assorted techniques to contain the burgeoning costs.

While reviewing all these trends, issues and dilemmas, two laws of physics came to mind.

Laws of Physics and Homecare

An oft quoted maxim says, "You just can't please everybody for trying." Newton's Third Law of Motion says the same thing in a more technical manner: for every action there is an equal and opposite reaction. Actually, the exact wording of the law is relevant: "Whenever one body exerts a force on a second body, the second body reacts on the first with a force opposite in direction but equal in magnitude" (Bolemon 1985). When HCFA exerts a force to reduce the Medicare home health benefit, NAHC, AFHHA, AARP and others react with an opposite force. When hospitals take actions to enhance their homecare activities, the freestanding HHAs react with an equal and opposite force to counter that intrusion. When nurses take action to achieve greater responsibility for establishing homecare plans, physicians react. And so it goes up and down the line, with adversaries moving in and out of the lineup as the issues twist and turn throughout the health care delivery system.

Despite the philosophical assumption that homecare is a humane, effective, and cost-efficient mechanism to meet a real need, the lack of a national homecare policy may continue to result in the "action and reaction" syndrome. That syndrome will keep issues and dilemmas such as those related to cost containment; the success or failure of PPS/DRG; the "Catch 22" of the "quicker and sicker" discharges creating a greater need for homecare services while the budget squeeze reduces funding at the same time; the fallout of the managed care explosion; the linking of long-term care and homecare; and the bottom line problem of evaluating the quality of care, churning the pressure cooker of policy decision-makers.

That pressure cooker image brings to mind another law of physics, Einstein's famous equation, E = MC2 wherein *E*nergy equals the *M*ass times *C*, the speed of light in a vacuum, squared. This formula was instrumental in the development of the atom bomb. Is there an atomic energy reaction coming up in the homecare industry? Will Califano's health revolution turn violent? Will there be peaceful coexistence?

Despite these tongue-in-cheek, dire expectations, it is obvious that the trends, issues and dilemmas will respond to a number of variables. Most experts predict continued rapid growth for the homecare industry, increased federal overall funding despite budget cuts, increased use of homecare by individuals covered by insurance, movement toward uniform definitions, action on standards, more accreditation programs, measureable common care units, and a host of related parts of the disparate homecare puzzle. If the pieces fit, homecare can coalesce into an integral part of the health care delivery system. Ultimately, that should be the end goal of all publicly minded organizations and individuals. It is hoped that men and women of good intentions working together will reduce the critical mass and harness the energy for the betterment of society.

References

American Association for Continuity of Care. 1986. Bridging the gap '86: changes, choices and challenges. Washington, DC.

American Federation of Home Health Agencies. 1986. Statement on the Medicare Quality Protection Act of 1986. Washington, DC (23 April).

American Medical News. 1986. House bill to address monitoring of home care. 29(31):33.

Antone, T. M., and G. L. Thietten. 1986. Statement of NAMES and AFHHA at oversight hearing on the Prompt Payment Act (P.L. 97-177). Washington, DC (19 June).

Azzarto, J. 1986. Medicalization of the problems of the elderly. *Health and Social Work* 11(3):189-195.

Benjamin, A. E., Jr. 1985. Community-based long-term care in *Long term care of the elderly. Public policy issues* edited by C. Harrington, R. J. Newcomer, C. L. Estes, et al. Beverly Hills, CA: Sage Publications.

Blumenthal, D., et al. 1986. The future of Medicare. *New England Journal of Medicine* 314:722-728.

Bolemon, J. S. 1985. *Physics: an introduction.* Englewood Cliffs, NJ: Prentice Hall.

Bowen, O. R. 1986. Cost control key to Medicare's future. *Provider* 12(6):9-10.

Brody, E. 1985. Parent care as a normative family stress. *The Gerontologist* 25(1):19-29.

Califano, J. A., Jr. 1986. A revolution looms in American health. *New York Times* (25 March).

Collier, E. M., Jr. 1986. Shaping a national policy for long-term care. *PRIDE Institute Journal* (Special issue):5-7.

Connaway, N. I. 1986. Should a home health nurse carry her own professional liability insurance? *Home Healthcare Nurse* 4(2):7-8.

Department of Health, Education, and Welfare. 1976. *Home health care: report on the regional public hearings. 9/20-*

10/1/76. Washington, DC: Government Printing Office. Pub. No. 76-135.

Ernst and Whinney. 1986. *Strategic responses to the managed care explosion for the medical device and diagnostic industry.* Washington, DC: Health Industry Manufacturers Association.

Fellner, B. A. 1986. *Americans needing home care.* Washington, DC: Government Printing Office. Pub. NO. (PHS) 86-1581 (March).

Flanagan, E. M. 1985. Some developments in home health law in the past year. Presentation at Health Law Update of the National Health Lawyers Association, Washington, DC (5 May).

Firshein, J. 1986. Prepaids' use of home health services booming. *Hospitals* 60(8):66,68.

Gallivan, M. 1986. Role of discharge planners draws scrutiny. *Hospitals* 60(13):108,110.

General Accounting Office. 1986. *Post-hospital care: efforts to evaluate Medicare prospective payment effects are insufficient.* Washington, DC: Government Printing Office. Pub. No. GAO/PEMD-86-10 (2 June).

Halamandaris, V. J. 1985a. The future of home care. *Caring* 4(10):5-11.

Halamandaris, V. J. 1985b. Caring thoughts. *Caring* 4(4):64.

Harnett, E. 1986. Editor's perspective. *PRIDE Institute Journal* (Special issue):2-3.

Heritage Foundation. 1984. *Mandate for leadership II.* Washington, DC (7 December).

Home Health Journal. 1986a. National association says Reagan out to dismantle Medicare home benefit. 7(4):5,8.

Home Health Journal. 1986b. Roper cites home health for change. 7(6):1,7.

House Select Committee on Aging. 1985. *Long term care in America: the people's call for federal action.* Washington, DC: Government Printing Office. Comm. Pub. No. 99-515.

House Subcommittee on Health and Long Term Care. 1984. *Long term care: need for a national policy.* Washington, DC: Government Printing Office. Comm. Pub. No. 98-444.

House Subcommittee on Health and Long Term Care. 1985. *Building a long term

care policy: home care data and implications.* Washington, DC: Government Printing Office. Comm. Pub. No. 98-484.

Knickman, J. R., and N. McCall. 1986. A prepaid managed approach to long-term care. *Health Affairs* 5(1):90-104.

Livengood, W. 1986. Deficit reduction: its impact on home health care. *Home Healthcare Nurse* 4(2):41-42.

Lukin, J. M. 1986. Nonmedical care for homebound elderly in peril. *New York Times* (3 January).

Marosy, J. P. 1985. Testimony before House Select Committee on Aging. Home Health Agency Assembly of NJ, Inc., Princeton, NJ (24 June).

McIlrath, S. 1986. Group raps cut in homecare benefits. *American Medical News* 29(14):2,53.

Medical World News. 1985. U.S. elderly's homecare in jeopardy. 26(15):30-31.

Mollica, R. L. 1986. Creating a national policy in long-term care: recommendations for a model bill. *PRIDE Institute Journal* (Special Issue Conference Proceedings):28-29.

National Association for Home Care. 1985. *Toward a national home care policy. Blueprint for action. A report.* Washington, DC (January).

National Association for Home Care. 1986a. High tech high touch focus of 1986 NAHC annual meeting. Washington, DC (August).

National Association for Home Care. 1986b. Key NAHC legislative and regulatory issues for 1986. Washington, DC (16 March).

O'Shaughnessy, C., R. Price, and J. Griffith. 1985. *Financing and delivery of long-term care services for the elderly.* Washington, DC: Congressional Research Service, Library of Congress, Pub. No. 85-1033 EPW(17 October).

Pear, R. 1986. Harvard study urges overhaul of Medicare. *New York Times* (13 March).

Pyles, J. C., and M. S. Philip. 1985. Current legal issues. Presentation at annual meeting of National Association for Home Care, Las Vegas, NV(16 October).

Ramage, N. B. 1985. In-home health care services: a policy perspective. *Family and Community Health* 8(2):11-21.

Rice, D. P. 1985. Health care needs of the elderly in *Long-term care of the elderly,* edited by C. Harrington, R. J. Newcomer, C. L. Estes, et al. Beverly Hills, CA: Sage Publications.

Ryder, C. F. 1967. *Changing patterns in homecare.* Washington, DC: Government Printing Office. Pub. No. PHS-1657 (June).

Sandrick, K. 1986. Home care: cutting health care's safety net. *Hospitals* 60(10):48-52.

Scheier, R. L. 1986. Innovative long-term care coverage to be marketed by Minnesota insurer. *American Medical News* 29(31):2,35.

Schutzer, A. I. 1985. Will the hospital cost squeeze produce an investor's bonanza? *Medical Economics* (7 Jan.).

Senate Special Committee on Aging. 1985. *Impact of Medicare's prospective payment system on the quality of care received by Medicare beneficiaries.* Staff report, Washington, DC (24 October).

Shaughnessy, P. W. 1985. Long-term care research and public policy. *Health Services Research* 20(4):489-499.

Shaw, S. 1985. 2001: a home care technology. *Caring* 4(10):20-22.

Smith, W. E. 1986. Ethical, economic and professional issues in home health care. *American Journal of Hospital Pharmacy* 43(3):695-698.

Spiegel, A. D., and F. Kavaler. 1986. *Cost containment and DRGs: a guide to prospective payment.* Owings Mills, MD: National Health Publishing.

Star-Ledger (Newark, NJ). 1986a. New age of medicine (editorial) (19 July).

Star-Ledger (Newark, NJ). 1986b. Bradley acts on health care (22 May).

Star-Ledger (Newark, NJ). 1986c. Medicare denials soar on home care claims (29 July).

Stoesz, D. 1986. Corporate health care and social welfare. *Health and Social Work* 11(3):165-172.

Sundwall, D. 1986. Federal legislation and initiatives in long-term care. *PRIDE Institute Journal* (special issue):7-14.

Thietten, G. L. 1986. Letter to Senator Proxmire on delays in Medicare reimbursement to homecare agencies. Washington, DC (27 May).

Trager, B. 1984. Testimony before House Subcommittee on Health and Long Term Care in *Long term care: need for a national policy.* Washington, DC: Government Printing Office. Comm. Pub. No. 98-444.

Turbo, R. 1986. Home health care encounters growing pains. *Medical World News* 27(3):76-88.

Vladeck, B. C. 1985. The static dynamics of long-term care policy in *The health policy agenda: some critical questions* edited by M. E. Lewin. Washington, DC: American Enterprise Institute.

Whitlow, J. 1985. Medicare cuts called threat to aged home care. *Star-Ledger* (Newark, NJ) (8 December).

Index

A Consumer Guide to Home Health Care, 14
A Model Curriculum and Teaching Guide for the Instruction of the Homemaker-Home Health Aide, 274
A Physician Guide to Home Health Care, 201, 275-276
Abuse, 410
Accident recovery, 31
Accounting, 52
Accreditation
    benefits, 244-245
    defined, 245
    homecare accreditation organizations, 246-253
Acquired immune deficiency syndrome, 45
Activities of daily living, 104
Activity limitation, age distribution, 104, 105
Age, 65, 114. *See also* Elderly
    need for homecare, 103-106
Ageism, 132
Agency. *See* Specific type
Aging
    biology of, 152
    population growth, 126-130
AID Atlanta, 45
Aid to Families with Dependent Parents, 34
Aide, 292
All About Home Care: A Consumer's Guide, 14
Allied Nursing Care, 44
Alternative Health Services Project, cost comparison, 229
Altruism, 241

Alzheimer's disease, 45-46, 317, 389
Ambulation, 114
Ambulatory visit group, 73
American Association for Continuity of Care, 30
American Association for Respiratory Therapists, 81-82
American Association of Retired Persons, 127, 238
American College of Health Care Administration, 148
American Federation of Home Health Agencies, Inc. 329, 336
American Hospital Association, 238
    Division of Ambulatory Care, 336
American Medical Association, 17, 23, 238
American Nurses Association, 17, 23, 238
American Physical Therapy Association, 296
American Society for Parenteral and Enteral Nutrition, 79
American Speech and Hearing Association, 306
Antibiotic therapy, 78, 382
    cost, 221-222
    intravenous, 74
    standards, 79
Anxiety, 14
Arthritis, 31, 388
Assembly of Ambulatory and Home Care Services of the American Hospital Association, 17, 23
Assessment instrument, 115

Association for Home Care, national survey, 41
Association of Medical Equipment Suppliers, 336
Attendant, 292
Audiologic services, 25
Audiologist
    business aspects, 307
    education, 306
    ethical issues, 307
    supply, 306
    utilization, 306-307

Baptist Medical Center, Oklahoma City, Oklahoma, 44
Barber-cosmetology services, 25
Baseline Assessment Instrument, 115-116
Bedsore, 31
Bereavement, 318
Bilirubin Phototherapy Program, 46-47
Bill of Rights, 14
    patient, 242-243
Blood pressure, high, 42
Blue Cross
    homecare funding, 201
    model plan, 24
    service structure, 22
Blue Cross/Blue Shield, 163
Blue Cross/Blue Shield of Maryland, Coordinate Home Care Program, 221
Boston Dispensary, 1-2
Bowel/bladder condition, 42

CAAST method, 114
Cancer, 14, 31
Cane, 80
Carcinoma, 42
Cardiology, 45
Care coordination, 20
Care level, 21-23
Caregiver, 112, 150-151. *See also*

Family
Caretaker, 18-19
    defined, 19
Caring Community, Inc., 149
Case assessment/case management, 287
Case management, 30, 379-380
Case manager, 26
Catastrophic insurance, 158, 166
Certificate of need, 260-261
Certification, 257-260
    defined, 257
    Medicare conditions of participation, 257-260
Charge, reasonable, usual, and customary, Medicare definition, 176
Chelsea-Village Program of New York City's St. Vincent's Hospital and Medical Center, cost comparison, 225-226
Chemotherapy, 78
    intravenous, 74
Cherkasky, Martin, 12
Chicago House and Social Service Agency, 45
Child abuse, 318
Chore service, 151
Circulatory condition, 31, 42
Cleaning service, heavy, 26
Coinsurance, 410
Colostomy, 318
Combined agency, 20
Commode, 80
Communication, continuity of care, 27
Communication services, 305-307
Community Health Services and Facilities Act, 5
Comorbidity, 65
Complex Care Team, 45
Complications, 65
Comprehensive care, 18
Computer, 55

Conference on Organized
   Homecare, 4
Congregate living arrangements, 34
Consumerism, 14
Continence, 114
Continuing care, 143-151
Continuing care community,
   139-140
Continuing education, 274
Continuity of care, 20, 26-30
   communication, 27
   obstacles, 27
   techniques, 27-28
Contractual arrangement, 20
Coordinated care, 26-30
Coordinated Homecare, 5
Copayment
   home health care, 179
   home visit, 179
Corporate reorganization, 51-53
   satisfaction with, 52-53
   variations, 52
Cost, 32-33
   elderly, 157
   home health care reimburse-
      ment, 166-167
   homecare, 163, 380-381
   impairment level, 217-219
   management aspects, 166-167
   medical diagnosis, 166
   nursing home, 147
   public health values, 167-168
   reimbursement variations, 202-
      203
Cost allocation, 52
Cost containment, 403-404
   evaluation, 369-370
   homecare, 211-233, 402
      basic premises, 212-213
      cost comparisons, 225-229
      cost evaluation problems,
         219-220
      cost-benefit analysis, 215-
         217

cost-effectiveness, 213-215
impairment level, 217-219
support, 211-212
vs. nursing home care, 224-
   232
Cost-benefit analysis, 215-217
   defined, 215
   dollar expenditures, 216
Cost-effectiveness, 213-215
   defined, 213
   measurement techniques, 213-
      214
   drawbacks, 214
Council for Homemaker Services, 7
Council of Home Health Agencies
   and Community Health Services of the National League
   for Nursing, 17, 23
Council on Accreditation of Services for Family and Children,
   252-253
Crutch, 80

Data collection, 375-377
   deterrents, 376-377
   uniform basic data set, 375-376
Day care, 34-35
Death, 377
Dementia, 317, 389
Demonstration project, 199
   government-funded, 199
Denial, 409
Dental care, 25, 312
Department of Health Education
   and Welfare, need assessment,
   108
Dependency, 19
   health services, 104
   household activity, 104
   mobility, 104
   personal care, 104
   types, 104
Depression, 32
Diabetes, 31, 42, 45, 389

Diagnosis related group, 65-73
  discharge planning, 70-71
  home health care, 68, 71-73
  long-term care, 66-67
  Medicare, 386-387
  as reason for discharge, 69
Diagnostic category, major, 65
Dialysis, home, 74-75
Diet therapy, 26
Dietitian, 309-311
  education, 310
  future, 311
  role, 309-310
Disability, 377
Discharge
  early, 403
  planned accelerated, 66-68
  premature, 66-68
Discharge needs, 385
Discharge planning, 66
  diagnosis related group, 70-71
  homecare, 70-71
Discharge recommendation, 38
Discomfort, 378
Disease, 377
Disease condition comparison, 388-389
Dissatisfaction, 378
Diversification, 51-52
Domiciliary patient care, comprehensive, 33
Dumping, 66-68

Education services, 26
Elderly, 125-158
  attitudes/culture, 125
  cost, 125, 157
  demographics, 125, 126-130
  epidemiology, 125
  impairment status, 130-132
  Medicaid, 136-137
  Medicare, 146-147, 157-158
  need planning, 155-157
  out-of-pocket homecare costs, 199-200
  physician education, 152-155
  population growth, 126-130
  public policy, 136-143
    recommendations, 141-143
  quality of life, 134-136
  research, 155-157
  scientific research, 125
  terminology, 132
Elderplan, Inc., 133
Enterostomal therapy, 45
Equipment
  durable medical, 80-97, 410
    alternative reimbursement, 95
    cost, 81
    defined, 80
    ethical issues, 86-88
    excess charges, 92
    federal budget activity, 92
    growth, 82, 86-88
    historical aspects, 81-82
    hospital referral, 86-88
    legal issues, 86-88
    marketing, 84-86
    Medicare, 81
    reasonable charge, 94-95
    referrals, 85-86
    reimbursement, 88-95
    rental, 88-92
    revenue, 83
Ethics, 57-58
Evaluation, 23, 24, 367-395
  comparison, 388-393
  constants, 393-394
  cost containment, 369-370
  data analysis, 386-387
  data collection, 375-377
  deterrents, 376-377
    uniform basic data set, 375-376
  death, 377
  defined, 371
  descriptive, 382-383

disability, 377
discomfort, 378
disease, 377
dissatisfaction, 378
literature review, 379-382
long-term care, 379
Medicare, 386-387
methods, 370-371
personal interview, 385-386
polling, 383-385
problems, 373-375
    political, 373-375
questions, 367-368
specific areas, 368-369
study characteristics, 371-373
survey, 383-385
typical, 378-393
Expenditure, 399-400

Family, 18, 112, 150-151, 314-320
full-time work and homecare,
    316-317
    corporate studies, 316-317
hospice, 318
need assessment, 112
public policy, 314-315
support group, 317-318
Financial planning, 53-54
Fiscal intermediary
Medicare definition, 175-176
regional, 175-176
Fraud, 410
Funding
federal, 28
fragmented, 28

Gateway II, cost comparisons, 225
Georgia Department of Human
    Resources, need assessment,
    108
Geriatric community nurse, 152
Geriatric nurse practitioner, 290
Geriatric nursing, 291
Geriatric social worker, 152

Geriatrician, 152
Geriatrics
education, 151-155
training, 151-155
Gerontological nurse, 291
Gerontological social work, 303
Gerontology, defined, 125
Geropsychiatric Outreach Team,
    382
Geropsychiatrist, 152
Gramm-Rudman-Hollings
    Balanced Budget and Emergen-
    cy Deficit Reduction Act, 163,
    404
Group living, 34-35
Growth factor, 76-77
Guidelines, 23-24
historical aspects, 4-5

Handyman services, 26
Health, defined, 31
Health Care Contractors Associa-
    tion, 81-82
Health Care Financing Administra-
    tion, 6, 163
Health care management consult-
    ant firm, 121
Health Industry Distributors As-
    sociation, 81-82, 86
Health Industry Manufacturers As-
    sociation, 336
    Home Care Products Commit-
    tee, 82
Health maintenance organization,
    133, 163
    homecare cost, 224
    homecare relationship, 50
Health promotion, 19
Health services, 104
Health Systems Agency of South-
    western Pennsylvania, Inc.,
    need assessment, 108
Healthcorp Affiliates, 43-44
Heart disease, 31, 42

Heart surgery, 318
Heavy cleaning service, 26
Heritage Foundation, 11-12
Home, 18-19
    suitable, characteristics, 15-16
Home birthing, 57
Home care intake coordinator, 66
Home equity conversion, 140-141
    reverse annuity mortgage, 140-141
    sales/leaseback plan, 140-141
Home health agency
    claim denial, 185-186
    growth, 345, 400
    hospital relations, 50
    Medicare definition, 171-172
    waiver of liability, 180
Home health aide, 20, 41, 42, 151, 292-296
    future, 295-296
    historical aspects, 6-7
    home help, 293
    model curriculum, 294-296
    personnel issues, 295-296
    tasks, 293
    titles, 293
    traits, 293-294
    typical, 294
Home health care
    1958 national survey, 7
    copayment, 179
    corporatization trend, 400-401
    cost limits, 177-179
    defined, 16-18
    diagnosis related group, 68, 71-73
    historical aspects, 1-6
    Medicare, 5
    prospective payment system, 65-73
    terminology, 16-17
    vs. homecare, 16
    vs. social care, 132-134
    women's issue, 150

Home Health Care: When a Patient Leaves the Hospital, 14
Home health care agency
    federal definitions, 5
    Medicare, 5
Home health care provider, 20
Home Health Care Services, Quarterly, 48
Home health nursing, 289
Home Health Services and Staffing Association, 336
Home infusion therapy, 77-78
Home nursing care
    historical aspects, 2
    patterns, 3
Home Nursing Care for the Elderly, 292
Home respiratory care, cost, 223
Home visit
    copayment, 179
    growth, 347-357
        geographic variability, 352
        by type of agency, 352-357
Home visiting, 33
Homebound, Medicare definition, 174
Homecare, 148-149, 400
    abuse, 203-206
    appropriate targeting, 212
    awareness effects, 329-330
    basic, 22
    business aspects, 49-55
    care level, 21-23
    concentrated, 21
    cost, 380-381
    cost containment, 211-233, 402, 403
        basic premises, 212-213
        cost comparisons, 220-224, 225
        cost evaluation problems, 219-220
        cost-benefit analysis, 215-217

cost effectiveness, 213-215
cost-saving strategies, 232-233
impairment level, 217-219
support, 211-212
vs. nursing home care, 224-232
cost-saving objectives, 213
defined, 16
demand, 406
diagnosis-specific, 46-47
cost, 223-224
discharge planning, 70-71
dismantling of benefits, 404-405
early discharge, 403
evaluation, literature review, 379-382
family advantages, 35
family problems, 316
fraud, 203-206
funding, 163-207
sources, 167
future, 399-423
group, referral, 362-363
growth, 329-363
barriers, 359-361
early, 344
home visits, 347-357
physician, 361-362
by state, 345-347
utilization as measure, 344-354
utilization impact, 357-359
growth factor, inhibiting, 331-332
growth rationales, 329-332
health maintenance relationships, 50
high technology, 74-80
clinical management, 76
defined, 74
equipment, 75
family education, 75
growth factors, 76-77

marketing analysis, 77-78
patient education, 75
patient selection, 75
psychological and sociological concerns, 75
quality assurance, 76
reimbursement, 76
safety, 79
standards, 79-80
supplies, 75
training, 79
hospital advantages, 36-37
hospital disadvantages, 37-38
hospital-based, 341-342
hospital-run, 43-44
agency contract, 44
coalition agency, 44
increased utilization, 69-70
institutional care service regulation, 212
intensive, 21, 21-22
intermediate, 21, 22
issues, 403-408
lower per capita cost, 213
maintenance, 21
management aspects, 31
marketing, 332-336
basic issues, 332-334
future, 335-336
place, 333
plan, 334
price, 333
product, 333
promotion, 333
rules, 335
Medicaid expenditures, 188-190
medical record, 272-273
national policy, 406
need, 406
patient advantages, 35, 39
patient selection, 30-31
pattern
current, 399-401

early, 399
future, 401-402
pediatric, 223
personal preference, 135-136
physician advantages, 38, 39
postinstitutional, 14
preferred provider arrangement, 50
private funding, 199-202
problems
  diagnosis related group, 408-412
  prospective payment system, 408-412
proprietary growth, 342-343
public awareness, 13
publicity, 329-330
recommendations, 407-408
reforms, 416-418
services defined, 24-26
societal advantages, 39
substitutability, 212
substitution or add-on service, 217
system characteristics, 262-264
tax incentives, 314
terminology, 16-17
trend, 399-402
  impact, 402
volunteer program, 312, 313
vs. home health care, 16
vs. hospice, 391
vs. hospice care cost, 230-232
vs. hospital, 391
vs. hostel, 391
vs. inpatient hospital care cost, 220-224
  diagnosis-specific, 223-224
  health maintenance organizations, 224
  high technology savings, 221-223
  insurance companies, 220-221

maternity, 223
pediatric, 223
vs. institutional care, 31-33
vs. nursing home care, 392
vs. nursing home care cost, 224-225
vs. social care, 132-134
women's issue, 319-320
as women's issue, 319-320
Homecare accreditation, 244-253
  accreditation organizations, 246-253
  benefits, 244-245
  future, 253
Homecare agency, professional judgment validation, 40-41
HomeCare Consumer, 329
Homecare industry, historical aspects, 1-2
Homecare program
  acquired immune deficiency syndrome, 48
  Alzheimer's disease, 45-46
  Chelsea-Village Program, 47-48
  Conference on Organized Homecare, 4
  disease/condition, 44-47
  elements, 4, 23-24
  examples, 41-49
  foreign, 48-49
  funding, 4
  long-term, 47-48
  Montefiore program services, 3-4
  pediatric, 47-48
  rural area, 48
  services, 4
  specific population group, 47-48
  standards, 4
Homecare Trade Association, 336-337
Homemaker, 41, 42, 151
  future, 295-296
  historical aspects, 6-7

home help, 293
  model curriculum, 294-295
  personnel issues, 295-296
  tasks, 293
  titles, 293
  traits, 293-294
  typical, 294
  vs. day care, cost comparison, 229
Hospice, 46, 134, 382-383
  family assurance, 232
  insurance coverage, 230-231
  licensed, 254
  medical record, 273
  national study, 231-232
  quality of care, 237
  social worker, 303
  volunteer, 313
Hospice Association of America, 336
Hospital
  durable medical equipment, 86-88
  extramural, 33
  historical aspects, 1
  home health agency relations, 50
Hospital Association of Pennsylvania, 68
Hospital bed, 80
Hospital coalition agency, 44
Hospital Home Care, Inc., 44
Hospital homecare program, examples, 43-44
Hospital need determination, 113-114
Hospital Without Walls, 33
Hospital-at-home, 33
Hospitalization-a-domicile, 33
House Select Committee on Aging, national survey, 41
House Subcommittee on Health and Long Term Care, national survey, 41

Household activity, 104
Housekeeping service, 26

Ileostomy, 318
Impairment
  classifications, 130
    extremely impaired, 130
    generally impaired, 130
    greatly impaired, 130
    moderately impaired, 130
    slightly/mildly impaired, 130
    unimpaired, 130
Impairment level, cost, 217-219
Independence, 19
Information and referral services, 26
In-Home Assessment, 115-116
In-Home Supportive Services Program, 150
Institutionalization
  inappropriate, 38-41
  need calculations, 116-119
Insurance, 163
  home nursing care, historical aspects, 2
  homecare funding, 201
  long-term care, 137-139
Interagency program conflict, 28
Intermittent care, Medicare definition, 172-174

John D. French Center for Alzheimer's Disease, 46
Joint Commission on Accreditation of Hospitals
  homecare accreditation, 246-248
  hospice accreditation, 248-249
  quality assurance, 261-262
Joint venture, 86-88, 337-341
  advantages, 337-338
  disadvantages, 337-338
  legal aspects, 340-341

physician role, 338
profitability, 338
risk, 339
typical, 339-340

Laboratory service, 26
Legal aspects, 56-57
Legal service, 26
Legislation
    federal, 419-420
    homecare priorities, 419
    reform, 418-420
Length of stay, 65-67
Liability, 56-57
Licensure, 253-257
    defined, 254
Life care community, 139-140
Living at Home Program, 48
Long Term Home Health Consulta-
    tion Service, 148-149
Long-term care, 143-151
    benefits, 416
    comparison, 389-391
    defined, 144
    eligibility, 416
    evaluation, 379
    financing, 415
    insurance, 137-139
    international prototypes, 146
    Medicare, 146-147
    problems, 144, 413-416
    public policy, recommenda-
        tions, 141-143
    reforms, 416-418
    service delivery, 415-416
Low Back Pain Program, 46-47
Low Income Elderly and Disabled
    Medicaid Amendments of
    1986, 136

Malpractice, 56-57, 421-422
    physicians, 56
Managed care, 400
Management

financial aspects, 53-54
    operational, 53-55
Management strategy, 55
Manager, development, 53
Market research forecast, 330-331
Marketing, 54-55
    durable medical equipment, 84-
        86
    referrals, 85-86
Marketing analysis, 77-78
Maternal and Child Health Home
    Visit Evaluation, 382
Maternity, early discharge, cost, 223
Meal service
    home-delivered, 26
    Meals on Wheels, 309
Meals on Wheels, 309
Medicaid, 5, 163, 167, 187-192
    elderly, 136-137
    homecare expenditures, 188-190
    overview, 187-188
    section 2176 waiver, 189-192
        cost comparison, 226-227
Medical education, homecare
    physician, 286-288
Medical procedure, 65
Medical Products Sales, 86
Medical record
    homecare, 272-273
    hospice, 273
    problem oriented, 265
    quality of care, 272-273
Medical social services, 20
Medical supplies and equipment, 26
Medicare, 65, 67-69, 163, 167, 169-
    187
    claim denial, 185-186
    conditions of participation, 257-
        260
    cost, budget stimulation, 176-
        179
    diagnosis related group, 386-
        387

durable medical equipment, 80-95
durable medical equipment, cost, 81-83, 88-95
elderly, 146-147, 157-158
evaluation, 386-387
expenditures, 180-184
    proprietary home health agency, 180
future, 186-187
home health care, 5
home health care agency, 5
hospice care, 134
long-term care, 146-147
nonreimbursable services, 169
occupational therapist, 302-303
overview, 169-171
problems, 412-413
reforms, 412-413
reimburseable services, 169
state reimbursement, 180
Medicare Partners, 133
Medicare Plus II, 133
Mended Hearts, 318
Mental deterioration, 32
Mental retardation, social worker, 305
Mobility, 104
Montefiore Hospital, prototype hospital-based homecare program, 3-4
Mutual aid self-help group, 317

National Association for Home Care, 13, 68, 285, 336
National Association for Homemaker-Home Health Aide Services, Inc., 17, 23
National Association of Medical Equipment Suppliers, 81-82
National Association of Retail Druggists, 81-82
National Council for Homemaker-Home Health Aide Services, 7

National Council on Aging, Inc., 69
National Foundation for Long Term Care, 68
National Health Council, 17, 23
National Health Interview Survey, 126
National Health Planning and Resources Development Act, 260
National HomeCaring Council, 7, 336
National HomeCaring Council Accreditation, 251
National Hospice Organization, 230, 336
National Hospice Study, 318, 391
National Intravenous Therapy Association, 79
National League for Nursing, 244-245
    need assessment, 108
National League for Nursing Accreditation, 249-251
National Long-Term Care Channeling Demonstration Program, 199
National Medical Enterprises, 46, 87
National Organization of Public Health Nursing, historical aspects, 2-3
National survey data, 41-43
Need assessment
    age, 103-106, 111
    consensus patterns, 111-112
    factors, 107, 111
    family, 112
    hospital-based, 113-114
    inappropriate placement, 116-119
    measurement, 103-107
    methods, 107-109
        application, 109, 111

patient assessment and classification, 115-116
physician, 114-115
public hearing, 106
techniques, 107-109
application, 109-111
Negligence
comparative, 57
contributory, 57
Nerve muscle disorder, 31
Neurology service, 113
Neuromuscular disease, 42, 393
Neurosurgery, 113
New York/Pennsylvania Health Systems Agency, need assessment, 109
Newborn-Family Care Program, 46-47
Nonprofit agency, 20
Nurse, 288-292
geriatric training, 154
licensed practical, 291-292
registered, 41, 42
in nursing home, 152
vocational, 291-292
Nursing
education, 289-292
independent practice, 291
responsibilities, 288-289
Nursing care, 20, 26
skilled, Medicare definition, 172
Nursing corporation, for-profit, independent, 291
Nursing Dynamics Corporation, 291
Nursing home, 104, 144, 147-148
abuse, 147-148
cost, 147
demographics, 147
fraud, 147-148
quality of care, 237
Nursing Home Without Walls, 33, 48
cost comparison, 227

Nutrition
enteral, 74, 78
parenteral, 383
problem, 42
standards, 79
total parenteral, 74, 78
cost, 222
Nutrition therapy, 26
Nutritionist, 20, 309-311
education, 310
future, 311
public health, 310-311
role, 309-310

Occupational therapist, 299-300
continuing education, 302
education, 300
functions, 299-300
future, 303
homecare problem-solving, 300-301
Medicare, 302-303
standards, 301-302
Occupational therapy, 20, 26
Ohio Department of Health and Battelle Laboratories, need assessment, 108
Older Americans Act, 6, 136, 163, 196-198
expenditures, 197-198
funding, 197
impact, 198
services, 196-197
Operational management, 53-55
Ophthalmologic services, 26
Orderly, 292
Orthopedic disability, 388
Outlier, 65
Oxygen regulator, 80

Parents Anonymous, 318
Park Nicollet Medical Center, 46-47
Participant observation, 393
Pastoral services, 26

Patient abuse, 15
Patient assessment, 115-116, 265
    computer-assisted, 115
Patient care management, 20
Patient education
    high technology homecare, 75
    postinstitutional homecare, 14-15
Patient rights, 242-243
Pediatric homecare, 223
Pennsylvania Assembly Quality Assurance Project, 264-265
Personal care, 104
Personal contact services, 25
Pharmacist, 307-309
    independent prescribing authority, 308-309
    reimbursement, 308
    role, 308
Physical deterioration, 32
Physical therapist, 296-299
    accreditation, 296
    defined, 296
    image, 298
    patient referral, 297
    quality assurance, 298-299
    undersupply, 299
Physical therapy, 20, 26
Physician, 284-288
    attitudes toward elderly, 153-154
    geriatric education, 152-155
    homecare advantages, 38, 39
    homecare growth, 361-362
    homecare role, 284-286
        indifference, 284-285
        legal aspects, 284
    malpractice, 56
    medical education, 286-288
    need assessment, 114-115
    quality of care, 275
    referral, 85
    services, 26
Plan of action, 23

Podiatry, 26
Population aging, 103
Portland Kaiser-Permanente Group, need assessment, 108
Postoperative recovery, 31
Pre-Admission Assessment Form, 115-116
Preferred provider arrangement, homecare relationship, 50
Prepaid group health plan, homecare funding, 202
Presbyterian Homes of Northern California, 139-140
Prescription drugs, 26
President's Commission for the Study of Ethical Problems in Medicine and Biomedical and Behavioral Research, 57
Preventive care, 3, 19, 23
Private practice, cost comparison, 229
Problem oriented medical record, 265
Productivity, 54
Professional disagreement, 38
Professional Review Organization, 239
Profit motivation, lack of, 241
Program administration, long-term care, 414
Proprietary agency, 20
Prospective payment system, home health care, 71-73
Prosthetics/orthotics, 26
Protective services, 26
Psoriasis Homecare Program, 46-47
Psychiatric patient, 389
Psychiatric services, 45
Psychologist, 20
Public agency, 20
Public health nursing service, 3
Public Health Service, 6
Pulmonary disorder, chronic, 45

Purchase agreement, durable medical equipment, 88-95

QT, Inc., 318
Quality assurance, 66, 76
    drawbacks, 262
    external review, 262
    internal review, 262
    Joint Commission on Accreditation of Hospitals, 261-262
    physical therapist, 298-299
Quality assurance program, 261-273
Quality Assurance Reform Act of 1985, 239
Quality Care, Inc., 343
Quality of care, 237-238, 238, 421-422
    criteria, 243-244
        defined, 243
    defined, 277-278
    disease type, 240
    fraud, 241
    impediments, 239-240
    input measure, 268-270
        defined, 268-270
    instruments, 240
    marketability, 276-277
    medical record, 272-273
    norms, 243-244
        defined, 243
    on-site monitoring, 239-240
    outcome measure, 268-270
        defined, 268-270
    personnel standards, 273-275
    physician, 275
    process measure, 268-270
        defined, 268-270
    standards, 241, 243-244
        defined, 243
    structure, 268-270
        defined, 268-270
    subjective elements, 240

Random clinical trial, 374
Reagan, Ronald, 11
Recreational service, 26
Recuperation, 19
Referral, 42, 362-363
    captive, 85
    durable medical equipment, 85-86
    physical therapist, 297-298
Regulation, certificate of need, 260-261
Regulatory process circumvention, NAHC's position, 409
Rehabilitation service, comprehensive, 388
Rehabilitative medicine, 113
Reimbursement, 20, 65. *See also* Cost
    durable medical equipment, 88-95
        federal budget activity, 92-94
        purchase, 88-92
        reasonable charges, 94-95
        rental, 88-92
    high technology homecare, 76
Relative intensity measures, 73
Religious agency, 163
Rental, durable medical equipment, 88-95
    Research project, 199
        government-funded, 199
Resource allocation, 119-121
Resource utilization group, 73
Respirator, 80
Respiratory ailment, 31, 42
Respiratory care, 74
Respiratory therapy, 26
Respite care, 384
    family, 318-319
    social worker, 305
Rx Home Care, 80

San Francisco General Hospital, 45

SCAN Health Plan, Inc., 133
Secondary care, domiciliary, 33
Section 2176 Waiver, 189-192
    cost comparison, 226-227
Self-monitoring, 330
Self-testing, 330
Senate Special Committee on
    Aging, 67, 127
Senior care network, 43
Shanti Project, 45
Skin problem, 42
Social Adjustment Assessment
    Form, 115-116
Social admission, 33
Social background, 114
Social care, 132-134
Social gerontologist, 152
Social Services Block Grant
    Title XX, 5, 136, 192-195
        expenditures, 193
        funding, 193
        impact, 195
        overview, 192-193
        services, 193
Social work services, 26
Social worker, 303-305
    education, 303-304
    function, 304
    hospice, 303
    mental retardation, 305
    planning, 305
    respite care, 305
Social/health maintenance organiza-
    tion, 133-134
Southern Piedmont (North
    Carolina) Health Systems
    Agency, need assessment, 108
Speech pathologist, 305-307
    business aspects, 307
    education, 306
    ethical issues, 307
    supply, 306
    utilization, 306-307
Speech pathology, 26

Speech therapy, 20
Stress management program, 54
Stroke, 31, 388
    recovery, 42
Supportive care, 23
Surgery, 65, 113

Teaching hospital, 65
Terminal illness, 19
The Home Health Care Profes-
    sional, 79-80
The Home Health Care Solution, 14
Therapeutic services, 23
Thought process, 114
Traction equipment, 80
Training, 274
Translation service, 26
Transportation and escort service,
    26

United Way organization, 163
University of California at
    Berkeley, need assessment, 109
Upjohn Health Care Services, 343
Utilization, 399-400
Utilization review, 66, 270-271
    defined, 270-271

Veterans Administration, cost com-
    parison, 229
Visiting housekeeper, 7
Visiting housewives, 6-7
Visiting Nurse Association, histori-
    cal aspects, 2
Visiting Nursing Service of New
    York, 87
VNS Med-Equip, 87
Vocational training, 26
Voluntary agency
    growth, 344
    historical aspects, 2
Volunteer, 312-313
    functions, 313

Volunteer--The National
    Center Accreditation, 253
Volunteers Organized in Com-
    munity Elderly Services, 313

Waiver of liability, 410
Walker, 80

Wheelchair, 80
Widows Anonymous, 318
World Health Organization, defini-
    tion of health, 31

X-ray services, 26